Contents

Appendices and index

Nutrition

X

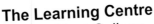

Lippincott Williams & Wilkins
a Wolters Kluwer business

Philadelphia · Baltimore
Buenos Aires · Hong Kong

Staff

Executive Publisher
Judith A. Schilling McCann, RN, MSN

Editorial Director
David Moreau

Clinical Director
Joan M. Robinson, RN, MSN

Senior Art Director
Arlene Putterman

Art Director
Mary Ludwicki

Senior Managing Editor
Jaime Stockslager Buss, ELS

Clinical Manager
Collette Bishop Hendler, RN, BS, CCRN

Clinical Project Manager
Mary Perrong, RN, CRNP, MSN, APRN,BC

Editors
Brenna H. Mayer, Libby Tucker, Susan Williams

Clinical Editors
Marcy Caplin, RN, MSN; Kathryn Henry, RN, BSN, CCRN

Copy Editors
Kimberly Bilotta, Jane Bradford Cortright, Pamela Wingrod

Illustrator
Bot Roda

Digital Composition Services
Diane Paluba (manager), Joyce Rossi Biletz

Associate Manufacturing Manager
Beth J. Welsh

Editorial Assistants
Megan L. Aldinger, Karen J. Kirk, Linda K. Ruhf

Design Assistant
Georg W. Purvis IV

Indexer
Barbara Hodgson

NUTRIE010606

Library of Congress Cataloging-in-Publication Data
Nutrition made incredibly easy.—2nd ed.
    p. ; cm.
    Includes bibliographical references and index.
    1. Diet in disease. 2. Nutrition. 3. Nursing. I. Lippincott Williams & Wilkins.
    [DNLM: 1. Nutrition—physiology. 2. Health Promotion. 3. Nutrition Assessment. 4. Patient Education. QU 145 N975355 2007]
RM216.N86156 2007
615.8'54—dc22
ISBN 1-58255-521-4 (alk. paper)   2006008352

Contributors and consultants

Liz Applegate, PhD, FACSM
Senior Lecturer, Nutrition Department
University of California, Davis

Jennifer Bueche, PhD, CDN, RD
Assistant Professor, Department of Human Ecology
SUNY College at Oneonta (N.Y.)

Nancy Collins, PhD, LD/N, RD
Consultant Dietitian
Weston, Fla.

Peggi Guenter, RN, PHD, CNSN
Managing Editor for Special Projects
American Society for Parenteral and Enteral
   Nutrition
Silver Spring, Md.

Alison H. Harmon, PhD, RD
Assistant Professor
Montana State University
Department of Health & Human Development
Bozeman

Cristen L. Harris, MS, LD/N, RD
Nutrition Consultant
Ft. Lauderdale, Fla.

Susan Luck, RN, BSN, MA, CCN, HNC
Clinical Nutritionist
Special Immunology Services
Mercy Hospital
Miami

Kathleen D. Meyer, LD, RD
Assistant Manager, Dietary
Fairfield Medical Center
Lancaster, Ohio

Sherry A. Parmenter, LD, RD
Clinical Dietitian
Fairfield Medical Center
Lancaster, Ohio

Alison J. Rigby, MPH, MS, PhD, CNSD, RD
Stanford University School of Medicine
Pediatric Endocrinology and Diabetes
Stanford, Calif.

Martine Scannavino, MS, LDN, RD
Assistant Professor
Associate Director—Allen Center for Nutrition
Cedar Crest College
Allentown, Pa.

Susan S. Swadener, PhD, RD
Dietetic Internship Director & Lecturer
California Polytechnic State University
San Luis Obispo

Kate Willcutts, MS, CNSD, RD
Assistant Nutrition Support Manager
University of Virginia Hospital
Instructor
School of Nursing
Charlottesville

Foreword

As you know, nutrition plays a major role in health promotion, disease prevention, and treatment in all patient care settings. To provide the best care for your patients, you must have a sound knowledge of nutritional principles. You must also be able to apply that knowledge in your practice and care and impart that knowledge to your patients so that they can better care for themselves. How do you do all of this? With the help of *Nutrition Made Incredibly Easy*, Second Edition—the resource that you need to take this challenging topic and make it more understandable, more practical, more digestible, more appetizing!

Do you have complete confidence in the nutritional care you provide to your patients? If not, it's probably because the nutrition classes you took in school were overwrought with bland, complex chemical equations and explanations that made your stomach turn and made you wonder how the information applied to your daily practice. Well, in this new edition of *Nutrition Made Incredibly Easy*, you won't find any drab drawings of chemical structures or drawn out descriptions of complex gastrointestinal processes. You'll find only clear descriptions of nutrition-related topics, simply explained.

Nutrition is a complex subject. Understanding how to provide the best nutritional care requires you to learn many concepts. Because nutrients come from food, you need to learn what foods should be eaten, how they should be prepared, and which portion sizes are appropriate. Your knowledge of anatomy and physiology is essential to helping you understand what happens to food in the digestive tract and how nutrients are absorbed and distributed throughout the body. You need to recall basic pathophysiology information to appreciate how diseases affect nutrition and how foods can be used in the treatment of various disorders. *Nutrition Made Incredibly Easy*, Second Edition, makes learning all of this information simple—and fun!

Offering comprehensive information on nutritional care throughout the lifespan, this one-of-a-kind reference is a fantastic tool for practitioners, students, faculty, and anyone interested in diet and nutrition. The text is organized into three square servings. Part I, Introduction to nutrition, offers a concise yet hearty review of such topics as nutrition basics, digestion and absorption, and essential nutrients. Fully updated, this second edition includes the *Dietary Guidelines for Americans 2005* as well as MyPyramid. Part II brings the topic of nutrition a little closer to your practice. It thoroughly covers nutritional assessment, including identifying at-risk patients, taking a dietary history, evaluating weight and body size, and documenting nutritional assessment findings. This section also has an entire chapter devoted to how nutritional considerations vary throughout the lifespan. In part III, Clinical nutrition, you'll find not only coverage of common nutritional and GI disorders, such as obesity, anorexia, dysphagia, GERD, and lactose intolerance, but also coverage of nutritional considerations for patients with cardiovascular, renal, and neurologic disorders; diabetes; HIV disease; and such special conditions as burns and trauma. In addition, you'll find the information on feeding patients that you'll need to use daily in your practice.

Sound boring? Hardly! You'll find plenty of features in *Nutrition Made Incredibly Easy* that make the complex study of nutrition simple, interesting, and fun. Characters that appear throughout the book reinforce important points and also spice up the text with a dash of humor. Objectives for each chapter help focus your study. In addition, special logos highlight important points and bolster learning throughout the book:

Lifespan lunchbox points out important age-related nutritional considerations.

Menu maven offers sample menus for special diets.

NutriTips gives pointers on nutritional care—many of which you can share with your patients.

Bridging the gap alerts you to practices and preferences of various cultures that may affect your nutritional care.

Memory jogger provides mnemonics and other ways to help you understand and remember difficult concepts.

To faculty in all health-related fields who are interested in using a well-organized reference to help their students grasp important nutrition concepts and to students who are looking for nutrition to be boiled down to the basics, I would highly recommend *Nutrition Made Incredibly Easy*, Second Edition. What might have been intimidating has been dissected, simplified, streamlined, and illustrated for easy application to daily practice. With the broad understanding of nutrition gained from this book, you'll be ready to make a valuable contribution to the nutritional health and well-being of patients. Bon appetit!

Lisa Pawloski, PhD
Associate Professor
George Mason University
Fairfax, Va.

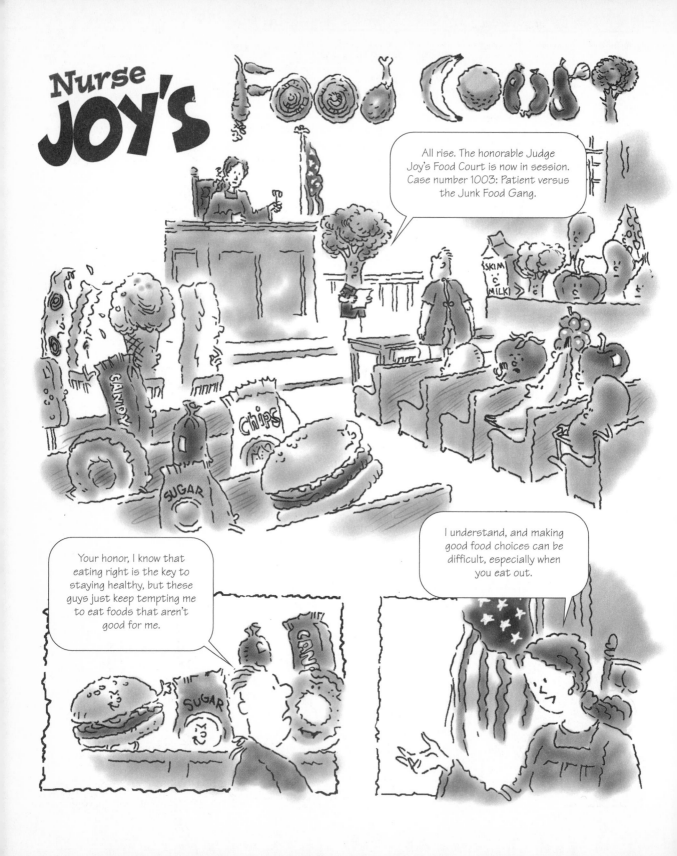

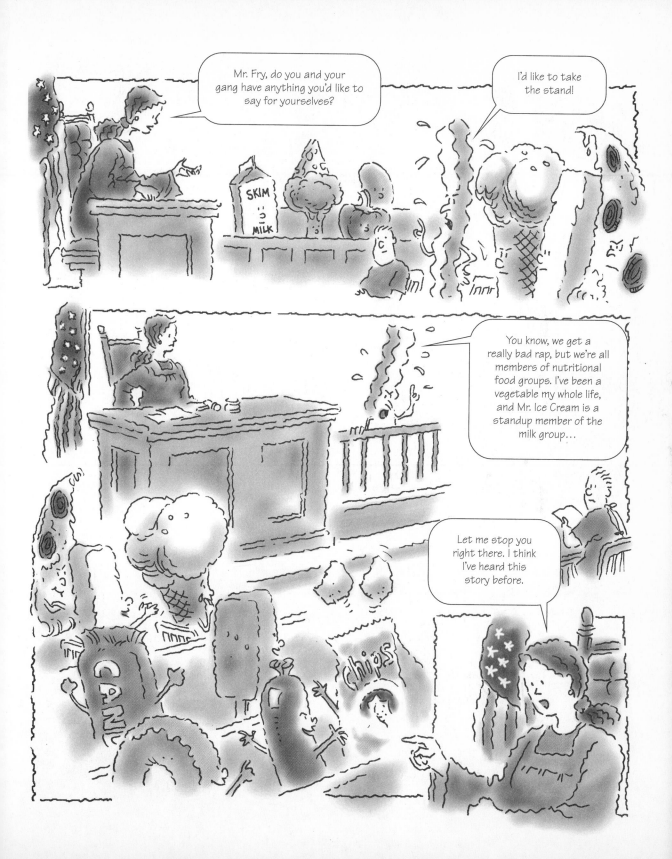

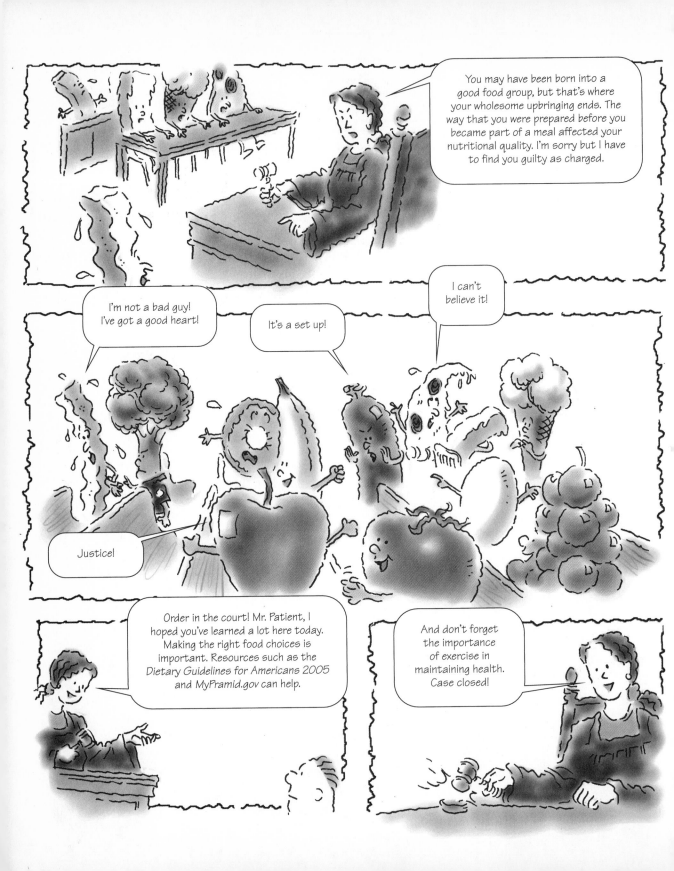

Part I   Introduction to nutrition

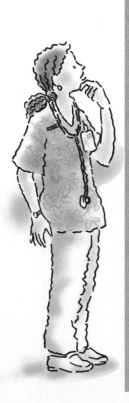

① Nutrition basics

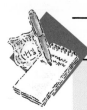

Just the facts

This chapter presents fundamental information about the key elements of nutrition. In this chapter, you'll learn:

♦ the role nutrients play in health promotion

♦ three levels of disease prevention

♦ the way to differentiate between good nutrition and poor nutrition

♦ techniques for ensuring that your patient eats a balanced diet

♦ the current nutrient standards for health promotion.

A look at nutrition

Nutrition refers to the processes by which a living organism ingests, digests, absorbs, transports, uses, and excretes nutrients (food and other nourishing material). Nutrition as a clinical area is primarily concerned with the properties of food that build sound bodies and promote health.

More than just a pretty process

Because good nutrition is essential to good health and disease prevention, any person involved in health care needs a thorough knowledge of nutrition and the body's nutritional requirements throughout the life span. What's more, the study of nutrition must focus on health promotion.

Each of us nutrients has his own special power, but we all work together to keep the body functioning.

Nutrients

For nutrition to be adequate, a person must receive certain *essential nutrients* — carbohydrates, fats, proteins, vitamins, minerals, and water. These nutrients must be present for proper growth and functioning; however, the body can't produce them on its own in adequate quantities, so they must be obtained through food. In addition, the digestive system must function properly to make use of these nutrients.

Each nutrient has a number of specific metabolic functions, but no nutrient works alone. Close metabolic relationships exist among all of the basic nutrients as well as with their metabolic products.

The nonessentials

A nonessential nutrient is one that isn't needed in the diet because it's manufactured by the body.

The nutrient breakdown dance

Nutrients can be used by the body for its immediate needs, or they can be stored for later use. The body breaks down nutrients into simpler compounds for absorption in the stomach and intestines in two ways:
• mechanical breakdown, which begins in the GI tract with chewing
• chemical breakdown, which starts with salivary enzymes in the mouth and continues with acid and enzyme action through the rest of the GI tract.

The role of a lifeline

Nutrients play a vital role in maintaining health and wellness. They have several important functions:
• providing energy, which can be stored in the body or transformed for vital activities
• building and maintaining body tissue
• controlling metabolic processes, such as growth, cell activity, enzyme production, and temperature regulation.

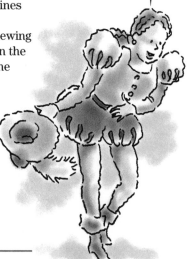

All the body's a stage…and all the nutrients play their roles, including providing energy, building tissue, and controlling metabolism.

Metabolism

Regulated mostly by hormones, metabolism is a combination of several processes by which energy is extracted from certain nutrients (carbohydrates, protein, and fat) and then used by the body. Vitamins and minerals don't directly provide us with energy, but they are an imporant part of the metabolic process.

Metabolism can be broken down into two parts:
• *Catabolism* is the breakdown of complex substances into simpler ones, resulting in the release of energy.
• *Anabolism* is the synthesis of simple substances into more complex substances. This process provides the energy necessary for tissue growth, maintenance, and repair.

Energy

Energy, in the form of adenosine triphosphate (ATP), is produced as a by-product of carbohydrate, fat, and protein metabolism. The amount of energy in food products is measured in kilocalories (kcal), which are commonly referred to as *calories*.

Through the processes of digestion and absorption, energy is released from food into the body. Small amounts of energy are stored within cells for immediate use. Larger amounts of energy are stored in glycogen and fat tissue to fuel long-duration activities. (For more information, see chapter 2, Digestion and absorption.)

Balancing act

In a healthy adult, the rate of anabolism equals the rate of catabolism, and energy balance is obtained. In other words, energy balance occurs when the caloric intake from food equals the number of calories expended. These calories may be used for voluntary activities (such as physical activity) or involuntary activities (such as basal metabolism).

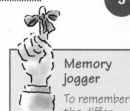

Memory jogger

To remember the difference between catabolism and anabolism, think **cut**abolism and **add**abolism. Catabolism cuts, or breaks down, substances in the body, whereas anabolism adds, or synthesizes, new substances.

Nutrition and health promotion

Many patients may consider themselves healthy because they don't feel sick. However, you must be concerned about a more holistic meaning of the term *health* — one that incorporates aspects of the patient's internal and external environments — in order to best care for your patients.

For you, health promotion must consider all of a patient's needs, including physical, emotional, mental, and social needs. Only when these needs are met can it be said that a person is healthy, or well. Furthermore, wellness implies a state of balance between a person's activities and goals. Maintaining this balance allows the patient to maintain his vitality and ability to function productively in society.

A nutritional diet provides the basis for health promotion and disease prevention, making it an important part of caring for any patient.

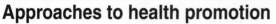

Approaches to health promotion

There are two main approaches to health promotion:
• The *traditional approach* is reactive; it focuses on treating symptoms after they present.

• The *preventive approach* involves identifying and eliminating risk factors to stop health problems from developing.

The current wellness and fitness movement in America is grounded in the preventive approach, with individuals educating themselves about maintaining health and preventing illness and disease. Most Americans, however, still don't get the recommended amount of physical activity, which can put them at greater risk for such disorders as heart disease, diabetes, and hypertension.

20/10 vision

The U.S. national health goals, which were originally published in the Department of Health and Human Services' report *Healthy People 2000* and have been updated for *Healthy People 2010*, also reflect this preventive wellness philosophy. Prominent themes in the latest report include:
• choosing a healthy diet
• maintaining weight control
• monitoring for and reducing high risk factors for disease.

How many ways can I serve it up? A nutritious diet provides the basis for health promotion and disease prevention.

Health promotion and disease prevention

Promoting health, establishing wellness, and preventing disease is a three-part process. (See *Three parts to prevention.*)

Nutrition and a balanced diet

You're part of a health care team that's responsible for making sure the patient maintains optimal nutritional health, even though he may be battling illness or recovering from surgery. It's also your job to stress to the patient the importance of good nutrition in maintaining health and recovering from illness, so that he can continue sound nutritional practices when he's no longer under your care.

Nutritional status

You must use your knowledge of nutrition to promote health through education and counseling of sick and healthy patients. This includes encouraging patients to consume appropriate types and amounts of food. It also means considering poor food habits as a contributing factor in a patient with chronic illness. Therefore, assessing nutritional status and identifying nutritional needs to meet the requirements of a balanced diet are primary activities

Three parts to prevention

Health promotion and disease prevention efforts can be categorized into three groups.

Primary prevention

Examples of primary prevention measures, which focus on health promotion, include:
- conducting nutrition classes to promote healthy eating patterns
- modifying menus in restaurants and offering low-fat alternatives
- offering fresh fruit and vegetables in workplace cafeterias.

Secondary prevention

Secondary prevention, which focuses on risk reduction, may include such measures as:
- screening for potential diseases (hypercholesterolemia, osteoporosis)
- nutritional counseling for people at risk for cardiovascular diseases and diabetes
- immunizations.

Tertiary prevention

Examples of tertiary prevention measures, which focus on disease treatment and rehabilitation, include:
- physical rehabilitation for the stroke patient
- cardiac rehabilitation for the cardiac patient
- diabetes education classes for the patient with newly diagnosed type 1 or type 2 diabetes.

> **Memory jogger**
>
> To remember the three parts to prevention, think **PST**:
>
> Primary = Health Promotion
>
> Secondary = Screening
>
> Tertiary = Treatment.

in planning patient care. (See *Religious practices and dietary restrictions,* page 8.)

Assessing nutritional status

A patient's nutritional status can influence the body's response to illness and treatment. Regardless of your patient's overall condition, an evaluation of his nutritional health is an essential part of your assessment. Assessment of the patient's nutritional status includes determining nutritional risk factors as well as individual needs.

Good nutrition

Good nutrition, or optimal nutrition, is essential in promoting health, preventing illness, and restoring health after an injury or illness. To achieve optimal nutrition, a person must eat a varied diet containing carbohydrates, proteins, fats, vitamins, minerals, water, and fiber in sufficient amounts. Although excesses of certain nutrients can be detrimental to a patient's health, intake of essential nutrients should be greater than minimum requirements to allow for variations in health and disease and to provide stores for later use.

> Balance is best! An assorted diet that provides all of the essential nutrients is a main ingredient of good nutrition.

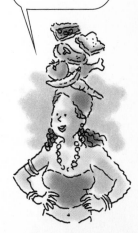

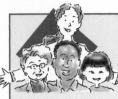

Poor nutrition

Poor nutrition, or malnutrition, is a state of inadequate or excess nutritional intake. It's most common among people living in poverty—especially those with greater nutritional requirements, such as elderly patients, pregnant women, children, and infants. It also occurs in hospitals and long-term care facilities, because the patients in these situations have illnesses that place added stress on their bodies, raising nutritional requirements.

Don't underestimate undernutrition

Undernutrition occurs when a patient consumes fewer daily nutrients than his body requires, resulting in a nutritional deficit. Typically, undernourished patients are at greater risk for physical illnesses. They may also suffer from limitations in cognitive and physical status.

Undernutrition can result from:
• inability to metabolize nutrients
• inability to obtain the appropriate nutrients from food
• accelerated excretion of nutrients from the body
• illness or disease that increases the body's need for nutrients.

Don't overdo it

In contrast, overnutrition occurs when a patient consumes an excessive amount of nutrients. For example, overnutrition may occur in patients who self-prescribe megadoses of vitamins and mineral supplements and in those who overeat. These practices can result in damage to body tissue or obesity.

Nutrient standards

To maintain healthy populations, most developed countries have established nutrition standards for major nutrients. These standards serve as guidelines for nutrient intake based on the nutritional needs of most healthy population groups.

U.S. standards

The U.S. nutrient standards, called Recommended Dietary Allowances (RDAs), were first published during World War II as a guide for planning and acquiring food supplies and promoting good nutrition. To keep up with increasing scientific information and social concerns about nutrition and health, these standards are revised and expanded approximately every 5 years.

Dietary Reference Intakes (DRIs) are the most recent version of the U.S. nutrient standards. Because DRIs consider an individual's sex and age-group and aren't limited to preventing deficiency diseases, these standards are more comprehensive than RDAs in measuring a patient's nutritional status and long-term health. (See *Dietary Reference Intakes*, page 10.)

Other standards

The published standards of other countries, such as Canada and Britain, are similar to U.S. standards. In impoverished countries, where quality of food and nutrition are lacking, standards are set by the Food and Agriculture Organization and the World Health Organization. No matter who sets the standards, the goal is the same: to promote good health and prevent disease through sound nutrition.

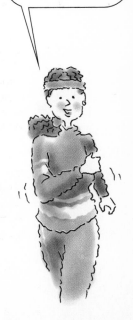

Most people need to step up their exercise. U.S. dietary guidelines recommend 30 minutes of moderate physical activity almost every day for adults.

Dietary guidelines

Dietary guidelines have been developed by governmental agencies, nutritionists, and special groups to provide recommendations that promote healthy eating habits. The U.S. dietary guidelines recommend that people age 2 and older eat a healthy assortment of foods from the basic food groups. They also emphasize the importance of:
• choosing foods that are low in added sugars and saturated and trans fats
• eating reasonable portions
• getting at least 30 minutes of moderate physical activity on most days for adults (the guidelines for children recommend at least 60 minutes of physical activity on most days of the week).

Dietary Reference Intakes

Dietary Reference Intakes (DRIs) comprise a set of four nutrient-based reference values being developed by the Food and Nutrition Board (FNB) of the National Academy of Sciences. These values, intended to replace and expand on the familiar Recommended Dietary Allowances (RDAs), can be used for planning and assessing diets. They include updated values for RDAs as well as values for Estimated Average Requirement (EAR), Adequate Intake (AI), and Tolerable Upper Intake Level (UL).

Recommended Dietary Allowance

The RDA of a nutrient is the average daily dietary intake needed to meet the requirements of virtually all healthy people in a given life stage or gender group. Critics have argued that RDAs merely prevent nutritional deficiencies rather than promote optimal health.

Estimated Average Requirement

The EAR of a nutrient is the average daily dietary intake needed to meet the requirements of half of all healthy people in a given life stage or gender group. Determination of this value isn't based solely on preventing nutritional deficiencies but also includes concepts related to risk reduction and bioavailability of a given nutrient.

Adequate Intake

An AI value is assigned to a nutrient if the FNB lacks sufficient information to establish an RDA and an EAR. The AI value is a recommended daily intake level based on estimates of nutrient intake by a group of healthy people.

Tolerable Upper Intake Level

The UL is the highest level of nutrient intake that doesn't cause adverse health effects in most individuals in the general population.

RDA...DRI... No wonder I have a craving for alphabet soup!

Dietary Guidelines for Americans 2005

The U.S. Department of Agriculture (USDA) and the Department of Health and Human Services released the first *Dietary Guidelines* and Food Guide Pyramid in 1980 to enable an individual to prepare a well-balanced diet through variety, balance, and moderation of choices. These guidelines have been revised several times, with the most recent *Dietary Guidelines* released in January 2005. *Dietary Guidelines for Americans 2005* introduces an updated food pyramid — called MyPyramid — that replaces the previous Food Guide Pyramid. These new guidelines promote an interactive and individualized approach to improving diet and lifestyle. MyPyramid helps people transfer the principles of the *Dietary Guidelines* into healthy eating and lifestyle choices. (See *Anatomy of MyPyramid*.)

Anatomy of MyPyramid

The U.S. Department of Agriculture's new food guidance system—called "MyPyramid: Steps to a Healthier You"—symbolizes a personalized approach to healthy eating and physical activity. Designed to be simple, the symbol has been developed to remind consumers to make healthy food choices and to be active every day. The different parts of the symbol are described below.

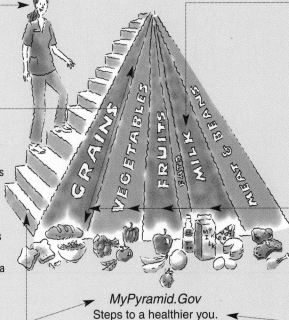

Activity

Activity is represented by the steps and the person climbing them, as a reminder of the importance of daily physical activity.

Moderation

Moderation is represented by the narrowing of each food group from the bottom to top. The wider base stands for foods with little or no solid fats or added sugars. These should be selected more often. The narrower top area stands for foods containing more added sugars and solid fats. The more active a person is, the more of these foods he can fit into his diet.

Personalization

Personalization is shown by the person on the steps, the slogan, and the URL. Personalized recommendations of the kinds and amounts of each food to eat can be found at *MyPryamid.gov.*

Proportionality

Proportionality is shown by the different widths of the food group bands. The widths suggest how much food a person should choose from each group. The widths are just a general guide, not exact proportions. To find out what proportion is right for your patient, visit the Web site (*www.mypyramid.gov*).

Variety

Variety is symbolized by the six bands representing the five food groups of the Pyramid and oils. This illustrates that foods from all groups are needed each day for good health.

Gradual improvement

Gradual improvement is encouraged by the slogan "Steps to a healthier you." It suggests that individuals can benefit from taking small steps to improve their diet and lifestyle each day.

MyPyramid.Gov
Steps to a healthier you.

Adapted from U.S. Department of Agriculture. Center for Nutrition Policy and Promotion. (2005). Anatomy of MyPyramid [Online]. *www.mypyramid.gov/downloads/mypyramid_anatomy.pdf*

What's new?

MyPyramid uses wedges of different widths and colors to represent the recommended amount of food a person should choose from a food group. Physical activity, represented by a figure climbing steps, has been added to the pyramid to emphasize the importance of regular exercise in achieving and maintaining good health.

Estimated daily calorie needs

To determine which food intake pattern to use for an individual, the following chart gives an estimate of individual calorie needs. The calorie range for each age and sex group is based on physical activity level, from sedentary to active.

Age (in years)	Calorie Range	
Children	*Sedentary*	*Active*
2 to 3	1,000	1,400
Females		
4 to 8	1,200	1,800
9 to 13	1,600	2,200
14 to 18	1,800	2,400
19 to 30	2,000	2,400
31 to 50	1,800	2,200
51+	1,600	2,200
Males		
4 to 8	1,400	2,000
9 to 13	1,800	2,600
14 to 18	2,200	3,200
19 to 30	2,400	3,000
31 to 50	2,200	3,000
51+	2,000	2,800

Sedentary means a lifestyle that includes only the light physical activity associated with typical day-to-day life.

Active means a lifestyle that includes physical activity equivalent to walking more than 3 miles per day at 3 to 4 miles per hour, in addition to the light physical activity associated with typical day-to-day life.

Adapted from U.S. Department of Agriculture. Center for Nutrition Policy and Promotion. (2005). Estimated Daily Calorie Needs [Online]. *www.mypyramid.gov/global_nav/pdf_food_intake.html*

The rainbow of colors in the new food pyramid represents one basic rule: Make sure that your patient's plate has a lot of color on it.

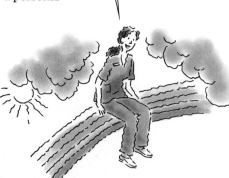

Another new feature of MyPyramid is that it promotes an online, interactive approach in which the individual obtains a personalized food plan and daily calorie intake level based on age, gender, and activity level. Daily amounts of food are recommended according to 12 different calorie levels, starting at 1,000 calories and increasing in 200-calorie increments, up to 3,200 calories.

The new food pyramid also makes recommendations based on health needs for specific populations, such as children and adolescents, women of childbearing age, pregnant and breast-feeding women, older adults, people with hypertension, and overweight children and adults. (See *Estimated daily calorie needs.*)

Food group recommendations

Each stripe on the food pyramid represents one of the six food groups: grains, vegetables, fruits, oils, milk, and meat and beans. The stripes are wider at the bottom and taper to the top, indicating that not all foods within a food group are of equal nutritional value. The following guidelines can help guide your patient to eat healthy. (See *Food group recommendations*, page 14.)

Grain group

Foods in the grain group are sources of complex carbohydrates, vitamins, minerals, and fiber. To help your patient make healthy food choices from this food group, suggest that he follow these recommendations:

- Consume 6 oz of grains each day, if following a 2,000-calorie diet.
- Make sure that one-half of all grains consumed each day (at least 3 oz) are whole grains, such as whole-grain cereals, breads, crackers, rice, or pasta.
- Be aware that 1 oz is approximately 1 slice of bread, 1 cup of breakfast cereal, or ½ cup of cooked rice, cereal, or pasta.
- Choose items made with little fat and sugar, such as bread, English muffins, rice, and pasta.
- Select several servings of food made from whole grains to add fiber.
- Avoid baked products that are high in fat and sugar, such as cakes and cookies.
- Use only one-half of the fat suggested when preparing package mixes.

Fruit group

The fruit group provides sources of vitamin A, vitamin C, and potassium. The foods in this group are naturally low in fat and sodium. To help your patient make the right choices from the fruit group, recommend that he follow these recommendations:

- Consume 2 cups of fruit each day, if following a 2,000-calorie diet.
- Select a variety of fruits. Although fruits can be consumed in various forms, including fresh, frozen, canned, or dried fruits, the use of fruit juices should be limited.
- When drinking fruit juice, choose 100% fruit juice over fruit-flavored juices.
- When choosing canned fruits, choose fruits that are canned in their own juice, not in syrup.

Vegetable group

Vegetables provide sources of vitamin A, vitamin C, folate, iron, magnesium, and fiber. To help your patient make healthy food

Food group recommendations

Because not all foods in a food group are created equal, the U.S. Department of Agriculture makes the following recommendations for choosing foods within a food group.

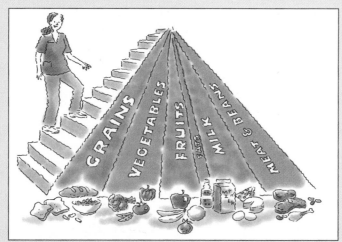

Find your balance between food and physical activity
• Be sure to stay within your daily calorie needs.
• Be physically active for at least 30 minutes most days of the week.
• About 60 minutes a day of physical activity may be needed to prevent weight gain.
• For sustaining weight loss, at least 60 to 90 minutes a day of physical activity may be required.
• Children and teenagers should be physically active for 60 minutes every day, or most days.

Know the limits on fats, sugars, and salt (sodium)
• Make the most of your fat sources from fish, nuts, and vegetable oils.
• Limit solid fats like butter, stick margarine, shortening, and lard, as well as foods that contain these.
• Check the Nutrition Facts label to keep saturated fats, trans fats, and sodium low.
• Choose food and beverages low in added sugars. Added sugars contribute calories with few, if any, nutrients.

Grains
• Make half your grains whole.
• Eat at least 3 oz of whole-grain cereals, breads, crackers, rice, or pasta every day.
• 1 oz is about 1 slice of bread, about 1 cup of breakfast cereal, or ½ cup of cooked rice, cereal, or pasta.

Vegetables
• Vary your veggies.
• Eat more dark-green veggies like broccoli, spinach, and other dark leafy greens.
• Eat more orange veggies, like carrots and sweet potatoes.
• Eat more dry beans and peas like pinto beans, kidney beans, and lentils.

Fruits
• Focus on fruits.
• Eat a variety of fruit.
• Choose fresh, frozen, canned, or dried fruit.
• Go easy on fruit juices.

Milk
• Consume calcium-rich foods.
• Go low-fat or fat-free when you choose milk, yogurt, and other milk products.
• If you don't or can't consume milk, choose lactose-free products or other calcium sources, such as fortified foods and beverages.

Meats & beans
• Go lean with protein.
• Choose low-fat or lean meats and poultry.
• Bake it, broil it, or grill it.
• Vary your protein routine; choose more fish, beans, peas, nuts, and seeds.

For a 2,000 calorie diet, you need the amounts below from each food group. To find the amounts that are right for you, go to *MyPyramid.gov*.

Grains	Vegetables	Fruits	Milk	Meats & beans
• Eat 6 oz every day.	• Eat 2½ cups every day.	• Eat 2 cups every day.	• Get 3 cups every day; for kids ages 2 to 8, 2 cups.	• Eat 5½ oz every day.

Adapted from U.S. Department of Agriculture. Center for Nutrition Policy and Promotion. (2005). MyPyramid Mini-Poster [Online]. http://www.mypyramid.gov/downloads/miniposter.pdf

choices from this group, suggest that he follow these recommendations:
• Consume 2½ cups of vegetables daily, if following a 2,000-calorie diet.
• Consume plenty of dark-green vegetables, such as broccoli, spinach, and other dark, leafy greens.
• Select orange vegetables, such as carrots and sweet potatoes.
• Eat dry beans and peas, such as pinto beans, kidney beans, and lentils.
• Vary the types of vegetables consumed, making sure to choose from all vegetable subgroups (dark green, orange, legumes, starchy vegetables, and other vegetables) several times per week.

Meat and bean group
Foods in the meat and bean group provide protein, vitamins, and minerals. To help your patient make healthy food choices from this group, suggest that he follow these recommendations:
• Consume low-fat or lean meats and poultry.
• Eat meats that are baked, broiled, or grilled.
• Vary selections among fish, beans, peas, nuts, and seeds.
• Trim away visible fat.
• Consume 5½ oz of meat and beans each day, if following a 2,000-calorie diet.

Milk group
Foods in the milk group provide protein, vitamins, and minerals. To help your patient make healthy choices from this group, suggest that he follow these recommendations:
• Eat or drink 3 cups of milk products each day, if following a 2,000-calorie diet.
• Pick low-fat or fat-free milk, yogurt, and other milk products.
• Choose lactose-free products or other calcium sources, such as fortified foods, if the patient doesn't or can't have milk.

Oils
Oils provide fat, sugar, and calories and have limited nutritional value. They should be used sparingly. To help your patient limit his intake of foods from this group, suggest that he follow these recommendations:
• Choose most sources of fats from fish, nuts, and vegetable oils.
• Cut back on solid fats, such as butter, stick margarine, shortening, and lard.

Be sure to tell your patient to choose low-fat or fat-free milk and milk products.

Vegetarian diets

For various reasons, including religious, environmental, ethical, and health reasons, people may choose to follow vegetarian diets. Typically, vegetarian diets are lower in saturated fat and cholesterol and higher in fiber, carbohydrates, magnesium, boron, folate, antioxidants, carotenoids, and phytochemicals. Vegetarians have a lower risk of obesity, cancer, heart disease, hypertension, dementia, type 2 diabetes mellitus and, possibly, kidney disease, gallstones, and diverticular disease. On the other hand, vegetarians are at risk for protein, iron, and vitamin B_{12} deficiencies. If they avoid dairy products, they are also at risk for calcium and vitamin D deficiencies.

The three basic types of vegetarian diets vary according to the needs or beliefs of the person following the diet:
• Lacto-ovo vegetarians include dairy products and eggs in their diet.
• Lacto-vegetarians include only dairy products as an animal food source in their diet.
• Vegans include no animal food sources in their diet. For patients on such a diet, the use of soybeans and its by-products, along with plant foods, can help provide a balanced diet.

Well-planned vegetarian diets can be nutritionally balanced diets for any patient, including a pregnant or nursing woman. (See *Tips for the vegetarian* and *Nutrient concerns for vegetarians.*)

To help a vegetarian patient meet all the nutrition recommendations of *Dietary Guidelines for Americans 2005*, offer the following suggestions:
• Eat a variety of foods to meet caloric needs.
• Plan meals around sources of protein that are low in fat. This includes beans, lentils, and rice. Avoid using cheeses that are high in fat to replace meat.
• Increase calcium intake by using calcium-fortified, soy-based beverages, which are typically low in fat and cholesterol.
• Prepare food dishes that are usually made with meat or poultry, such as lasagna or pizza, as vegetarian dishes. This increases the number of servings of vegetables while reducing saturated fat and cholesterol.
• Consider vegetarian products that look, and often taste, like meat dishes, such as soy-based sausages and "veggie burgers." These vegetable products are usually low in saturated fat and cholesterol-free.

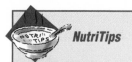

Tips for the vegetarian

If your patient is a vegetarian, suggest these tips to help ensure that he's meeting his daily protein requirements:
• Eat a variety of foods from all food groups, being sure to include all nutrients.
• Consume adequate calories for your lifestyle to prevent your body from using amino acids for fuel.
• Use low-fat or nonfat products and moderately consume nuts and seeds to maintain a low-fat diet.
• Select whole grains whenever possible to increase fiber and iron content.
• Include a vitamin C source at every meal to aid iron absorption.
• Use vitamin supplements, especially vitamin B_{12} (for strict vegans).

Nutrient concerns for vegetarians

It's important to emphasize to vegetarians that they include all nutrients in their diet. Here are some nutrients that are commonly lacking in vegetarian diets as well as suggestions for incorporating them into the diet.

Calcium

Calcium intake is comparable to or higher than that of the nonvegetarian diet. Found in dairy products and dark leafy vegetables, calcium can also be obtained by consuming calcium-fortified products, such as orange juice, or calcium supplements.

Iron

Iron can be incorporated into the diet through the consumption of fortified breads or grains, legumes, and soy products. Dried fruits and foods prepared in cast iron or stainless steel cookware also provide iron.

Iron deficiency anemia isn't prevalent in the vegan population. This may be because vegans consume large amounts of vitamin C, which enhances iron absorption.

Linolenic acid

Linolenic acid is a true dietary fatty acid that aids tissue strength, muscle tone, blood clotting, cholesterol metabolism, and heart function. Usually obtained in fish or eggs, linolenic acid can also be obtained in walnuts, flaxseeds, and soybean and canola oils.

Vitamin B$_{12}$

Vitamin B$_{12}$ occurs naturally only in animal products. It may be used as an additive to such products as cereal or it may be taken as a supplement.

Vitamin D

Vitamin D intake is typically low in the vegan diet because of the lack of milk and milk products; vitamin D can't be obtained in adequate quantities in plants alone. Milk is the largest source of vitamin D because it is fortified with the vitamin.

Vitamin D can also be found in fortified soy milk and ready-to-eat cereal, or it can be obtained by spending about 10 minutes in the sun each day.

Zinc

Vegetarians typically eat fewer foods that contain zinc. Despite this, most maintain adequate levels in the body because there are some plant sources of zinc. The zinc found in plants isn't as easily absorbed as zinc from animal sources. Zinc can also be found in whole grains, soy products, nuts, and seeds.

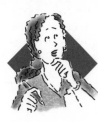

Quick quiz

1. Which of the following activities would be considered a secondary prevention measure?

    A.   Promotion of health behaviors
    B.   Implementation of screenings for disease
    C.   Conduction of classes for patients with diabetes
    D.   Rehabilitation of a stroke patient

Answer: B. Secondary prevention focuses on risk reduction, which may include screening for disease.

2.   Through metabolism, energy is extracted from which nutrients?
   A.   Carbohydrates, proteins, and fats
   B.   Carbohydrates, fats, and sodium
   C.   Fats, adenosine triphosphate, and minerals
   D.   Vitamins, minerals, and electrolytes

Answer: A. Energy is produced through the metabolism of carbohydrates, proteins, and fats.

3.   Essential nutrients are supplied to the body by:
   A.   vitamin or mineral supplements.
   B.   certain food combinations.
   C.   body functions.
   D.   food in many different combinations.

Answer: D. Essential nutrients are supplied by the many combinations of food consumed.

4.   Which of the following populations is most at risk for poor nutrition?
   A.   Young adults
   B.   Adult men
   C.   Adult women
   D.   Elderly people

Answer: D. Elderly people are a high-risk population for poor nutrition due to the aging process.

Scoring

☆☆☆   If you answered all four questions correctly, treat yourself to a fresh salad or a juicy apple! You've earned a tasty reward for knowing the basics of nutrition so well.

☆☆   If you answered three questions correctly, good for you. You have a well-balanced knowledge of nutrient essentials.

☆   If you answered fewer than three questions correctly, don't give up! There's still plenty of time to climb the food guide pyramid and energize your nutrient know-how.

If you thought this chapter was tasty, wait 'til you feast on chapter 2!

crackle crackle

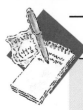

2

Digestion and absorption

Just the facts

The processes of digestion and absorption are fundamental to nutrition. In this chapter, you'll learn:

♦ the purpose of digestion and absorption

♦ structures of the GI tract wall, digestive organs, and accessory organs as well as their functions in digestion and absorption

♦ the mechanical and chemical processes of digestion.

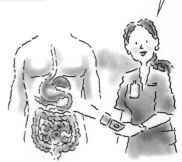

Chew on this fact: Digestion, absorption, and excretion of waste products are the GI tract's major functions.

A look at digestion and absorption

The basic purpose of digestion and absorption is to deliver essential nutrients to the cells in order to sustain life. To break food down into these essential nutrients, the body sends it through various mechanical and chemical processes in the GI tract, or *alimentary canal*. Successful digestion and absorption depend on the coordinated function of the GI tract wall's muscles and nerves, the GI tract organs, and the accessory organs of digestion. (See *Structures of the GI system*, page 20.)

GI tract wall structures

The wall of the GI tract consists of four major layers:

     visceral peritoneum

     tunica muscularis

     submucosa

     mucosa.

Structures of the GI system

The GI system includes the alimentary canal (pharynx, esophagus, stomach, and small and large intestines) and the accessory organs (liver, biliary duct system, and pancreas).

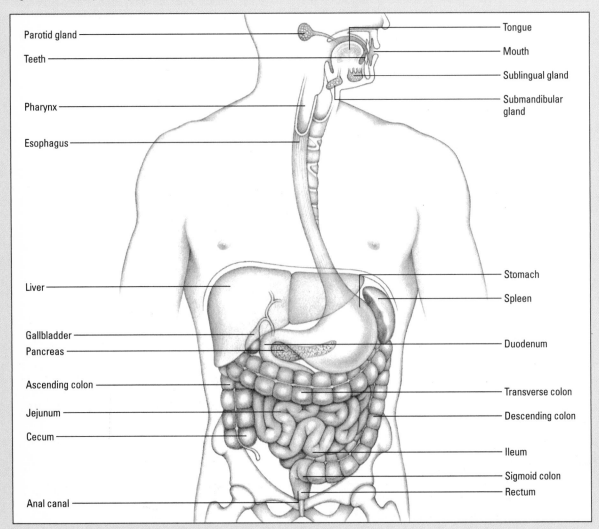

Parotid gland — Teeth — Pharynx — Esophagus — Liver — Gallbladder — Pancreas — Ascending colon — Jejunum — Cecum — Anal canal

Tongue — Mouth — Sublingual gland — Submandibular gland — Stomach — Spleen — Duodenum — Transverse colon — Descending colon — Ileum — Sigmoid colon — Rectum

Visceral peritoneum

The *visceral peritoneum* is the GI tract's outer covering. It covers most of the abdominal organs and lies next to an identical layer, the *parietal peritoneum*, which lines the abdominal cavity.

To serve and protect

The main job of this outer layer of the GI tract wall is to protect the blood vessels, nerves, and lymphatics. It also attaches the jejunum, ileum, and transverse colon to the posterior abdominal wall to prevent twisting.

Many names, one layer

The visceral peritoneum has many names. In the esophagus and rectum, it's called the *tunica adventitia.* Elsewhere in the GI tract, it's called the *tunica serosa.*

Tunica muscularis

The *tunica muscularis,* which lies within the visceral peritoneum, is a layer composed of skeletal muscle in the mouth, pharynx, and upper esophagus.

Elsewhere in the tract...

The tunica muscularis is made up of longitudinal and circular smooth-muscle fibers. At points along the tract, circular fibers thicken to form sphincters.

Pucker pouches

In the large intestine, these fibers gather into three narrow bands (*taeniae coli*) down the middle of the colon and pucker the intestine into characteristic pouches (*haustra*).

Nerve network

Between the two muscle layers lies a nerve network—the *myenteric plexus,* also known as *Auerbach's plexus.* The stomach wall contains a third muscle layer made up of oblique fibers.

Submucosa

The *submucosa,* also called the *tunica submucosa,* lies under the tunica muscularis. It's composed of loose connective tissue, blood and lymphatic vessels, and another nerve network called the *submucosal plexus,* or *Meissner's plexus.*

Mucosa

The *mucosa,* the innermost layer of the GI tract wall, is also called the *tunica mucosa.* This layer consists of epithelial and surface cells and loose connective tissue. Villi from surface cells secrete gastric and protective juices and absorb nutrients.

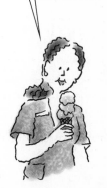

Past the lips, past the gums...look out mucosa, here it comes!

GI tract wall functions

The nerves and muscles of the GI tract wall work jointly to ensure that food moves spontaneously through the digestive system (motility). GI tract functions include innervation and secretion.

GI tract innervation

Distention of the submucosal plexus in the submucosa or myenteric plexus in the tunica muscularis stimulates transmission of nerve signals to the smooth muscle, which initiates contraction and relaxation of these muscles, or *peristalsis*. During peristalsis, longitudinal fibers of the tunica muscularis shorten the lumen length and circular fibers reduce the lumen diameter.

GI tract secretion

Five major substances secreted by the GI tract contribute to the chemical process of digestion:

 Mucus protects the lining of the GI tract and aids in motility.

 Enzymes are proteins that break down nutrients.

Acid and various buffer ions contribute to the level of alkalinity or acidity (pH) needed to activate digestive enzymes.

Electrolytes and water carry nutrients through the GI tract and aid in the absorption process.

Bile emulsifies fat to promote intestinal absorption of fatty acids, cholesterol, and other lipids.

How digestion and absorption work

The organs of the GI tract play the major role in mechanical and chemical digestion and absorption of food and fluid. (See *Functions of the digestive system organs*.) Aided by the GI tract wall and accessory organs, the organs of the GI tract process nutrients in three phases of digestion:

 cephalic

 gastric

 intestinal.

Functions of the digestive system organs

This chart lists the digestive system organs and their primary functions.

Organ	Function
Mouth	• Breaks down food into smaller particles • Releases saliva to promote chewing and swallowing • Secretes amylase (ptyalin) to begin breaking down starch
Esophagus	• Propels food downward into the stomach
Stomach	• Acts as a food reservoir • Mixes food with gastric secretions (hydrochloric acid, pepsin, mucus, intrinsic factor) • Begins protein digestion • Absorbs water, alcohol, and some drugs
Liver	• Produces bile • Metabolizes carbohydrates, protein, and fat • Stores nutrients • Detoxifies drugs and waste products
Gallbladder	• Concentrates and stores bile • Releases bile into the duodenum
Pancreas	• Produces and secretes insulin and glucagon • Produces and secretes digestive enzymes: proteases, lipase, and amylase
Small intestine	• Secretes hormones to stimulate the secretion of pancreatic juices, bile, and intestinal enzymes • Secretes digestive enzymes: peptidases, disaccharidases • Absorbs iron, magnesium, and calcium (duodenum) • Absorbs water-soluble vitamins and simple sugars (jejunum) • Absorbs amino acids, peptides, fat-soluble vitamins, fats, cholesterol, bile salts, and vitamin B_{12} (ileum)
Large intestine	• Absorbs water, sodium, potassium, and vitamin K formed by colonic bacteria • Eliminates solid waste

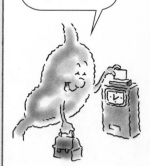

I'd better punch in! All of us GI organs have a lot of work to do.

Cephalic phase

The cephalic phase of digestion uses the GI tract organs of the mouth, pharynx, and esophagus to begin the mechanical processes of digestion. Mechanical digestion breaks down food into smaller particles, which increases the surface area on which digestive enzymes can work.

Mouth

Digestion begins in the mouth (also called the *buccal cavity* or *oral cavity*). Ducts connect the mouth with the three major pairs of salivary glands:
- parotid
- submandibular
- sublingual.

These glands secrete the enzyme *ptyalin* (a salivary amylase) to moisten food during chewing (mastication) and begin breaking down starch into maltose. (See *Causes of dry mouth in older adults.*)

Pharynx

The *pharynx* is a cavity extending from the base of the skull to the esophagus. The pharynx aids swallowing by grasping food and propelling it toward the esophagus.

Esophagus

A muscular tube, the *esophagus* extends from the pharynx through the mediastinum to the stomach.

Down the hatch

When a person swallows, the cricopharyngeal sphincter in the upper esophagus relaxes, allowing food to enter the esophagus. In the esophagus, the glossopharyngeal nerve activates peristalsis, which moves the food bolus down toward the stomach.

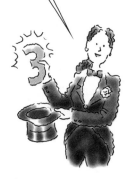

And the magic number is…3. The three major pairs of salivary glands are the parotids, submandibulars, and sublinguals.

Lifespan lunchbox

Causes of dry mouth in older adults

As people age, salivation decreases, leading to dry mouth and a reduced sense of taste. Certain drugs, such as anticholinergics, antihistamines, tricyclic antidepressants, phenothiazines, clonidine, and opioid analgesics, can also decrease salivation. Be sure to take a drug history for older adults. Other causes of dry mouth in older adults include facial nerve paralysis, salivary duct obstruction, Sjögren's syndrome, and radiation of the mouth or face.

One slippery bolus

As food passes through the esophagus, glands in the esophageal mucosal layer secrete mucus, which lubricates the bolus and protects the mucosal membrane from damage caused by poorly chewed foods.

Stomach express

Because food is only in the mouth for a short time, digestion of starch is limited. The salivary amylase that's swallowed continues to work for another 15 to 30 minutes in the stomach before it's inactivated by gastric acids. By the time the food bolus is traveling toward the stomach, the stomach has begun secreting digestive juices (hydrochloric acid [HCl] and pepsin).

Digestive juices are secreted in response to stimuli aroused by smelling, tasting, chewing, or thinking about food.

Gastric phase

When food enters the stomach, the gastric phase of digestion begins.

Stomach

Chemical digestion, which occurs as food mixes with digestive enzymes, begins in the stomach. The stomach acts, in part, as a temporary storage area for food and has four main regions:

 cardia

 fundus

 body

antrum.

Cardia

The *cardia* lies near the junction of the stomach and esophagus. Relaxation of the cardiac sphincter in this region allows food to pass from the esophagus to the stomach.

Fundus

The *fundus* is an enlarged portion above and to the left of the esophageal opening into the stomach. Continued peristaltic activity in this region propels the intact food bolus toward the stomach body.

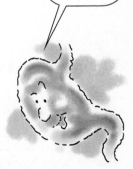

I can't help it. Just thinking about food makes me gush!

Body

The *body* is the middle portion of the stomach. In this region, distention of the stomach wall due to the food bolus stimulates secretion of gastrin.

Gassing up with gastrin

Gastrin, in turn, stimulates the stomach's motor functions and release of digestive secretions by the gastric glands. Highly acidic (pH of 0.9 to 1.5), these secretions consist mainly of HCl, intrinsic factor (which helps the body absorb vitamin B_{12}), and proteolytic enzymes (which help the body use proteins). (See *GI system changes in older adults* and *Sites and mechanisms of gastric secretion.*)

HCl helps absorb calcium and iron and activates gastric enzymes that kill most foodborne bacteria. HCl is also needed to convert the enzyme pepsinogen into pepsin.

Enzyme with pep

Pepsin, a major protein-splitting enzyme, activates the secretion of the gastric mucus that protects the gastric lining. The mucus also helps move the food bolus along the path to the small intestine.

Not much at all but alcohol

Normally, except for alcohol, little food absorption occurs in the stomach. Peristaltic contractions in the stomach body churn the food into tiny particles and mix it with gastric juices, forming *chyme.*

Antrum

The *antrum* is the lower portion of the stomach, lying near the junction of the stomach and duodenum. Stronger peristaltic waves move the chyme from the stomach body into the antrum. Here, it backs up against the pyloric sphincter before being released into the small intestine and triggering the intestinal phase of digestion. (See *Stomach emptying,* page 28.)

Intestinal phase

The majority of absorption occurs during the intestinal phase of digestion, which involves the small and large intestines.

Small intestine

The longest organ of the GI tract, the *small intestine* is a tube measuring about 20′ (6 m) long. It performs most of the work of

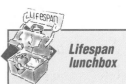

Lifespan lunchbox

GI system changes in older adults

Age-related changes in the GI system can lead to conditions that impact nutrition. Reduced gastric acid secretion in older adults can result in pernicious anemia, iron deficiency anemia, and reduced calcium absorption. Reduced production of bile acid, enlargement of the common bile duct, and increased output of cholecystokinin can lead to biliary stasis, cholelithiasis, and reduced appetite.

Sites and mechanisms of gastric secretion

Between the lower esophageal sphincter (LES), or cardiac sphincter, and the pyloric sphincter lie the fundus, body, antrum, and pylorus of the stomach. These areas have a rich variety of mucosal cells that help the stomach carry out its tasks.

Glands and gastric secretions
Cardiac glands, pyloric glands, and gastric glands secrete 2 to 3 L of gastric juice daily through the stomach's gastric pits.
• Both the cardiac gland (near the LES) and the pyloric gland (near pylorus) secrete thin mucus.
• The gastric gland (in body and fundus) secretes hydrochloric acid (HCl), pepsinogen, intrinsic factor, and mucus.

Protection from self-digestion
Specialized cells line the gastric glands, gastric pits, and surface epithelium. Mucous cells in the necks of the gastric glands produce thin mucus. Mucous cells in the surface epithelium produce an alkaline mucus. Both substances lubricate food and protect the stomach from self-digestion by corrosive enzymes.

Other secretions
Argentaffin cells produce gastrin, which stimulates gastric secretion and motility. Chief cells produce pepsinogen, which breaks proteins down into polypeptides.

Large parietal cells scattered throughout the fundus secrete HCl and intrinsic factor. HCl degrades pepsinogen, maintains an acid environment, and inhibits excess bacteria growth. Intrinsic factor promotes vitamin B_{12} absorption in the small intestine.

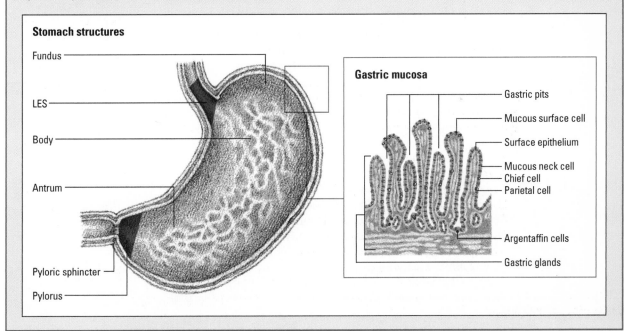

Stomach structures

Fundus

LES

Body

Antrum

Pyloric sphincter

Pylorus

Gastric mucosa

Gastric pits

Mucous surface cell

Surface epithelium

Mucous neck cell
Chief cell
Parietal cell

Argentaffin cells

Gastric glands

digestion and absorption. (See *Digestion and absorption in the small intestine*, page 29.)
The small intestine has three major divisions:
• The *duodenum* is the longest and most superior division.
• The *jejunum*, the middle portion, is the shortest segment.
• The *ileum* is the most inferior portion.

Break it down, please

In the small intestine, intestinal wall contractions and digestive enzymes break down carbohydrates, proteins, and fats so the intestinal mucosa can facilitate absorption of these nutrients into the bloodstream (along with water and electrolytes). These nutrients are then available for use by the body.

The great intestinal wall

The intestinal wall has structural features that significantly increase its absorptive surface area. These features include:
• *plicae circulares* — circular folds of the intestinal mucosa, or mucous membrane lining
• *villi* — fingerlike projections on the mucosa
• *microvilli* — tiny cytoplasmic projections on the surface of epithelial cells.

Secretion police

The small intestine also releases hormones that help control the secretion of bile, pancreatic juice, and intestinal juice.

Large intestine

The main tasks of the large intestine are absorption of body water and elimination of digestive waste. In addition, the large intestine harbors the bacteria *Escherichia coli*, *Enterobacter aerogenes*, *Clostridium perfringens*, and *Lactobacillus bifidus*. All of these bacteria help synthesize vitamin K and break down cellulose into usable carbohydrates. Bacterial action also produces *flatus*, which helps propel stool toward the rectum.

Protection from bacterial action

The mucosa of the large intestine also produces *alkaline secretions* from tubular glands composed of goblet cells. This alkaline mucus lubricates the intestinal walls as food pushes through, protecting the mucosa from acidic bacterial action.

The *large intestine* extends from the ileocecal valve (the valve between the ileum of the small intestine and the first segment of the large intestine) to the anus. The large intestine has five segments:

 cecum

 ascending colon

 transverse colon

 descending and sigmoid colons

 rectum.

Stomach emptying

The rate of stomach emptying depends on several factors, including gastrin release, neural signals generated when the stomach wall distends, and the *enterogastric reflex*.

Enterogastric reflex
The enterogastric reflex is a response in which the duodenum releases secretin and gastric-inhibiting peptide, and the jejunum secretes cholecystokinin. Both reactions decrease gastric motility.

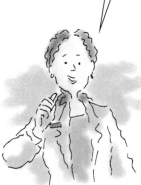

There's nothing small about the job of the small intestine. It does most of the digesting and absorbing!

Digestion and absorption in the small intestine

The small intestine performs most of the work of digestion and absorption. Here's a summary of the small intestine's major tasks.

Mechanical digestion
- Small muscles mix chyme.
- Peristaltic motions propel the food mass over the length of the intestine.
- Surface villi mix chyme at the intestinal wall, enhancing absorption.
- Long muscle moves the food mass in a circular motion, providing new surface sites for absorption.
- Segmentation rings from circular muscle mix the food into soft masses and then mix it with secretions.

Chemical digestion
- Lipase breaks fats into fatty acids and glycerides.
- Amylase converts starch to the disaccharides maltose and sucrose.
- Enterokinase activates trypsinogens, which become trypsin.
- Trypsin and chymotrypsin split protein molecules into small peptides and then into individual amino acids.

- Disaccharidases convert their respective disaccharides to monosaccharides.
- Bile from the liver helps to digest and absorb fat.
- Carbohydrate foods are changed into simple sugars.
- Fats are changed into fatty acids and glycerides.
- Proteins are changed into amino acids.
- Vitamins and minerals are also released.

Absorption
- Microvilli, villi, and mucus absorb essential nutrients.
- Absorption is controlled by diffusion — passive for the small materials and carrier-assisted for larger items.
- Digestive contents are mostly water soluble and can be absorbed directly into the circulation.
- Fatty contents aren't water soluble; they must pass through the villi, then into the lymph system, and finally into the bloodstream.

Cecum

The *cecum*, a saclike structure, makes up the first few inches of the large intestine. The cecum is connected to the ileum of the small intestine by the ileocecal pouch.

Ascending colon

The *ascending colon* rises on the right posterior abdominal wall, then turns under the liver at the hepatic flexure. By the time chyme passes through the ileocecal valve and enters the ascending colon of the large intestine, it has been reduced to mostly indigestible substances.

Transverse colon

The *transverse colon* is located above the small intestine, passing horizontally across the abdomen and below the liver, stomach, and spleen. It proceeds to turn downward at the left colic flexure. Through blood and lymph vessels, the large intestine has absorbed all but about 100 ml of water from the chyme by the time it leaves the transverse colon. It also absorbs large amounts of sodium and chloride at this point.

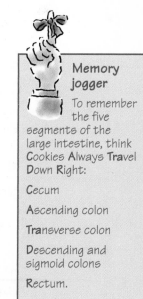

Memory jogger

To remember the five segments of the large intestine, think Cookies Always Travel Down Right:

Cecum

Ascending colon

Transverse colon

Descending and sigmoid colons

Rectum.

Got to have your fiber

Because dietary fiber isn't digested, it travels through the large intestine unabsorbed and contributes to the formation of feces.

Descending and sigmoid colons

The *descending colon* starts near the spleen and extends down the left side of the abdomen into the pelvic cavity. The *sigmoid colon* descends through the pelvic cavity, where it becomes the rectum. The descending and sigmoid colons are responsible for evacuation. Contents move slowly along the tract, enabling water and electrolytes to be absorbed.

Rectum

The *rectum*, the last few inches of the large intestine, terminates at the anus.

Mass movement

In the lower colon, long and relatively sluggish contractions cause propulsive waves, or *mass movements*. Normally occurring several times per day, these movements propel intestinal contents into the rectum and produce the urge to defecate.

Accessory organs of digestion and absorption

Accessory organs of the digestive system—the liver, biliary duct system, and pancreas—contribute hormones, enzymes, and bile vital to digestion and absorption.

Liver

The body's largest gland, the highly vascular liver, is enclosed in a fibrous capsule in the right upper quadrant of the abdomen.

The *lesser omentum*, a fold of peritoneum, covers most of the liver and anchors it to the lesser curvature of the stomach. The *hepatic artery* and *hepatic portal vein* as well as the common bile duct and hepatic veins pass through the lesser omentum.

Functioning features

The liver's functional unit, the *lobule*, consists of a plate of hepatic cells, or *hepatocytes*, that encircle a central vein and radiate out-

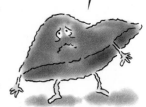

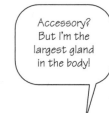

Accessory? But I'm the largest gland in the body!

ward. Separating the hepatocyte plates from each other are *sinusoids*, the liver's capillary system. Reticuloendothelial macrophages (Kupffer's cells) lining the sinusoids remove bacteria and toxins that have entered the blood through the intestinal capillaries.

Go with the blood flow

The sinusoids carry oxygenated blood from the hepatic artery and nutrient-rich blood from the portal vein. Unoxygenated blood leaves through the central vein and flows through hepatic veins to the inferior vena cava.

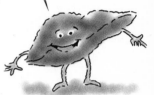

My role in carbohydrate metabolism is very important. I also detoxify plasma.

All that and a bag of chips

The liver performs many important functions in the processes of digestion and absorption. The liver:
• aids in carbohydrate metabolism
• detoxifies various endogenous and exogenous toxins, such as drugs and alcohol
• synthesizes plasma proteins, nonessential amino acids, and vitamin A
• stores essential nutrients, such as vitamins K, D, B_{12}, and iron
• removes ammonia from body fluids, converting it to urea for excretion in urine
• converts glucose to glycogen and stores it as fuel for the muscles
• produces and secretes bile to aid in digestion
• stores fats and converts the excess sugars to fats to store in other parts of the body
• removes naturally occurring ammonia from body fluids, converting it to urea for excretion in the urine.

Biliary duct system

The biliary duct system consists of a network of ducts and includes the gallbladder.

Ducts

Think of ducts as a subway system transporting bile through the GI tract. *Bile* is a greenish liquid composed of water, cholesterol, bile salts, and phospholipids. From the liver, bile travels via the common bile duct to the small intestine, entering through the duodenum.

When bile salts are MIA

When bile salts are absent from the intestinal tract, lipids are excreted and fat-soluble vitamins are absorbed poorly.

Report on bile production

The liver recycles about 80% of bile salts into bile, combining them with bile pigments (biliverdin and bilirubin, the breakdown products of red blood cells) and cholesterol. The liver secretes this alkaline bile continuously. Bile production may increase from stimulation of the vagus nerve, release of the hormone secretin, increased blood flow in the liver, and the presence of fat in the intestine. (See *GI hormones: Production and function.*)

Gallbladder

The *gallbladder* is a pear-shaped organ joined to the ventral surface of the liver by the cystic duct. The gallbladder:

• stores and concentrates bile produced by the liver

• releases bile into the common bile duct for delivery to the duodenum in response to the contraction and relaxation of the sphincter of Oddi.

The secretion of the hormone cholecystokinin causes the gallbladder to contract. This allows the release of bile into the common bile duct for delivery to the duodenum.

> They got us on charges of accessories to digestion. Who says chyme doesn't pay?

Pancreas

The *pancreas* is a somewhat flat organ that lies behind the stomach. Its head and neck extend into the curve of the duodenum and its tail lies against the spleen. The pancreas performs both exocrine and endocrine functions.

Exocrine function

The pancreas' exocrine function involves scattered cells that secrete more than 1,000 ml of digestive enzymes every day. Lobules and lobes of the clusters (*acini*) of enzyme-producing cells release their secretions into ducts that merge into the pancreatic duct. The pancreatic duct runs the length of the pancreas and joins the bile duct from the gallbladder before entering the duodenum. The vagus nerve stimulates the production and release of secretin and cholecystokinin, which are the two hormones responsible for regulating the rate and amount of pancreatic secretions.

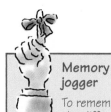

Memory jogger

To remember the difference between exocrine and endocrine, just remember that **exo**crine refers to **ex**ternal, so **endo**crine refers to **in**ternal.

GI hormones: Production and function

When stimulated, GI structures secrete four hormones. Each hormone plays a different part in digestion.

Hormone and production site	Stimulating factor or agent	Function
Gastrin Produced in pyloric antrum and duodenal mucosa	• Pyloric antrum distention • Vagal stimulation • Protein digestion products • Alcohol	Stimulates gastric secretion and motility
Gastric inhibitory peptides Produced in duodenal and jejunal mucosa	• Gastric acid • Fats • Fat digestion products	Inhibits gastric secretion and motility
Secretin Produced in duodenal and jejunal mucosa	• Gastric acid • Fat digestion products • Protein digestion products	Stimulates secretion of bile and alkaline pancreatic fluid
Cholecystokinin Produced in duodenal and jejunal mucosa	• Fat digestion products • Protein digestion products	Stimulates gallbladder contraction and secretion of enzyme-rich pancreatic fluid

Endocrine function

The endocrine function of the pancreas involves the islets of Langerhans. Two types of cells formulate the islets of Langerhans, alpha and beta cells.

The ABCs of alpha and beta cells

Over 1 million of these alpha and beta cells are in the islets. Alpha cells secrete *glucagon*, a hormone that stimulates glycogenolysis in the liver; beta cells secrete insulin to promote carbohydrate metabolism. Both hormones flow directly into the blood. Their release is stimulated by blood glucose levels.

Pancreatic duct

Running the length of the pancreas, the *pancreatic duct* joins the bile duct from the gallbladder before entering the duodenum. Vagal stimulation and release of the hormones secretin and cholecystokinin control the rate and amount of pancreatic secretion.

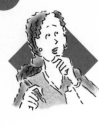

Quick quiz

1. Which of the following functions is characteristic of the stomach?
    A. Breaks down carbohydrates for absorption
    B. Mixes food with gastric secretions
    C. Completes food digestion
    D. Helps synthesize vitamin K

Answer: B. The stomach mixes food with gastric secretions to aid digestion.

2. Which GI hormone stimulates gastric secretion and motility?
    A. Gastrin
    B. Gastric inhibitory peptides
    C. Secretin
    D. Pepsinogen

Answer: A. Gastrin is produced in the pyloric antrum and duodenal end mucosa and stimulates gastric secretion and motility.

3. In which phase of digestion does the stomach secrete the digestive juices hydrochloric acid and pepsin?
    A. Cephalic
    B. Gastric
    C. Intestinal
    D. Mastication

Answer: A. By the time the food is traveling toward the stomach, the cephalic phase — during which the stomach secretes digestive juices — has begun.

Scoring

☆☆☆ If you answered all three questions correctly, bravo! You've passed through the GI system and absorbed this material with the greatest of ease.

  ☆☆ If you answered two questions correctly, super. You've chewed the fat of this system, and it's time to move on.

    ☆ If you answered fewer than two questions correctly, keep at it! Take a few more minutes to digest this material.

Carbohydrates

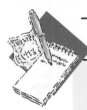

Just the facts

This chapter reviews carbohydrates, one of the essential nutrients that must be consumed in the diet. In this chapter, you'll learn:

♦ classification of carbohydrates

♦ carbohydrate functions

♦ the ways in which carbohydrates are digested, absorbed, and metabolized

♦ food sources of carbohydrates.

A look at carbohydrates

Carbohydrates are organic compounds of carbon, hydrogen, and oxygen that are stored in muscles and in the liver and can be converted quickly when the body needs energy. Carbohydrates are made through photosynthesis—the process by which the sun's energy allows chlorophyll-containing plants to take in carbon dioxide through their roots and release oxygen into the air. Carbon and water that remain in the plant form carbohydrates.

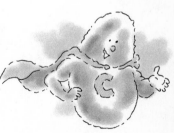

Carbohydrates are organic compounds that can be quickly converted to energy.

Classification of carbohydrates

Carbohydrates are classified according to the number of sugar units, or *saccharides*, that make up their structure:
• Simple carbohydrates are sugars with a simple structure of on (*monosaccharides*) or two (*disaccharides*) sugar units.
• Complex carbohydrates, or starches, consist of many sugar units (*polysaccharides*).

Singled out

Monosaccharides, also known as *simple sugars*, are carbohydrates that can be absorbed through the small intestine into the blood, where they then travel to the liver. Monosaccharides aren't broken down in the digestive process.

Examples of monosaccharides include:
• glucose (dextrose), which comes from the digestion of starch and circulates in the blood; it's the primary fuel for cells
• fructose (fruit sugar), which is found in fruits and in honey
• galactose, which comes from the digestion of lactose and is the sweetest of the sugars.

Two sweet

Disaccharides consist of two monosaccharides (one of which is glucose) minus a water molecule. These simple carbohydrates must first be digested into their component monosaccharides before being absorbed.

Important disaccharides include:
• sucrose — common table sugar that occurs naturally in minimal amounts in some fruits and vegetables
• lactose — nonsweet sugar found in milk that aids calcium absorption and helps manufacture bacteria that are necessary for vitamin K production in the intestines
• maltose — sugar found in germinating grains that's also a by-product of stomach digestion.

Poly want a cracker?

Polysaccharides, or complex carbohydrates, consist of larger, more complex molecules of carbohydrates that contain many sugar units. Polysaccharides are ingested and broken down into simple sugars so that they can later be used as fuel.

Examples of polysaccharides include:
• starch, which is found primarily in plant foods and is most abundant in grains, legumes, and starchy vegetables (such as potatoes and corn)
• glycogen, which is formed within the body's tissues and is then converted as needed to glucose for metabolism and energy balance
• fiber, commonly referred to as *roughage*, which is found in fruits, vegetables, legumes, and grains (it can't be digested and, therefore, is vital to good dietary health). (See *Poor oral health effects in older adults*.)

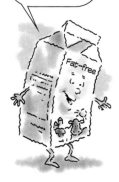

The lactose found in milk aids calcium absorption and vitamin K production.

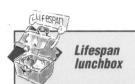

Lifespan lunchbox

Poor oral health effects in older adults

Older adults with dental problems or ill-fitting dentures might have trouble chewing fruits, vegetables, and whole grains. Older adults who avoid these foods are at increased risk for nutritional deficiencies. Moreover, poor oral health may result in ineffective chewing, increasing the risk of choking.

Functions of carbohydrates

The metabolic processes of anabolism and catabolism keep the body's carbohydrate supply in constant flux, ensuring that adequate supplies are available for both energy needs and the production of other necessary compounds.

Other functions of carbohydrates include:
• conserving protein during energy production
• helping to burn fats more efficiently and completely
• providing a quick source of energy (glucose)
• aiding in the normal functioning of the intestines (fiber)
• providing laxative action and aiding in the absorption of calcium (lactose).

Although the body can make glucose from amino acids and glycerol, carbohydrates serve as the body's primary energy source. The Recommended Dietary Allowance (RDA) is based on the role of carbohydrates as a primary energy source for the brain. The Acceptable Macronutrient Distribution Range, the percentage of total calories for energy nutrients, is based on the role of carbohydrates as a source of calories to maintain body weight and to reduce the risk of chronic disease and should be 45% to 65% of total calories.

Function 1: Energy

The primary function of carbohydrates is to meet the body's specific needs for energy. Each gram of carbohydrates yields 4 kilocalories (kcal) of energy. Because glucose burns more efficiently and completely than protein or fat and because it has no end products that must be excreted, it's the body's primary fuel source. Within cells, glucose molecules are partially broken down to produce energy in the form of adenosine triphosphate (ATP). To function properly, the body must have a continuous supply of glucose available to all cells. (See *Tracking the glucose pathway*, page 38.)

Brains constantly crave carbs

Carbohydrates are also the primary source of energy for the central nervous system, especially the brain. Because the brain can't store carbohydrates, it must have an uninterrupted source of carbohydrates to function properly.

Preventing the misappropriation of protein

Adequate carbohydrate intake is also essential to protein function. To meet the high energy demands of the body, dietary protein is converted to glucose when the supply of carbohydrates is inade-

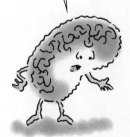

If you want me to function properly, keep the carbs coming!

Tracking the glucose pathway

All ingested carbohydrates are converted to glucose, the body's main energy source. Glucose catabolism generates energy in three phases: glycolysis, the Krebs cycle, and the electron-transport chain. The flowchart shown here summarizes the first two phases.

Glycolysis
Glycolysis, the first phase, breaks apart one molecule of glucose to form pyruvate, which yields energy in the form of adenosine triphosphate (ATP) and acetyl coenzyme A (acetyl CoA).

Krebs cycle
The second phase, the Krebs cycle, continues carbohydrate metabolism. Fragments of acetyl CoA join to oxaloacetic acid to form citric acid. The CoA molecule breaks off from the acetyl group and may form more acetyl CoA molecules. Citric acid is first converted into intermediate compounds, and then back into oxaloacetic acid. The Krebs cycle also liberates carbon dioxide (CO_2).

Electron-transport chain
In the third phase of glucose catabolism, molecules on the inner mitochondrial membrane attract electrons from hydrogen atoms and carry them through oxidation-reduction reactions in the mitochondria. The hydrogen ions produced in the Krebs cycle then combine with oxygen (O_2) to form water (H_2O).

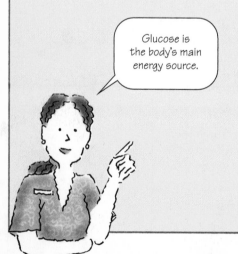

Glucose is the body's main energy source.

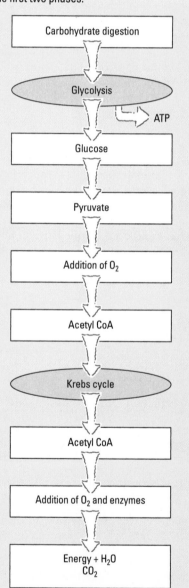

Carbohydrate digestion

Glycolysis

ATP

Glucose

Pyruvate

Addition of O_2

Acetyl CoA

Krebs cycle

Acetyl CoA

Addition of O_2 and enzymes

Energy + H_2O
CO_2

quate. Protein used for energy is then unavailable for other protein functions, such as replenishing enzymes, hormones, and blood cells. When the supply is extremely low, the body begins to break down its own protein tissue. This results in the production of energy as well as a reduction in energy needs. Adequate carbohydrate intake is especially important when the body's protein needs are high, such as for wound healing and during pregnancy and breast-feeding.

Fat's not good

The body also breaks down stored fat to meet its fuel needs when carbohydrate levels are low. When partially broken down fats accumulate in the blood, they form ketones. Although muscles and other body tissues can use ketones for energy, they're normally produced only in small quantities. Rising ketone levels lead to ketosis, which may result in fatigue, nausea, and lack of appetite. If the condition becomes severe, coma and death may result.

Function 2: Other compounds

After the body's energy demands are met, excess glucose can be converted to glycogen, used to produce nonessential amino acids and other compounds, or converted to fat and stored.

Conversion version

Liver and muscle cells pick up unused glucose molecules and join them together to form glycogen, which is stored in the liver and in muscles. Liver glycogen stores can quickly be converted to glucose in times of need. Between meals, glycogen breaks down and releases glucose into the bloodstream to maintain normal blood glucose levels and provide fuel for tissues. Muscle glycogen stores are available only for use by the muscles.

Essentials of nonessentials

If an adequate supply of essential amino acids is available, the body can use them and glucose to make nonessential amino acids. Nonessential amino acids are necessary for protein synthesis and metabolism (tissue and cellular). Because the body can synthesize nonessential amino acids with the use of nitrogen, they don't have to be consumed in the diet.

Fat figures

When body energy requirements are met, glycogen reserves are full, and body compounds are made, liver cells convert the remaining glucose into triglycerides, which are stored in body fat. Liver cells do so by combining acetate molecules to form fatty acids, which then are combined with glycerol to make triglycerides.

How the body handles carbohydrates

Carbohydrates move through the body via the processes of digestion, absorption, and metabolism.

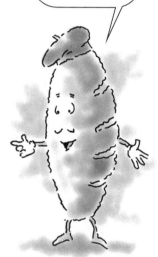

Zut alors! In order for the starches found in me to be absorbed, they must first be broken down into simple sugars.

Digestion

Monosaccharides are the only carbohydrates that the body can absorb intact. All other forms of digestible carbohydrates must be broken down into monosaccharides before they can be absorbed:
• Disaccharides must be split, in one step, into their two component sugar molecules for digestion.
• Starches require a step-by-step breakdown of complex sugar molecules into simple ones for digestion.

Too much to swallow?

Carbohydrate digestion begins in the mouth, where food is chewed and broken down into smaller particles. The food mass, now known as *chyme,* is moved by peristalsis to the small intestines, where most carbohydrate digestion occurs. In the small intestine, pancreatic amylase breaks down complex carbohydrates into disaccharides. Disaccharide enzymes (maltase, sucrase, and lactase) finish digestion by splitting maltose, sucrose, and lactose into monosaccharides, which are the only form of carbohydrates the body can absorb. (See *Carbohydrate digestion.*)

Fiber foibles

The GI tract lacks the enzymes to digest fiber; however, fiber is important because it can speed up the digestive process. Insoluble fiber isn't soluble and can't be dissolved in water; soluble fiber dissolves or forms a gel in water. Soluble fibers delay gastric emptying. Most fibers react with bacteria in the large intestine to form gas, water, short-chain fatty acids, and other compounds. Short-chain fatty acids are an energy source for the mucosal lining of the colon.

Absorption

The monosaccharides glucose, fructose, and galactose are absorbed through the intestinal mucosa and travel to the liver through the portal vein. Small amounts of starch and fiber that haven't been fully digested are excreted in feces. Soluble fiber slows the absorption of glucose, delaying the rise in serum glucose that occurs after eating.

Carbohydrate digestion

This chart explains how carbohydrates are digested in the body.

Organ	Action
Mouth	• Chewing action breaks down food into smaller particles. The salivary enzyme amylase acts on starch to break it down first into dextrins and then into maltose.
Stomach	• Peristalsis mixes food particles with gastric secretions.
Small intestine	• The pancreatic enzyme amylase continues the breakdown of starch to maltose. • The intestinal enzyme sucrase acts on sucrose to produce fructose. • The intestinal enzyme lactase acts on lactose to produce galactose. • The intestinal enzyme maltase acts on maltose to produce glucose.

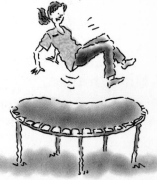

What goes up must come down. Insulin and glucagon regulate rising and falling glucose levels.

Metabolism

In the liver, fructose and galactose are converted to glucose. The liver then releases glucose into the bloodstream, where its level is maintained by the actions of hormones. A rise in serum blood glucose stimulates insulin, which moves glucose out of the bloodstream and into the cells.

Leveling off

Eventually, the body uses up the energy from the most recent meal and blood glucose levels start to fall. Even a slight drop in glucose stimulates the pancreas to release glucagon, which causes the liver to release glucose from its supply of glycogen. The result is that blood glucose levels again rise to normal.

Sources of carbohydrates

Carbohydrates are found in all of the food groups. The amounts and types of carbohydrates vary considerably between food groups and among selections within each group.

Grain group

Grains include bread, cereal, rice, and pasta. They provide complex carbohydrates and some protein; some grain selections also contain fat. Fiber content is low in refined products, moderate in whole grains, and highest in bran products. At least half of the recommended servings of grains should be whole grains. Grains represent the foundation of a healthy diet.

For many selections in this group, one serving provides approximately 15 g of carbohydrates. A serving is equal to:

- 1 slice of bread
- ½ c cooked pasta or rice
- ½ c cooked cereal
- ½ English muffin or small bagel.

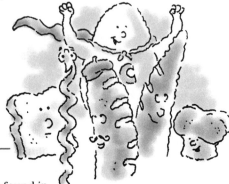

The best place to find me is in breads, cereals, rice, and pasta.

Vegetable group

Most of the carbohydrates in the vegetable group are found in starchy vegetables, such as peas, corn, potatoes, and legumes.

Fruit group

The fruit group contains many foods that are mostly sugar. Dried fruits have a higher sugar content than fresh fruits because the removal of water increases the sugar concentration. In addition, eating whole fruits rather than drinking fruit juice increases fiber intake.

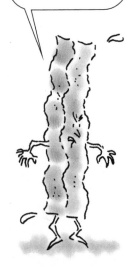

There's at least one of us in every group. Most of the carbs in the vegetable group are found in starchy vegetables such as potatoes.

Milk group

The milk, yogurt, and cheese (or dairy) group contains the sugar lactose. Such dairy products as chocolate milk, strawberry yogurt, and ice cream are flavored or have added sugar, which increases the amount of carbohydrates per serving. Cheese, however, is a selection from the dairy group that's low in lactose and, therefore, low in carbohydrates.

Meat and beans group

The foods in the meat and beans group are mostly protein. However, dried beans, which are a plant source of protein, are also high in carbohydrates, such as starch and fiber. In addition, the majority of the calories in nuts come from fats, but most varieties of nuts have 4 to 8 g of carbohydrates per 1-oz serving.

Legumes belong to both the vegetable and meat and beans group because they contain nutrients and both groups are high in fiber.

Carbohydrates in health promotion

Carbohydrates should provide 45% to 65% of the total calories in a person's diet, with the majority coming from complex carbohydrates (starches). Foods with added sugar, such as soft drinks, candy, cookies, and fruit drinks, should be limited. The RDA of carbohydrates for children and adults is 130 g/day.

Balancing act

Each type of carbohydrate has its own benefits to a person's health. The key to a healthy diet is balance, consuming selections from each food group in moderation. At least 50 g/day of carbohydrates are necessary to prevent the physical symptoms of ketosis and muscle wasting.

Fiber

Fiber, which has numerous health benefits, is a polysaccharide that may be soluble or insoluble:
• Soluble fiber dissolves in water and forms a gel. It's primarily found in fruits, vegetables, oats, barley, and legumes and the grain psyllium. Soluble fiber binds bile acids so they can't be reabsorbed in the colon, which aids in their excretion. This reduces serum cholesterol, a risk factor for cardiovascular disease. Soluble fiber also helps delay blood glucose concentration in diabetic patients by slowing glucose absorption in the small intestine.
• Insoluble fiber doesn't dissolve in water. It is found primarily in the bran layers of cereal grains and in certain vegetables (such as cabbage and brussel sprouts). Insoluble fiber increases fecal bulk and decreases free radicals in the GI tract. The recommended intake of dietary fiber is 13 to 14 g for every 1,000 calories consumed. (See *Tips for increasing fiber intake* and *Constipation in older adults*, page 44.)

Fantastic fiber facts

Because humans lack the enzymes necessary to digest fiber, it can't be broken down by the body for fuel. However, this inability to be digested gives fiber unique benefits, including:
• preventing or relieving constipation (insoluble)
• protecting against colon and rectal cancer (insoluble)

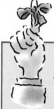

Memory jogger

The benefits of fiber are easy to "C." It prevents:

Constipation

Cancer

Colonic diverticulitis.

It also Causes a feeling of fullness and reduces Cholesterol.

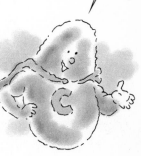

Approximately 45% to 65% of a healthy person's total caloric intake should come from carbohydrates.

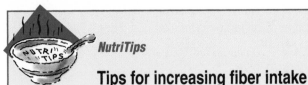

NutriTips

Tips for increasing fiber intake

Here are some easy ways to increase your daily fiber intake:
- Choose whole fruits or vegetables over juice.
- Eat a variety of fruits and vegetables daily.
- Eat foods with whole grains instead of refined grains, such as whole wheat breads, brown rice, and whole wheat English muffins.
- Read the fiber content on cereal boxes and choose one that has at least 5 g of fiber per serving.
- Eat foods that include beans, such as chili, bean burritos, and minestrone soup.

- preventing diverticulitis (insoluble)
- reducing serum cholesterol (soluble)
- aiding weight management by causing a feeling of fullness, which leads to reduced intake (insoluble)
- decreasing blood glucose (soluble).

Sugar

Even though sugar isn't an independent risk factor for any particular disease, limiting sugar is wise, especially for patients with diabetes mellitus, obesity, or cardiovascular disease. Excess sugar intake is associated with an increased risk of dental caries, which may be a predictor of heart disease.

How much is enough?

Added sugars provide minimal or no essential nutrients. They include the sugars and syrup added to foods and beverages that are not naturally occurring. Encourage your patient to select foods without added sugars to meet his nutritional needs while reducing the amount of calories. Even if he consumes only nutrition-dense foods (those low in fat and without added sugars), only a small amount of calories are left for added sugars and other low nutrition-dense foods, such as fats and alcohol. This is called *discretionary calorie allowance*.

For example, according to the *Dietary Guidelines for Americans 2005*, if a patient consumes a 2,000-calorie diet, only about 267 discretionary calories remain. If 29% of discretionary calories

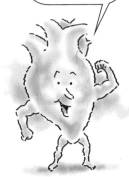

Increasing fiber intake helps to reduce cholesterol levels and keeps a heart healthy!

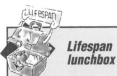

Lifespan lunchbox

Constipation in older adults

Constipation is a concern in as much as 20% of adults older than age 65. Encourage older adult patients to eat foods high in dietary fiber, such as fresh fruits and vegetables, bran, and other whole grain products. Recommend that they drink plenty of fluids each day unless contraindicated by a medical condition. Also be sure to emphasize the importance of regular exercise.

come from total fat, that leaves just 8 tsp of added sugar to consume each day.

Here are some tips you can give your patient to help him decrease his daily sugar intake:
• Select foods with no added sugars.
• Drink fewer soft drinks; replace with unsweetened beverages, milk, or water.
• Choose 100% juice rather than sugar-sweetened juices.
• Reach for fruits instead of candy, cakes, and cookies. ·
• Plan and prepare snacks ahead of time so there's no need to visit high-calorie vending machines.
• Use sugar alternatives (especially if you're diabetic or obese)
• Read the ingredients to figure out whether food contains added sugars. (See *Recognizing added sugars.*)
• Compare food choices by looking at the Nutrition Facts label and choosing products with the least sugar. Remind the patient that the sugars listed on the Nutrition Facts label include both naturally occurring and added sugars.

Sugar substitutes

Sugar alcohols, such as sorbitol, mannitol, and hydrogenated starch hydrolyses, are low-calorie alternatives to sugar. Nonnutritive sweeteners, such as saccharin, aspartame, and sucralose, have virtually no calories and are much sweeter than sugar, requiring smaller amounts for flavor. However, patients with phenylketonuria must limit their intake of aspartame because they can't metabolize the phenylalanine it contains, which increases the risk of toxic blood levels.

> Although I may go by a pseudonym to disguise my identity on food labels, sugar is still sugar.

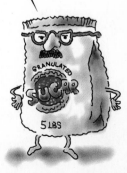

Recognizing added sugars

Help your patient avoid added sugars in foods by teaching him to look for "hidden" sources of sugar on food labels. Examples include:
• corn sweetener
• corn syrup (especially high-fructose)
• dextrose
• fructose
• fruit juice concentrates
• glucose
• honey
• lactose
• maltose
• malt syrup
• molasses
• sucrose
• sugar (brown, invert, raw)
• syrup.

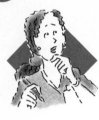

Quick quiz

1. Carbohydrates are composed of all of the following elements except:

- A. carbon.
- B. hydrogen.
- C. nitrogen.
- D. oxygen.

Answer: C. Carbohydrates are organic compounds that are composed of carbon, hydrogen, and oxygen.

2. Which substance is a type of carbohydrate?

- A. Monosaccharide
- B. Amino acid
- C. Lipid
- D. Albumin

Answer: A. Monosaccharides, or simple sugars, are carbohydrates that aren't broken down in the digestive process.

3. Which hormone regulates the blood glucose level?

- A. Insulin
- B. Cortisol
- C. Epinephrine
- D. Thyroxine

Answer: A. Insulin is the only hormone that significantly reduces blood glucose by aiding glucose entry into the cells, stimulating glycogenesis, and promoting glucose catabolism.

4. Carbohydrates are found in which of the following food groups?

- A. Vegetable
- B. Milk
- C. Grain
- D. All of the above

Answer: D. Carbohydrates can be found in all food groups.

Don't try to worm your way out of reading the next chapter. It's packed with protein power!

Scoring

☆☆☆ If you answered all four questions correctly, excellent! It looks like you've been carb-loading the right information.

☆☆ If you answered three questions correctly, you're getting the essentials! Move on to the next chapter.

☆ If you answered fewer than three questions correctly, don't worry! Your body is just craving more carbohydrates. Go back and review the chapter.

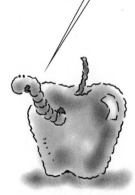

Protein

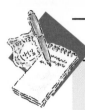

Just the facts

This chapter explains the importance of the essential nutrient protein to the body. In this chapter, you'll learn:

♦ classification of protein

♦ protein functions

♦ the ways in which proteins are digested, absorbed, and metabolized

♦ food sources of protein.

A look at protein

Proteins, which are components of every living cell, are large, complex molecules composed of individual building blocks known as *amino acids*. Like carbohydrates, amino acids are organic compounds made from carbon, hydrogen, and oxygen atoms. Unique to amino acids is their nitrogen component, which distinguishes them from other energy nutrients. Proteins come in various sizes and shapes and are composed of different amino acids joined in various proportions and sequences. The shape of a protein molecule determines how it functions.

Protein is required for normal growth and development. It's broken down by the body as a source of energy when the supply of carbohydrates and fats is inadequate. Protein is stored in muscle, bone, blood, skin, cartilage, and lymph.

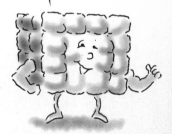

Protein is the body's backup generator. I'm used for energy after carbs and fats.

Amino acids

All amino acids have a carbon atom core with four bonding sites: one site holds a hydrogen atom, one an amino group (NH_2), and one an acid group (COOH). Attached to the fourth bonding site is a side group (R group), which contains the atoms that give each amino acid its distinct identity.

Essential and nonessential amino acids

Amino acids are the structural units of proteins. Here's a list of the 22 amino acids required by the body. They're divided into two classes: essential (can't be synthesized and must be obtained from the diet) and nonessential (can be synthesized and therefore don't need to be obtained from the diet).

Essential
- Arginine
- Histidine
- Isoleucine
- Leucine
- Lysine
- Methionine
- Phenylalanine
- Threonine
- Tryptophan
- Valine

Nonessential
- Alanine
- Asparagine
- Aspartic acid
- Cystine
- Glutamic acid
- Glutamine
- Glycine
- Hydroxylysine
- Hydroxyproline
- Proline
- Serine
- Tyrosine

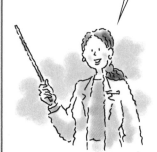

There are 22 common amino acids: 10 essential and 12 nonessential.

Reviewing the essentials

There are 22 common amino acids. Ten of them are classified as essential amino acids because they can't be made by the body and therefore must be consumed through food. The remaining 12 are nonessential amino acids because they can be synthesized in the liver if nitrogen and other precursors are available. (See *Essential and nonessential amino acids*.)

Classification of food protein

Food proteins are classified as complete or incomplete. This classification depends on their amino acid compositions.

Complete proteins

Complete proteins are foods that contain all of the essential amino acids in the correct proportions. They must contain enough of each amino acid to meet the body's needs. Meat, milk, cheese, and eggs are considered complete proteins. Soy is the only plant source that's considered a complete protein.

Incomplete proteins

If a food source is deficient or has limited amounts of one or more essential amino acids, it's considered an incomplete protein. With the exception of soybeans, all plant proteins are incomplete.

The buddy system

It's possible to combine two different incomplete proteins to make a complete protein. In other words, one source may be lacking a particular amino acid; if that amino acid is found in another source, together they can create a complete protein. Examples of foods that contain complementary proteins include:

- black beans and rice
- bean taco
- pea soup with toast
- peanut butter sandwich
- french toast
- vegetable quiche
- cereal and milk.

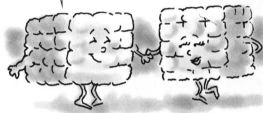

Two incomplete proteins that can be combined to obtain sufficient quantities and proportions of all essential amino acids are called complementary proteins.

That's what friends are for!

Functions of protein

Protein performs many functions in the body:

- The primary function of protein is the growth, repair, and maintenance of body structures and tissue. The body's cells are always making proteins to replace those that are broken down from normal wear.
- Proteins are involved in the manufacture of hormones, such as insulin and epinephrine.
- Proteins may act as enzymes that help bring about certain chemical reactions, such as digestion or protein synthesis.
- Plasma proteins (such as albumin) aid in maintaining fluid and electrolyte balance by attracting water and causing changes in osmotic pressure.
- Amino acids contain an acid and a base; therefore, they can neutralize excesses of either acids or bases in the body, thereby maintaining a normal pH.
- Proteins help transport other substances through blood. For example, hemoglobin transports oxygen and lipoproteins transport lipids.
- Proteins function within the immune system by helping to create lymphocytes and antibodies that protect the body from infection and disease.

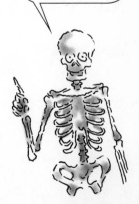

A continuous supply of protein maintains body structures, such as bones, muscles, tendons, skin, and hair.

- Protein is a component of numerous body compounds, including thrombin, which helps blood to clot.
- Proteins can be used as a source of energy (providing 4 cal/g) when intake of carbohydrates and fats is inadequate.

How the body handles protein

Protein moves through the body via the processes of digestion, absorption, and metabolism.

Digestion

The digestion of protein begins in the stomach, where hydrochloric acid (HCl) works on protein to make it more susceptible to the action of enzymes. HCl converts pepsinogen to the enzyme pepsin. Pepsin begins to break down proteins into smaller polypeptides and some amino acids.

The bulk of protein digestion takes place in the small intestines with the help of enzymes secreted by the pancreas. These pancreatic enzymes (trypsin, chymotrypsin, and carboxypeptidase) are responsible for breaking down proteins into simpler substances (tripeptides, dipeptides, and amino acids). Enzymes located on the surface of the intestinal wall (aminopeptidase and dipeptidase) complete the digestive process. (See *Protein digestion*.)

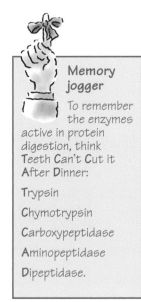

Memory jogger

To remember the enzymes active in protein digestion, think Teeth Can't Cut it After Dinner:

Trypsin

Chymotrypsin

Carboxypeptidase

Aminopeptidase

Dipeptidase.

Absorption

Amino acid absorption takes place in the mucosa of the small intestines through active transport, with the aid of vitamin B_6. Intestinal cells release amino acids into the bloodstream for transport to the liver through the portal vein.

Metabolism

Protein metabolism is a constant two-part process. Proteins are broken down by the body into amino acids through the process of catabolism and then resynthesized into tissues as needed through anabolism. This continuous conversion is needed to maintain overall protein balance within the body.

Leave it to liver

The liver serves many important functions related to protein metabolism:

Protein digestion

Active enzymes in the stomach and intestine break protein down into various substances, as shown below.

Organ	Active enzymes	Digestive action
Stomach	Pepsin	• Breaks protein into polypeptides
Intestine	Trypsin-pancreatic enzyme	• Breaks protein and polypeptides into tripeptides and dipeptides
	Chymotrypsin-pancreatic enzyme	• Breaks protein and polypeptides into tripeptides and dipeptides
	Carboxypeptidase	• Breaks polypeptides into simpler peptides and amino acids
	Aminopeptidase	• Breaks polypeptides into peptides, dipeptides, and amino acids
	Dipeptidase	• Breaks dipeptides into amino acids

• It uses the amino acids that it needs and releases those that aren't needed elsewhere.
• It retains amino acids to make liver cells, nonessential amino acids, and plasma proteins, such as heparin, prothrombin, and albumin.
• It regulates the release of amino acids into the bloodstream and removes excess amino acids from the circulation.
• It regulates energy metabolism by removing nitrogen from amino acids so that they can be burned for energy and by converting amino acids into glucose or fat, as necessary.

Waiting pool

Unlike excess glucose and fat, the body can't store excess protein for later use. However, a limited supply of free amino acids exists within cells in a metabolic pool that accepts and donates amino acids as needed. This metabolic pool is constantly changing in response to the ongoing buildup and breakdown of body proteins and the influx of amino acids from food.

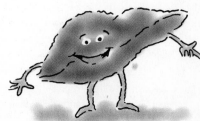

I regulate the release of amino acids in the bloodstream and remove excess amino acids from the circulation.

Neutral nitrogen balance is best

When the amount of protein made is equal to the amount used, as in healthy adults, the body has a neutral nitrogen balance. If protein synthesis exceeds protein breakdown, such as during growth, pregnancy, or recovery from injury, a positive nitrogen balance exists. A negative nitrogen balance exists when protein breakdown exceeds protein synthesis, such as during starvation.

Protein turnovers

The body's supply of amino acids comes from food (exogenous) and its own protein tissue (endogenous). Amino acids released from protein breakdown may be recycled to build new proteins or burned for energy. This continuous process of protein synthesis and breakdown is called *protein turnover*.

The rate of turnover varies throughout the body. For example, turnover in the GI system (pancreas, liver, and stomach) is rapid, and turnover in muscles is slower.

Sources of protein

Proteins can be found in both plant and animal sources. In each food group, the protein quantity and quality vary among the items, with the meat and bean group (chicken, dry beans, steak, peanut butter) and milk group (cottage cheese, yogurt, hard cheese) having the greatest amounts of protein. The grain group (oatmeal, crackers, whole grain bread) and vegetable group (dark green and deep yellow vegetables) contain lesser amounts of protein, whereas the fruit group has minimal amounts of protein. (See *Lactose intolerance link to race*.)

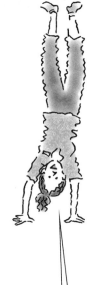

Protein synthesis and breakdown happens continuously in a process called *protein turnover*.

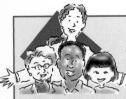

Bridging the gap

Lactose intolerance link to race

As much as 90% of black adults have lactose intolerance. Other ethnic groups with a high incidence of lactose intolerance include Mexican-Americans, some Native American tribes, Asians, and Ashkenazic Jews. When caring for patients from these ethnic groups, ask about a family history of lactose intolerance and question them about its signs and symptoms.

Proteins in health promotion

The Recommended Dietary Allowance (RDA) of protein in a healthy diet is 0.8 g/kg of recommended body weight per day, or approximately 10% of total recommended daily calories. This protein allowance is based on the minimum requirements needed to maintain nitrogen balance and the mixed quality of proteins typically consumed. The recommended protein allowance per kilogram of body weight is higher for children (from infancy to adolescence) and for pregnant and breast-feeding women.

Other factors also determine how much protein the body needs. Emotional or physical stress, infection, and high environmental temperatures increase protein needs. Protein requirements also increase during times when the body must heal itself, such as after surgery, trauma, or burn injuries.

Building up the body

Protein needs are also higher for people with large muscle mass because muscle tissue is metabolically active and requires protein to maintain itself. Many bodybuilders believe that consuming large amounts of protein will help increase their muscle strength and size. Some even utilize protein supplements. It's important to remind your patient that muscles are built and maintained through a combination of caloric intake and strength training. (See *Supplement setbacks*, page 54.) A bodybuilder should consume 60% to 65% of his total calories as carbohydrates and should consume adequate amounts of protein, 1 g to 1.5 g of protein per kilogram of body weight.

Hi-pro, hi-pro...

Despite the importance of protein in forming muscle, protein intake shouldn't exceed twice the RDA, or 1.6 g/kg of body weight for adults. High protein intake:
• increases the excretion of calcium, which may increase the risk of osteoporosis
• increases excretion of nitrogen by the kidneys, which may play a role in the loss of renal function
• increases the risk of atherosclerosis and colon and prostate cancers.

Building muscle requires adequate amounts of carbohydrates and protein.

Supplement setbacks

Single amino acid supplements can offer more of one amino acid than another. When this occurs, it may have adverse effects in the body. For example, an excess of the amino acid tryptophan, which promotes sleep, has been linked to cases of permanent brain damage and even death.

If your patient is a bodybuilder, advise him not to use supplements to build and maintain muscle mass; instead, suggest that he:

▪ consume tuna, eggs, and milk as protein sources rather than protein powders and liquids to provide an adequate supply of protein in the diet.

▪ drink adequate fluids because exercise increases the body's fluid requirements.

▪ eat a variety of foods from all food groups.

▪ consume calories appropriate for his lifestyle, which may mean larger or more frequent meals.

Vegetarian variations

For most Americans, protein intake isn't a concern because the amounts of proteins and calories consumed are more than adequate. Most vegetarian diets also meet or surpass the RDA for protein; however, these diets contain less protein than nonvegetarian diets. To obtain adequate daily protein intake, a vegan should consume adequate amounts of the essential amino acids from plants. Soy protein, which is found in such foods as tempeh (fermented soybeans), tofu (soybean curd), textured soy products (soy flour altered to look like ground beef on rehydration), and meat analogs (soy hot dogs), is a meat alternative that's also a good source of protein.

Although most vegetarian diets aren't lacking in protein, some don't meet the minimum requirements for other important nutrients. For example, calcium, iron, linolenic acid, vitamins B_{12} and D, and zinc are important nutrients that can't be obtained in adequate quantities from plants and, therefore, are commonly lacking in vegetarian diets.

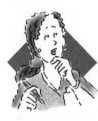

Quick quiz

1. Two incomplete proteins that combine to make a complete protein are known as:
- A.   combination proteins.
- B.   complementary proteins.
- C.   common proteins.
- D.   core proteins.

Answer: B. When two incomplete proteins combine to make a complete protein, they're known as complementary proteins. Examples include peanut butter sandwiches and bean tacos.

2. Essential amino acids are:
- A.   the structural units of proteins that must be obtained from the diet.
- B.   the structural units of proteins that don't need to be obtained from the diet.
- C.   organic compounds that don't dissolve in water but do dissolve in alcohol and other organic compounds.
- D.   inorganic compounds.

Answer: A. Essential amino acids are protein units that can't be synthesized in the body and therefore must be obtained from the diet.

3. The primary function of protein in the body is:
- A.   maintenance of fluid and electrolyte balance.
- B.   transportation of lipids.
- C.   growth, repair, and maintenance of body structures and tissue.
- D.   maintenance of normal pH.

Answer: C. The primary function of protein is growth, repair, and maintenance of body structures and tissue.

4. Which of the following hormones is protein responsible for manufacturing?
- A.   Insulin
- B.   Thyroxine
- C.   Oxytocin
- D.   Estrogen

Answer: A. Protein is responsible for the manufacture of insulin for the body.

5.   Which of the following amino acids is considered an essential amino acid?

    A.   Cystine
    B.   Glutamine
    C.   Tyrosine
    D.   Lysine

Answer: D. Lysine is an essential amino acid that can't be synthesized by the body and, therefore, must be obtained in the diet.

Scoring

☆☆☆   If you answered all five questions correctly, you're a protein pro! Don't be shy about moving onto the chapter about fat.

☆☆   If you answered four questions correctly, you don't have to worry about your protein intake. You've thoroughly digested the information in this chapter.

☆   If you answered fewer than four questions correctly, don't be discouraged. Go take a dip in your metabolic pool and then come back and review the chapter.

5

Fat

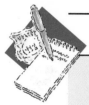

Just the facts

This chapter presents information about dietary fat. In this chapter, you'll learn:

♦ classification of fat

♦ fat functions

♦ the ways in which fats are digested, absorbed, and metabolized

♦ food sources of fat.

A look at fat

Fats (lipids) are organic compounds that dissolve in alcohol and other organic solvents but don't dissolve in water. Fats are composed of the elements carbon, hydrogen, and oxygen. Although these are the same elements that make up carbohydrates, the proportions of oxygen to carbon and hydrogen are lower in fats. Because fats have less oxygen, they provide more than double the amount of calories than the same amount of carbohydrates. The body gets many fats from consumed food, but it also manufactures some fats.

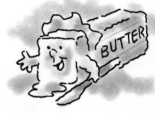

Fats are like supersized carbs — they're double the calorie count.

Classification of fat

There are three kinds of fats: triglycerides, trans fats, phospholipids, and sterols.

Triglycerides

Triglycerides account for approximately 95% of the fat in foods and are the major storage form of fat in the body. The basic structural unit of triglycerides is one molecule of glycerol joined to three fatty acid chains.

The chain gang

A fatty acid is composed of a chain of carbon atoms with hydrogen and a few oxygen atoms attached. The fatty acid chains joined to the glycerol molecule vary in length and composition. The different taste, smell, and physical appearance of each fat results from the variety of fatty acids and their physical arrangements in the fat molecule. The length of the chain, which can be between 2 and 24 carbon atoms long, determines how the body transports and absorbs the fat. Short-chain fatty acids have 2 to 4 carbon atoms, medium-chain fatty acids contain 6 to 12 carbon atoms, and long-chain fatty acids include more than 12 carbon atoms. Long-chain fatty acids are found in most food fats.

Saturation explanation

Saturation of fatty acids depends on how many hydrogen atoms bond to the four potential bonding sites of each carbon atom. If all four sites have a hydrogen atom bond, it's *saturated.* Because all of the carbon atoms are bonded to as many hydrogen atoms as they can hold, no double bonds between carbon atoms exist.

Saturated fats are found in meat, poultry, full-fat dairy products, and tropical oils, such as palm and coconut oils. Most saturated fats:
- originate from animal sources
- remain solid at room temperature
- have high melting points
- are less likely to become rancid.

Unsaturation explanation

An *unsaturated* fatty acid is a fatty acid that isn't completely filled with all the hydrogen atoms it can hold. This results in the formation of double bonds between carbon atoms.

In general, unsaturated fats:
- originate from plant fat and oils
- are soft or liquid at room temperature
- have lower melting points than saturated fats
- can become rancid when exposed to extended periods of light and oxygen.

There are two types of unsaturated fatty acids, monounsaturated (MUFA) and polyunsaturated (PUFA). MUFA are found mostly in vegetable oils, such as olive, canola, and peanut oils. PUFA are found in nuts and vegetable oils, such as sunflower, safflower, and soybean oils and in fatty fish. (See *Comparing saturated and unsaturated fats.*)

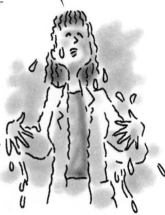

I'm saturated! I guess that means all of my carbon atoms are bonded to hydrogen atoms. No double carbon bonds here!

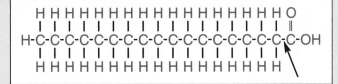

Comparing saturated and unsaturated fats

The saturation of fatty acids depends on how many hydrogen atoms bond to the four potential bonding sites of each carbon atom and the number of resulting double carbon bonds.

Saturated
A saturated fatty acid has no carbon-carbon double bonds.

Unsaturated
A monounsaturated fatty acid has only one double carbon bond.

A polyunsaturated fatty acid has more than one double carbon bond.

Trans fats

In a process called *hydrogenation*, manufacturers add hydrogen to polyunsaturated oils to make them solid at room temperature. The hydrogenation process improves the shelf-life of foods, making them less likely to become rancid. Oils that are lightly hydrogenated remain liquids but are more stable than polyunsaturated fats because they don't have as many double carbon bonds. Partially hydrogenated oils, however, are solid at room temperature.

Factory fat

Trans fat is produced by the hydrogenation process and is found in vegetable shortening, certain margarines, crackers, cookies, snack foods, and other foods made with hydrogenated oils. Small amounts of trans fat occur naturally, mostly in dairy products but also in some meats and other animal foods.

Phospholipids

Phospholipids are a group of compound fats that are similar to triglycerides. They contain a glycerol molecule but only two fatty acid chains. Instead of the third fatty acid, phospholipids have a phosphate group and another nitrogen-containing compound. Phospholipids occur naturally in almost all foods.

Sterols

Sterols are complex molecules in which carbon atoms form four cyclic structures attached to various side chains. Sterols don't contain glycerol or fatty acid molecules. Cholesterol is one example of a sterol.

Cholesterol

Cholesterol, the most common sterol, is a fatlike substance that's manufactured daily by the body. The liver produces cholesterol and filters out excess cholesterol to eliminate it from the body. Cholesterol also is a component of the foods that we eat. It occurs naturally in all animal foods.

Cholesterol has several important functions:
- It's a vital component of bile salts that help in fat digestion.
- It's an essential part of all cell membranes. It's also found in brain and nerve tissue and in the blood.
- It's necessary for the production of several hormones, including cortisone, adrenaline, estrogen, and testosterone.

Functions of fat

Most people are all too aware that fats contribute flavor, satiety, and palatability to food in the diet. They also supply texture to food, intensify its flavor, and enhance its odor. In addition, these nutrients serve many functions in the body. Different fats have specific functions. For example, phospholipids work as emulsifiers to keep fats suspended in the blood and in body fluids. They also serve as an integral part of cell membranes and help to transport nutrients, metabolites, and fat-soluble substances across cell membranes.

Fats perform six general functions in the body:

- providing energy for the body
- facilitating absorption of fat-soluble vitamins
- supplying essential fatty acids
- supporting and protecting internal organs
- aiding in temperature regulation
- lubricating body tissue.

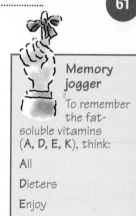

Memory jogger

To remember the fat-soluble vitamins (A, D, E, K), think:

All

Dieters

Enjoy

Kale.

It may not be true, but it will help you remember!

Fat as fuel

Fat is a concentrated form of energy that provides 9 cal/g—double the amount of calories of either a carbohydrate or protein. Yet fat isn't the body's preferred fuel source because it's more difficult to metabolize. Stored fat in adipose cells represents the body's largest and most efficient energy reserve. Adipose cells have a virtually limitless capacity to store fat.

Taking in your vitamins

Dietary fat facilitates the absorption of the fat-soluble vitamins—A, D, E, and K.

Suppliers of essential fatty acids

Dietary fat supplies the essential fatty acids: linoleic acid and alpha-linolenic acid. These are considered essential fatty acids because the body can't manufacture them. Essential fatty acids are important for maintaining healthy skin, promoting normal growth in children, and maintaining healthy immune function. They may also play a role in the prevention of age-related chronic diseases, such as heart disease and Alzheimer's disease.

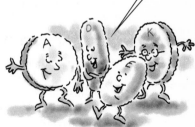

Dietary fat helps us become absorbed.

People padding

Fatty tissue cushions and protects vital organs by providing a supportive fat pad that absorbs mechanical shocks. Examples of organs supported by fat are the eyes and kidneys.

Body insulation

Fat layers insulate the skin, helping to protect the body from excessive heat or cold. A sheath of fatty tissue surrounding nerve fibers provides insulation to help transmit nerve impulses.

Pretty slick

Fats also lubricate the body tissue. The human body manufactures oil in structures called *sebaceous glands*. Secretions from sebaceous glands lubricate the skin to slow the loss of body water to the outside environment.

How the body handles fat

Fat moves through the body via the processes of digestion, absorption, and metabolism. To be transported throughout the body, fats must combine with plasma proteins to form lipoproteins.

Digestion

A minimal amount of fat digestion occurs in the mouth and stomach. General muscle action mixes the fat with the stomach contents. As fat enters the duodenum, it stimulates the release of the hormone cholecystokinin, which stimulates the gallbladder to release bile. Bile is an emulsifier that breaks fat into small particles and reduces the surface tension so that enzymes can penetrate the fat and work more effectively.

The pancreas provides a punch

Most fat digestion occurs in the small intestine. Pancreatic lipase, a powerful fat enzyme, breaks off one fatty acid at a time from the triglyceride molecule until only two free fatty acids and a monoglyceride are left. Each step of this process requires more energy. The end products of digestion are mostly monoglycerides with free fatty acids and some glycerol, which are absorbed into the intestinal cells. Small amounts of fat (4 to 5 g) escape digestion and are excreted in the feces.

The digestion of phospholipids is similar; however, the end products are two free fatty acids and a phosphorous fragment. Cholesterol isn't digestible; rather, it's absorbed unaltered.

Absorption

In the duodenum and jejunum, 95% of consumed fat is absorbed. Small fat particles are absorbed directly through the mucosal cells into the capillaries leading to the portal vein and liver.

Back to the beginning

Larger fat particles (monoglycerides and long-chain fatty acids) are dissolved into a compound called *micelles*, which are created from the bile salts that encircle the fat particles to aid their diffusion into the intestinal cells. After delivering the fat to the intestinal cells, the released bile salts are reabsorbed in the terminal ileum, travel back to the liver, and are then recycled. Once inside the intestinal cells, monoglycerides and long-chain fatty acids combine to form triglycerides. These triglycerides, along with phospholipids and cholesterol, become encased in protein to form chylomicrons (a class of lipoproteins). Chylomicrons transport absorbed fats from the intestinal cells through the lymph system and eventually into the bloodstream for distribution throughout the body.

Metabolism

In the bloodstream, triglycerides in the chylomicrons are broken down into glycerol and fatty acids by lipoprotein lipase, a fat-digesting enzyme located on the surface of adipose cells and other body cells. These fatty acids and glycerol enter cells, where they can be broken down for energy or rebuilt into triglycerides for storage. Fat metabolism is regulated by the hormones adrenocorticotropin, epinephrine, glucagon, glucocorticoids, and thyroxine, which also promote fat mobilization (catabolism). Insulin, another hormone, stimulates fat synthesis (anabolism).

Until required for use as energy fuel, lipids are stored in adipose tissue within cells. When needed for energy, each fat molecule is hydrolyzed to glycerol and three molecules of fatty acids. Glycerol can be converted to pyruvic acid and then to acetyl coenzyme A (CoA), which enters the Krebs cycle.

Ketone body formation

The liver normally forms ketone bodies from acetyl CoA fragments, derived largely from fatty acid catabolism. Acetyl CoA molecules yield three types of ketone bodies:

acetoacetic acid — results from the combination of two acetyl CoA molecules and subsequent release of CoA from these molecules

beta-hydroxybutyric acid — forms when hydrogen is added to the oxygen atom in the acetoacetic acid molecule; *beta* indicates the location of the carbon atom containing the hydroxyl (OH) group

acetone — forms when the carboxyl (COOH) group of acetoacetic acid releases carbon dioxide; muscle tissue, brain tissue, and other tissues oxidize these ketone bodies for energy.

More than enough

Under certain conditions, the body produces more ketone bodies than it can oxidize for energy. Such conditions include fasting, starvation, and uncontrolled diabetes (in which the body can't break down glucose). The body must then use fat instead of glucose as its primary energy source.

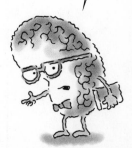

Along with other tissues, I oxidize ketone bodies for energy.

Ketone cops

Use of fat instead of glucose for energy leads to an excess of ketone bodies. This condition disturbs normal acid-base balance and homeostatic mechanisms, leading to ketosis.

Lipid formation from proteins and carbohydrates

Excess amino acids can be converted to fat through keto acid–acetyl CoA conversion. Glucose may be converted to pyruvic acid and then to acetyl CoA, which is converted into fatty acids and then fat (in much the same way that amino acids are converted into fat).

Lipid carriers

Lipoproteins are a group of compounds made by the body that transport lipids through the bloodstream to various parts of the body. All lipoproteins contain both lipids and protein but in different ratios. As the protein concentration increases, the density of the lipoprotein increases. There are four types of lipoproteins:

 very low-density lipoproteins (VLDLs)

 low-density lipoproteins (LDLs)

 high-density lipoproteins (HDLs)

 chylomicrons.

Each type of lipoprotein has a different function. (See *Types of lipoproteins.*)

Sources of fat

The type and amount of fat in each food group vary. Some fat is visible, such as butter and the fat surrounding a piece of steak. However, most fat is invisible, such as the fat in milk, cheese, and nuts and the fat that's intertwined in the steak. Animal sources account for approximately 57% of total fat intake; plant sources account for the rest. (See *Dietary sources of trans fats*, page 66.)

The top five sources of saturated fat in the diet of an American adult are:

 beef

 butter or margarine

Types of lipoproteins

The various types of lipoproteins are detailed here.

Very low-density lipoproteins (VLDLs)

VLDLs are produced and secreted by the liver cells. They contain 50% triglycerides, some cholesterol, phospholipids, and protein. VLDLs transport the lipids made in the liver to body tissues. They
also lose triglycerides to body cells and gain cholesterol from other body tissues. When present in
large concentration, VLDLs may increase the risk of atherosclerosis.

Low-density lipoproteins (LDLs)

LDLs are the major carrier of cholesterol in the blood. They contain 50% cholesterol, lesser
amounts of protein and phospholipids, and a small amount of triglycerides. LDLs are responsible for transporting cholesterol from the liver to the tissues. Commonly called "bad" cholesterol, LDLs are the major contributor to atherosclerosis.

High-density lipoproteins (HDLs)

Referred to as "good" cholesterol, HDLs are made by the liver and contain 50% protein, with
lesser amounts of cholesterol, phospholipids, and triglycerides. HDLs carry cholesterol from
body tissues to the liver, where it's recycled or degraded. High HDL levels decrease the risk of
atherosclerosis.

Chylomicrons

Chylomicrons are composed of triglycerides absorbed from food and contain little protein, phospholipids, and cholesterol. They transport dietary fats from the intestine to the liver and other
body cells. Chylomicrons are the least dense and the largest of the lipoproteins.

 salad dressings, including mayonnaise

 cheese

 milk.

Major sources of trans fat in the diet include french fries,
doughnuts, and other commercially fried foods. Other sources of
trans fat include cookies, crackers, and other baked goods.

Grain group

Grains naturally contain very little fat. However, prepared foods
within this group, such as granola cereals, pancakes, doughnuts,
cakes, cookies, and pies, contain significant added fat. These
foods may also be sources of trans fat.

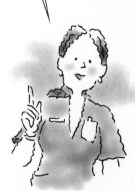

Most of
the fat we
consume is
invisible. Too
bad it shows
up later!

Dietary sources of trans fat

Instruct your patient to reduce his intake of trans fat as much as possible. The major dietary sources of trans fat are listed here in decreasing order.

Food group	Contribution (percent of total trans fats consumed)
Cakes, cookies, crackers, pies, bread etc.	40
Animal products	21
Margarine	17
Fried potatoes	8
Potato chips, corn chips, popcorn	5
Household shortening	4

Adapted from U.S. Department of Agriculture. Center for Nutrition Policy and Promotion. (2005). Dietary Guidelines for Americans 2005 [Online]. *www.health.gov/dietaryguidelines/dga2005/document/*

Vegetable and fruit groups

With the exception of avocado, coconut, and olives, fruits don't contain appreciable amounts of fat. Unadulterated vegetables contain little or no fat. Vegetables that are fried, creamed, served with cheese, or mixed with mayonnaise contain significantly more fat.

Milk group

Items within the milk group come in fat-free, reduced-fat, and whole-fat varieties. To reduce your patient's risk of high-fat intake among foods in this group, advise him to read labels and compare different varieties and brands. Because dairy foods originate from animals, also have him watch cholesterol levels in these products.

Meat and beans group

The plant items in this group (beans and nuts) are cholesterol-free and contain little or no saturated fat. In general, untrimmed meats are higher in fat than lean portions and white meat is lower in fat than dark meat (chicken). Shellfish, such as crab, lobster, and shrimp, are high in cholesterol but low in fat and saturated fat. (See *Mercury warning*.)

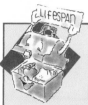

Lifespan lunchbox

Mercury warning

Because some fish contain high levels of mercury that could be harmful to the nervous system of an unborn or developing child, pregnant women, women who are nursing, and young children should avoid fish known to be high in mercury. According to a Food and Drug Administration (FDA) advisory, these populations should avoid shark, swordfish, king mackerel, and tilefish. The FDA recommends eating up to 12 oz of fish and shellfish that are lower in mercury each week. Popular fish and shellfish that are low in mercury include shrimp, canned light tuna, salmon, pollock, and catfish. Tuna steaks contain higher levels of mercury than canned light tuna.

Fat in health promotion

The American Heart Association, Surgeon General, American Cancer Society, and American Diabetes Association all suggest that consumers choose diets low in fat, saturated fat, trans fat, and cholesterol and moderate in total fat.

The *Dietary Guidelines for Americans 2005* also recommend a diet low in saturated fat, trans fat, and cholesterol and moderate in total fat. However, this diet isn't recommended for everyone, particularly children and people who need to consume calorie-dense foods, such as elderly patients and those with chronic renal failure. (See *Fat intake for children.*)

Don't spend your fat allowance all in one place

For healthy adults, the *Dietary Guidelines for Americans 2005* recommend a total fat intake of 20% to 35% of total calories, with most fat calories coming from polyunsaturated and monounsaturated fats. To help your patient meet this recommended guideline, make these suggestions:
• Reduce intake of trans fats as much as possible.
• Limit saturated fat to less than 10% of total calories. (See *Maximum daily amounts of saturated fats*, page 68.)
• Limit cholesterol to 300 mg or less daily.
See also *Tips to reduce dietary fat*, page 69.

Stress to your patient that a low-fat diet needs to be centered on the right types of fat. For example, high levels of polyunsaturated fat has been shown to lower "good" and "bad" cholesterol levels. High levels of monounsaturated fats and low levels of saturated and trans fats in the diet may produce the right changes in

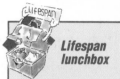

Lifespan lunchbox

Fat intake for children

The American Academy of Pediatrics recommends no restriction of fat or cholesterol for children ages 2 years and younger, when rapid growth and development require high energy levels. The Dietary Guidelines for Americans 2005 recommend that total fat intake in children ages 2 to 3 years should be 30% to 35% of calories, 25% to 35% is recommended for children between ages 4 and 18. The majority of fats should come from polyunsaturated and monounsaturated fats.

As children begin to consume fewer calories from fat, they should replace these calories by eating more grain products, fruits, vegetables, low-fat milk products or other calcium-rich foods, beans, lean meat, poultry, and fish or other protein-rich foods.

Maximum daily amounts of saturated fats

As recommended by the Dietary Guidelines for Americans 2005, instruct your patient to limit saturated fat intake to less than 10% of total daily calorie intake. The following table lists maximum daily amounts by total calorie intake.

Total calorie intake	Limit of saturated fat intake
1,600	18 g or less
2,000	20 g or less
2,200	24 g or less
2,500	25 g or less
2,800	31 g or less

Source: U.S. Department of Agriculture. Center for Nutrition Policy and Promotion. (2005). Dietary Guidelines for Americans 2005 [Online]. *www.health.gov/dietaryguidelines/dga2005/document/*

HDL and LDL levels; however, if the diet is too high in fat, weight gain may result, increasing the risk of heart disease.

Read the writing

The Food and Drug Administration established new nutritional label laws that go into effect in January 2006 and require manufacturers of conventional foods and some dietary supplements to list trans fat on the Nutrition Facts panel in addition to total fat grams, saturated fat grams, milligrams of cholesterol, and percentage of daily value from fat. This change can help patients make healthier food decisions to reduce their intake of trans fat and lower their risk of heart disease. As part of this new ruling, trans fat must be listed on a separate line, directly below saturated fats on the nutrition panel. If total fat content is under 0.5 g, this listing isn't required. (See *Understanding new nutrition labeling,* page 70.)

Food product labels also make fat content claims such as "93% fat-free." However, these claims are usually based on the weight of the product and not the number of calories. Therefore, these products don't necessarily fall within dietary guidelines for 20% to 35% of calories from fat. (See *Translating fat terminology,* page 71.)

Calling in the replacements

Fat replacers are utilized to substitute for the characteristics of fat without the calories and saturation. Replacers can be made from carbohydrates, protein, or even fat:

• Olestra, which is made from vegetable oil, fatty acids, and sugar molecules, doesn't provide calories because the body can't absorb

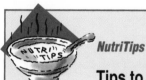

NutriTips

Tips to reduce dietary fat

Here are some additional tips that can help your patient reduce fat in his diet:
• Use fats and oils sparingly in cooking and at the table.
• Use low-fat or fat-free salad dressings.
• Choose vegetable oil and soft margarines most often because they're lower in saturated fat than solid shortenings.
• Choose low-fat sauces with pasta, rice, and potatoes.
• Season foods with herbs, spices, lemon juice, and fat-free or low-fat salad dressings.
• Eat meats labeled "lean" or "extra lean" and trim visible fat from meat. Remove the skin from poultry before eating it.
• Eat lean fish, poultry, meats, or other protein-rich foods, such as beans, each day.
• Limit intake of organ meats (liver).
• Drink two to three servings of low-fat or fat-free milk and milk products daily.
• Choose monounsaturated fats (such as olive and canola oils) and polyunsaturated fats (such as soybean oil, corn oil, sunflower oil, nuts, and fish) over saturated and trans fats.
• Choose fish that contain omega-3 fatty acids and may reduce the risk of heart disease, such as mackerel, sardines, and salmon.

Memory jogger

To reduce fat intake, advise your patient not to fry foods. Instead, encourage him to remember the three **Bs** of cooking:

Bake

Boil

Broil.

it. It may cause GI upset, such as cramping and diarrhea, and may decrease the absorption of fat-soluble vitamins.
• Lighter Bake is a carbohydrate-based fat replacer made from starch, gels, and grain- or fruit-based fibers. It may have a laxative effect if taken in large amounts.
• Simplesse is a protein-based replacer made by converting proteins in milk, egg, or corn using a cooking and blending process. It isn't effective in products that require a high cooking temperature.
    Fat replacers should be used only as part of an overall plan for healthy eating.

Disease prevention

More than any other nutrient, fat is identified as playing a leading role in several chronic diseases. Evidence is overwhelming that high-fat diets increase the risk of cardiovascular disease, obesity, and certain cancers.

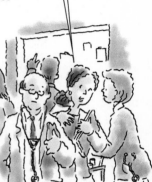

Not enough room to work? That's what fat can do to arteries — plaques of fat narrow artery lumens, reducing blood flow.

Understanding new nutrition labeling

According to new guidelines that went into effect in January 2006, trans fat must be listed separately on Nutrition Facts labels. When selecting food choices, look at the number of grams of saturated fat and trans fat as well as the percentage of daily value (%DV) of cholesterol. Choose products with the lowest combined number of grams of saturated fat and trans fat and the lowest %DV of cholesterol. When looking at saturated fat and cholesterol, a %DV of 5% or less is considered low, while a %DV of 20% or more is considered high. Note that no reference value for %DV is provided for trans fat. That's because health experts recommend that people keep intake of trans fats as low as possible to reduce the risk of coronary heart disease.

Nutrition Facts

Serving Size: Approx. 14 crackers (32g)
Servings Per Container: about 9

Amount Per Serving

Calories 150	Calories from Fat 60

	% Daily Value*
Total Fat 6g	**9**%
Saturated Fat 0.5g	**3**%
Trans Fat 0g	
Polyunsaturated Fat 2g	
Monounsaturated Fat 3.5g	
Cholesterol 0mg	**0**%
Sodium 300mg	**13**%
Potassium 60mg	**2**%
Total Carbohydrate 21g	**7**%
Dietary Fiber 3g	**12**%
Sugars 3g	
Protein 2g	

Vitamin A 0%	•	Vitamin C 0%
Calcium 2%	•	Iron 6%

* Percent Daily Values are based on a 2,000 calorie diet. Your daily values may be higher or lower depending on your calorie needs:

	Calories	2,000	2,500
Total Fat	Less Than	65g	80g
Sat Fat	Less than	20g	25g
Cholesterol	Less than	300mg	300mg
Sodium	Less than	2,400mg	2,400mg
Total Carbohydrate		300g	375g
Dietary Fiber		25g	30g

Calories per gram
Fat 9   •   Carbohydrate 4   •   Protein 4

Cardiovascular disease

Coronary artery disease caused by atherosclerosis is the leading cause of death among Americans. In this condition, fatty fibrous plaques progressively narrow the coronary artery lumens, reducing the volume of blood that can flow through them. Plaque develops as a result of a complex series of events that seem to be initiated by increased amounts of LDLs. Eating a diet high in saturated fats, trans fats, and cholesterol raises LDL level, increasing the risk of heart disease.

Obesity

Obesity — which is defined as a body mass index greater than 30 — occurs from taking in more calories than the body requires. Fats contribute more calories to the diet than carbohydrates and

Translating fat terminology

Here's a guide you can give your patients to help them decipher terms used to describe the amount and type of fats listed in food products.

Terms	
Saturated fat-free	One serving containing less than 0.5 g of fat, with the level of trans-fatty acids not exceeding 1% of total fat
Low fat	3 g of fat or less
Reduced or less saturated fat	At least 25% less fat than the reference food (but not necessarily "low fat")
Light	One-third fewer calories or 50% less fat than the reference food
Low cholesterol	20 mg or less of cholesterol and 2 g or less of saturated fat
Reduced or less cholesterol	At least 25% less cholesterol than the reference food and less than 2 g of saturated fat

protein, which the body can burn more easily. Weight gain results when excess fats are stored.

Cancer

Although dietary fat hasn't been shown to cause cancer, it may help promote certain cancers. The American Cancer Society Guidelines state that following a high-fat diet can increase the risk of colon, rectal, prostate, and endometrial cancers.

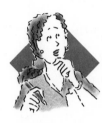

Quick quiz

1. Fat is composed of all of the following elements except:
   A. carbon.
   B. oxygen.
   C. hydrogen.
   D. potassium.

   Answer: D. Fats are organic compounds that are composed of carbon, hydrogen, and oxygen.

2.   An unsaturated fat is:

    A.   a fatty acid that isn't completely filled with hydrogen atoms.

    B.   a fatty acid that's completely filled with hydrogen atoms.

    C.   a fatty acid that's highly concentrated and heavy.

    D.   a fatty acid that originates from animals.

Answer: A. An unsaturated fatty acid isn't completely filled with hydrogen atoms and, therefore, is less concentrated and lighter.

3.   In which organ does the digestion of fats primarily occur?

    A.   Stomach

    B.   Large intestine

    C.   Liver

    D.   Small intestine

Answer: D. Fat digestion occurs in the small intestine, where the enzymatic processes occur.

4.   Which lipoprotein contributes to the development of atherosclerosis and is termed the "bad" cholesterol?

    A.   LDL

    B.   HDL

    C.   VLDL

    D.   Chylomicrons

Answer: A. LDL levels contribute to atherosclerosis. They're the major source of cholesterol in the blood.

5.   When using the Nutrition Fact labels to make healthy food selections, choose foods with:

    A.   the lowest combined number of grams of saturated fat and trans fat.

    B.   the highest percent daily value of cholesterol.

    C.   the lowest percent daily value of trans fat.

    D.   the highest amount of total fat.

Answer: A. To select healthy foods, choose foods with the lowest combined number of grams of saturated fat and trans fat and the lowest percent daily value of cholesterol.

Scoring

☆☆☆   If you answered all five questions correctly, way to go! You're saturated with information on fats!

☆☆   If you answered four questions correctly, good job! Your mind bonded with the information on fats.

☆   If you answered fewer than four questions correctly, don't worry! You apparently didn't absorb fats well. That isn't always a bad thing, but you should probably look over the chapter again.

Vitamins and minerals

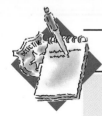

Just the facts

This chapter presents essential information about vitamins and minerals. In this chapter, you'll learn:

♦ classification of vitamins and minerals

♦ functions of vitamins and minerals

♦ the ways in which vitamins and minerals are digested, absorbed, and metabolized

♦ food sources of vitamins and minerals.

A look at vitamins

Vitamins are organic compounds of carbon, hydrogen, oxygen and, occasionally, nitrogen or other elements that are needed in small quantities for normal metabolism, growth, and development. Because they're needed only in small quantities, they're referred to as micronutrients. With few exceptions, the body can't produce vitamins, so they must be consumed in the diet.

Contrary to popular belief, vitamins don't directly provide energy to the body. As catalysts, they're part of the enzyme system that's required to release energy from protein, fat, and carbohydrates. Vitamins are also needed to form red blood cells, hormones, and genetic material and to maintain proper functioning of the nervous system. Many vitamins exist in more than one active form, and each of these forms has a different function in the body.

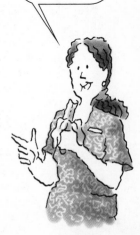

Eat up! Vitamins are essential in the diet because they can't be made by the body or are produced by the body in inadequate amounts.

Classification of vitamins

Vitamins are classified as water soluble or fat soluble. (See *Guide to vitamins*, pages 75 and 76.)

Daily duty

Water-soluble vitamins are absorbed into the bloodstream directly and move freely within cells. Because storage of these vitamins in the body is limited, they must be consumed daily in the diet. When excess amounts are consumed, they're excreted in urine.

Examples of water-soluble vitamins are:
- vitamin B_1 (thiamine)
- vitamin B_2 (riboflavin)
- vitamin B_3 (niacin)
- vitamin B_6 (pyridoxine)
- vitamin B_{12} (cobalamin)
- vitamin C (ascorbic acid)
- biotin
- folate (folic acid)
- pantothenic acid.

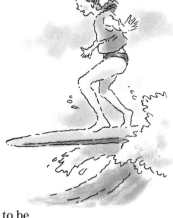

Zowee! Excess water-soluble vitamins are excreted in urine...

On layaway

Fat-soluble vitamins are absorbed with fat into the lymphatic system and the bloodstream. Once in the bloodstream, these vitamins need to attach to lipoproteins to be transported. Excess amounts of fat-soluble vitamins are stored in the liver and adipose tissue; therefore, these vitamins don't need to be consumed daily in the diet.

The fat-soluble vitamins are:
- vitamin A (retinol)
- vitamin D (calciferol)
- vitamin E (tocopherol)
- vitamin K (menadione).

...while excess fat-soluble vitamins are stored in the liver and adipose tissue.

Functions of vitamins

Vitamins have four main functions. They may work as:
- antioxidants
- coenzymes
- food additives
- pharmacologic agents.

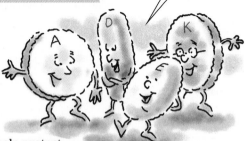

Fighting free radicals

Some vitamins function as antioxidants, which help protect the body from the instability of free radicals. Free radicals are unstable molecule fragments with one or more unpaired electrons that are produced in cells as they burn oxygen during metabolism. Other factors, such as ultraviolet radiation, smoking, and air pollu-

Guide to vitamins

Good health requires intake of adequate amounts of vitamins to meet the body's metabolic needs. A vitamin excess or deficiency, although rare, can lead to various disorders. The chart below reviews major functions and food sources of vitamins.

Vitamins	Major functions	Food sources
Water-soluble vitamins		
Vitamin B_1 (thiamine)	Appetite stimulation, blood building, carbohydrate metabolism, circulation, digestion, growth, learning ability, muscle tone maintenance	Meat, fish, poultry, pork, molasses, brewer's yeast, brown rice, nuts, wheat germ, whole and enriched grains
Vitamin B_2 (riboflavin)	Antibody and red blood cell (RBC) formation; energy metabolism; cell respiration; epithelial, ocular, and mucosal tissue maintenance	Meat, fish, poultry, milk, molasses, brewer's yeast, eggs, fruit, green leafy vegetables, nuts, whole grains
Vitamin B_3 (niacin)	Circulation, cholesterol level reduction, growth, hydrochloric acid production, metabolism (carbohydrate, protein, fat), sex hormone production	Eggs, lean meat, milk products, organ meat, peanuts, poultry, seafood, whole grains
Vitamin B_6 (pyridoxine)	Antibody formation, digestion, deoxyribonucleic acid and ribonucleic acid synthesis, fat and protein utilization, amino acid metabolism, hemoglobin production	Meat, poultry, bananas, molasses, brewer's yeast, desiccated liver, fish, green leafy vegetables, peanuts, raisins, walnuts, wheat germ, whole grains
Vitamin B_{12} (cobalamin)	Blood cell formation, cellular and nutrient metabolism, iron absorption, tissue growth, nerve cell maintenance	Beef, eggs, fish, milk products, organ meat, pork
Vitamin C (ascorbic acid)	Collagen production, digestion, fine bone and tooth formation, iodine conservation, healing, RBC formation, infection resistance	Fresh fruits and vegetables, especially citrus fruits and green leafy vegetables
Biotin	Cell growth, fatty acid production, metabolism, vitamin B utilization, skin, hair, nerve, and bone marrow maintenance	Egg yolks, legumes, organ meats, whole grains, yeast, milk, and seafood
Folate (folic acid)	Cell growth and reproduction, hydrochloric acid production, liver function, nucleic acid formation, protein metabolism, RBC formation	Citrus fruits, eggs, green leafy vegetables, milk products, organ meat, seafood, whole grains
Pantothenic acid	Antibody formation, cortisone production, growth stimulation, stress tolerance, vitamin utilization, conversion of carbohydrates, fats, and protein	Eggs, legumes, mushrooms, organ meats, salmon, wheat germ, whole grains, fresh vegetables, yeast

(continued)

Guide to vitamins *(continued)*

Vitamins	Major functions	Food sources
Fat-soluble vitamins		
Vitamin A (retinol)	Body tissue repair and maintenance, infection resistance, bone growth, nervous system development, cell membrane metabolism and structure	Fish, green and yellow fruits and vegetables, milk products
Vitamin D (calciferol)	Calcium and phosphorus metabolism (bone formation), myocardial function, nervous system maintenance, normal blood clotting	Bonemeal, egg yolks, organ meat, butter, cod liver oil, fatty fish
Vitamin E (tocopherol)	Aging retardation, anticoagulation, diuresis, fertility, lung protection (antipollution), male potency, muscle and nerve cell membrane maintenance, myocardial perfusion, serum cholesterol reduction	Butter, dark green vegetables, eggs, fruits, nuts, organ meat, vegetable oils, wheat germ
Vitamin K (menadione)	Liver synthesis of prothrombin and other blood-clotting factors	Green leafy vegetables, safflower oil, yogurt, liver, molasses

tion, can also create free radicals in the body. Each of these free radicals attempts to become stable by gaining an electron. While doing so, they cause damage by oxidizing body cells and deoxyribonucleic acid. These damaged cells are believed to contribute to aging and such health problems as cancer and heart disease.

Antioxidants are substances that yield electrons to free radicals, helping to stabilize them and protect cells from damage. Vitamin C, vitamin E, and beta-carotene (a precursor to vitamin A) are all important antioxidants. Because antioxidants complement each other and each antioxidant has a slightly different role, an excess or deficiency of one may impair the action of others.

> Radical, man! Some vitamins are antioxidants, which donate electrons to free radicals to stabilize them.

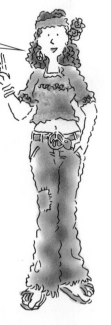

Catalysts for change

Enzymes are proteins that catalyze chemical reactions within the body without changing themselves in the process. Many enzymes aren't active without a coenzyme, an organic molecule that makes up the nonprotein portion of the enzyme. Vitamins work as coenzymes, facilitating many important chemical reactions throughout the body.

Food boosters

Vitamins are also used as additives in some foods to boost their nutritional content. Examples include vitamin-fortified cereals and juices. As additives, vitamins may also be used to preserve foods, such as fish, luncheon meats, and oils.

Vitamin therapy

Certain vitamins have been found to have pharmacologic uses. For example, large doses of niacin have been used to help lower the levels of serum cholesterol, low-density lipoproteins, and triglycerides in patients with elevated levels. In addition, retinoic acid, a form of vitamin A, has been used to treat acne vulgaris.

How the body handles vitamins

Vitamins move through the body via the processes of digestion, absorption, and metabolism.

Digestion

Digestion of vitamins occurs mainly in the small intestine and requires the breakdown of food into its constituent parts. Contractions of the intestinal wall and the secretion of digestive enzymes break down food to facilitate absorption of nutrients through the intestinal wall.

Absorption

Absorption of vitamins is accomplished through active transport and diffusion across cell membranes. A number of vitamins require a specific carrier or transport system. For example, vitamin B_{12} isn't absorbed in the absence of intrinsic factor, which is secreted by the parietal cells of the stomach.

Fat-soluble vitamins are absorbed in different portions of the small intestine. For example, vitamin A is absorbed in the duodenal and upper jejunal areas of the small intestine. The process of their absorption is similar to that of fats and, like fats, these vitamins can be stored in the body. Consequently, excessive intake of fat-soluble vitamins can be fatal.

Water-soluble vitamins are generally absorbed throughout the GI tract. For example, folic acid is absorbed in the ileum. Because excess amounts of water-soluble vitamins are typically excreted in urine, one of these vitamins is less likely to be toxic to the body.

Metabolism

All vitamins are metabolized independently of one another. The process differs for each vitamin.

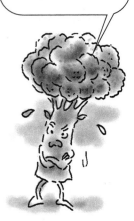

Boy, am I steamed! Overcooking us vegetables can cause our vitamins to vacate before we're even eaten.

Sources of vitamins

Vitamins can be found in all the major food groups:
• Bread, cereal, rice, and pasta may be enriched with niacin, riboflavin, and thiamine and fortified with folic acid. Whole-grain items also contain vitamin E.
• Fruits and fruit juices, particularly orange and grapefruit juices, are high in vitamin C and beta-carotene and are also significant sources of folate. Some juices are also fortified with calcium. Juices that contain 100% fruit juice are recommended.
• Vegetables are good sources of beta-carotene, vitamin C, folic acid, and vitamin K. Because cooking and soaking can destroy vitamins, minimal preparation of vegetables is recommended.
• Milk, yogurt, and cheese may contain riboflavin, some B vitamins, and vitamins A and D.
• Meat contains niacin, riboflavin, and vitamins B_6 and B_{12}; pork is also rich in thiamine. Dry beans contain folate, nuts and seeds supply vitamin E, and eggs are good sources of vitamin A.
• Vegetable oils supply vitamin E. Margarine contains vitamins A, D, and E.

A basic principal of the *Dietary Guidelines for Americans 2005* is that vitamins should come mainly from foods. (See *Nutritional needs of breast-feeding vegans.*)

Vitamins in health promotion

The recommended dietary intake necessary to meet the nutrient requirements of adults varies for each vitamin. (See *Vitamin requirements, deficiencies, and toxicities.*)

Recently, an intensive consumer interest in vitamin therapy and supplementation has grown in conjunction with public interests in defying aging and changing eating patterns.

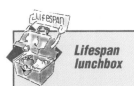

Lifespan lunchbox

Nutritional needs of breast-feeding vegans

Breast milk contains all the vitamins needed for an infant's growth and development. However, the milk of breast-feeding mothers who are vegans may be deficient in vitamin B_{12} and vitamin D. Breast-fed infants of these mothers may need vitamin B_{12} supplementation.

Vitamin requirements, deficiencies, and toxicities

This table lists the daily requirements of common vitamins as well as the signs and symptoms of deficiency and toxicity for each.

Vitamins	Adult requirements	Signs and symptoms of deficiency	Signs and symptoms of toxicity
Water-soluble vitamins			
Vitamin B$_1$[†] (thiamine)	*Men:* 1.2 mg *Women:* 1.1 mg	Beriberi (fatigue, muscle weakness, confusion, edema, enlarged heart, heart failure)	None
Vitamin B$_2$[†] (riboflavin)	*Men:* 1.3 mg *Women:* 1.1mg	Ariboflavinosis (dermatitis, glossitis, photophobia)	None
Vitamin B$_3$ (niacin)[†]	*Men:* 16 mg *Women:* 14 mg	Pellagra (dermatitis, diarrhea, dementia, death)	Flushing, gastric ulcers, low blood pressure, nausea, vomiting, diarrhea, liver damage
Vitamin B$_6$ (pyridoxine)[†]	*Men:* 1.3 mg (< age 50) 1.7 mg (> age 50) *Women:* 1.3 mg (< age 50) 1.5 mg (> age 50)	Dermatitis, glossitis, seizures, anemia	Depression, irritability, headaches, fatigue
Vitamin B$_{12}$ (cobalamin)[†]	2.4 mcg	Indigestion, diarrhea or constipation, weight loss, macrocytic anemia, fatigue, poor memory, irritability, paresthesia of the hands and feet	None
Vitamin C (ascorbic acid)[†]	*Men:* 90 mg *Women:* 75 mg	Scurvy (bleeding gums, delayed wound healing, hemorrhaging, softening of the bones, easy fractures)	Diarrhea, nausea, headaches, fatigue, hot flashes, insomnia
Biotin*	30 mcg	Anorexia, fatigue, depression, dry skin, heart abnormalities	None
Folate (folic acid)[†]	400 mcg	Diarrhea, macrocytic anemia, confusion, depression, fatigue	Masks vitamin B$_{12}$ deficiency
Pantothenic acid[†]	5 mg	General failure of all body systems	None

*Adequate intake   †Recommended dietary allowance

(continued)

Vitamin requirements, deficiencies, and toxicities (continued)

Vitamins	Adult requirements	Signs and symptoms of deficiency	Signs and symptoms of toxicity
Fat-soluble vitamins			
Vitamin A (retinol)[†]	*Men:* 960 mcg retinol equivalents *Women:* 700 mcg retinol equivalents	Night blindness, bone growth cessation, dry skin, decreased saliva, diarrhea	Headaches, vomiting, double vision, hair loss, liver damage
Vitamin D (calciferol)*	5 mcg (age 50) 10 mcg (ages 51 to 70) 15 mcg (> age 70)	Rickets (retarded bone growth, bone malformations, decreased serum calcium, abdominal protrusion); osteomalacia (softening of bones, decreased serum calcium, muscle twitching)	Kidney stones, kidney damage, muscle and bone weakness, excessive bleeding, headache, excessive thirst
Vitamin E (tocopherol)[†]	15 mg	Red blood cell hemolysis, edema, skin lesions	None
Vitamin K (menadione)*	*Men:* 80 mcg *Women:* 65 mcg	Hemorrhaging	None

*Adequate intake   [†]Recommended dietary allowance

Vitamin supplements

Vitamin supplements can prevent such deficiency diseases as scurvy and beriberi, which can occur when dietary intake is inadequate. Research is still needed, however, to determine if vitamin supplements can help prevent chronic disease.

Health and nutrition authorities agree that the best way to get nutrients is through food and not through supplements. Vitamin supplements are limited in what they offer and hardly compare with the array of vitamins, minerals, and fibers found in foods. Vitamins also lack the natural chemicals produced by plants needed to protect against bacteria, viruses, and fungi.

Currently, there isn't a pill that can sufficiently substitute for a healthy diet, but taking a balanced multivitamin supplement that provides no more than 100% of the daily requirement for each vitamin is harmless. Some special populations and people whose food choices fall short of the ideal diet may benefit from taking a multi-

Target populations for vitamin supplementation

Even though vitamin supplements can't compete with the array of vitamins, minerals, and fibers found in foods, special populations, such as those listed here, may benefit from vitamin supplements:

- Alcoholics—Alcohol alters vitamin absorption, metabolism, and excretion. Nutrients that may be affected include riboflavin, niacin, thiamine, folate, and pantothenic acid.
- Elderly patients—Vitamin requirements may be increased due to chronic disease, adverse effects of medication, illness, poor chewing and swallowing, physical limitations, or a decreased sense of smell or taste. Absorption of vitamin B_{12} and synthesis of vitamin D decreases with aging. Research has shown that a multivitamin and mineral supplement may improve immune function.
- Smokers—Smokers require more vitamin C than nonsmokers. If these patients consume an adequate amount of vitamin C in the diet, a supplement may not be needed.
- Dieters and particular eaters—If intake is less than 1,200 calories per day, it's difficult to obtain the necessary nutrients for a healthy diet. People who eliminate specific food groups from their diet, such as vegans and people with food intolerances or allergies, also may not obtain the needed nutrients.
- Pregnant and breast-feeding women and women of childbearing age—Folate is vital to prevent neural tube defects. All childbearing women are encouraged to take synthetic folate through supplements or fortified foods. Prenatal vitamins are routinely given to safeguard against a poor diet.

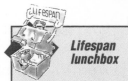

Lifespan lunchbox

Folic acid needs in women of childbearing age

Folate deficiency increases the risk of spina bifida and neural tube defects in unborn children. Therefore, women of childbearing age should consume 400 mcg/day of synthetic folic acid from fortified foods and supplements, in addition to food forms of folate from a varied diet. Pregnant women should consume 600 mcg/day of synthetic folic acid from fortified foods and supplements, in addition to food forms of folate from a varied diet. Rich sources of dietary folate include dark-green, leafy vegetables; dried peas; beans; citrus fruits; peanuts; and organ meat.

vitamin. (See *Target populations for vitamin supplementation* and *Folic acid needs in women of childbearing age*.)

A look at minerals

Minerals are simple inorganic substances that are widely distributed in nature. They play a role in promoting growth and maintaining health. Minerals represent 4% of body weight and are found in all body fluids and tissues.

Classification of minerals

Minerals are classified as major minerals (macrominerals) or trace minerals (microminerals). Major minerals are present in the body in amounts larger than 5 g (the equivalent of 1 tsp) and are needed in large quantities. Trace minerals are present in the body in amounts less than 5 g and are only needed in small amounts.

Guide to minerals

This chart reviews major functions and food sources of major and trace minerals.

Minerals	Major functions	Food sources
Major minerals		
Calcium	Blood clotting, bone and tooth formation, cardiac rhythm maintenance, cell membrane permeability, muscle growth and contraction, nerve impulse transmission	Bonemeal, cheese, milk, molasses, yogurt, whole grains, nuts, legumes, green leafy vegetables
Chloride	Fluid, electrolyte, acid-base, and osmotic pressure balance	Fruits, vegetables, table salt
Magnesium	Acid-base balance, metabolism, protein synthesis, muscle relaxation, cellular respiration, nerve impulse transmission	Green leafy vegetables, nuts, seafood, cocoa, whole grains
Phosphorus	Bone and tooth formation, cell growth and repair	Eggs, fish, grains, meats, poultry, yellow cheese, milk, milk products
Potassium	Muscle contraction, nerve impulse transmission, rapid growth, fluid distribution, osmotic pressure balance, acid-base balance	Seafood, bananas, peaches, peanuts, raisins, oranges, tomatoes, peas, beans, green leafy vegetables, milk products
Sodium	Cellular fluid level maintenance, muscle contraction, acid-base balance, cell permeability, muscle function, nerve impulse transmission	Seafood, cheese, milk, salt
Sulfur	Collagen synthesis, vitamin B formation, enzyme and energy metabolism, blood clotting	Milk, meats, legumes, eggs
Trace minerals		
Chromium	Carbohydrate and protein metabolism, serum glucose level maintenance	Clams, meats, cheese, corn oil, whole grains
Cobalt	Vitamin B_{12} formation	Beef, eggs, fish, milk products, organ meats, pork
Copper	Bone formation, hair and skin color, healing processes, hemoglobin and red blood cell formation, maintenance of nerve fibers, iron metabolism	Organ meats, raisins, seafood, nuts, molasses
Fluoride	Bone and tooth formation	Drinking water

Guide to minerals *(continued)*

Minerals	Major functions	Food sources
Trace minerals *(continued)*		
Iodine	Energy production, metabolism, physical and mental development	Kelp, salt (iodized), seafood
Iron	Growth (in children), hemoglobin production, stress and disease resistance, cellular respiration, oxygen transport	Eggs, organ meats, poultry, wheat germ, liver, potatoes, enriched breads and cereals, green leafy vegetables
Manganese	Enzyme activation, fat and carbohydrate metabolism, reproduction and growth, sex hormone production, vitamin B_1 metabolism, vitamin E utilization	Bananas, egg yolks, green leafy vegetables, liver, soybeans, nuts, whole grains, coffee, tea
Molybdenum	Body metabolism	Whole grains, legumes, organ meats
Selenium	Immune functions, mitochondrial adenosine triphosphate synthesis, cellular protection, fat metabolism	Seafood, meats, liver, kidneys
Zinc	Burn and wound healing, carbohydrate digestion, metabolism, prostate gland function, reproductive organ growth and development	Liver, mushrooms, seafood, soybeans, spinach, meat

Choose a major

There are seven major minerals:
- calcium
- chloride
- magnesium
- phosphorus
- potassium
- sodium
- sulfur.

Leaving a trace

Trace minerals essential to health maintenance include chromium, cobalt, copper, fluoride, iodine, iron, manganese, molybdenum, selenium, and zinc. (See *Guide to minerals.*)

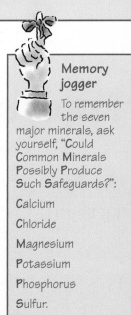

Memory jogger

To remember the seven major minerals, ask yourself, "Could Common Minerals Possibly Produce Such Safeguards?":

Calcium

Chloride

Magnesium

Potassium

Phosphorus

Sulfur.

Functions of minerals

Minerals have many roles in the body, including:
- providing structure to body tissues
- regulating body processes.

A disruption of the body's balance in any one mineral can be life threatening.

Structure

Minerals play a major role in several elements of body structure. For example, calcium, phosphorus, magnesium, and fluoride combine to give bones and teeth their hardness. Sulfur is a fundamental constituent of skin, hair, and nails.

Minerals are also components of vitamins, hormones, and enzymes. For example, iodine becomes part of thyroid hormones.

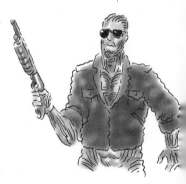

Ask the governator: Minerals play an important role in muscle contraction.

Processes

Minerals also help to regulate various bodily processes. For example, they help to maintain osmotic pressure in body compartments. Sodium, potassium, and calcium have important functions in nerve cell transmission and muscle contraction. Sodium is also essential for maintaining fluid balance.

Potassium and phosphorus play a role in fluid and acid-base balance. Minerals also maintain normal hemoglobin levels, play a role in the function of the nervous system, and are involved in hormone activity and skeletal development and maintenance.

How the body handles minerals

Minerals move through the body via the processes of digestion, absorption, and metabolism.

Digestion

Minerals must be digested in the GI tract by enzymes that split large units into smaller ones. The process, called *hydrolysis*, consists of a compound uniting with water and then splitting into simpler compounds. The smaller units are then absorbed from the small intestine and transported to the liver through the portal vein system.

Absorption

Minerals are absorbed in the small intestine. How much of a mineral is absorbed depends on three factors:

☞ tissue health — because tissue that's affected by disease has decreased absorptive capability

☞ food form — because minerals obtained from animal foods are more easily absorbed than those obtained from plant foods

☞ body requirements — because the body will absorb more of a mineral to compensate for a deficiency in that mineral.

For some minerals, absorption isn't regulated, which can lead to problems. For example, the body doesn't regulate sodium absorption, which can lead to sodium overload in patients who can't excrete the mineral properly.

Metabolism

Minerals are metabolized independently of one another. Metabolism occurs according to body need, and the process differs for each mineral. For example, because calcium is absorbed according to body requirements and must be aided by vitamin D, calcium metabolism is hindered by excess fiber ingestion.

Sources of minerals

Minerals are obtained in a variety of ways. Most are found in unrefined or unprocessed foods. Trace minerals vary with the mineral content of the soil in which the the food is grown. Processed foods are high in chloride and sodium. Drinking water contains different amounts of magnesium, calcium, and other minerals. Sodium is added to soften the water, and fluoride can be an added or a natural component.

Minerals are found in all the major food groups:
• Enriched and whole grain breads and cereals provide magnesium, iron, chromium, and manganese. Bran contains potassium.
• Vegetables provide iron, potassium, and magnesium. Green leafy vegetables provide calcium.
• Fruits aren't good sources of minerals, except for potassium, which is found in bananas and oranges.
• Milk, yogurt, and cheese may contain phosphorus and potassium. They're also the richest source of calcium.

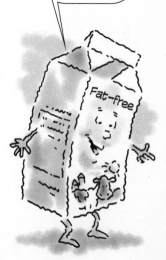

Got milk? Me and the guys in my gang are the richest sources of calcium you can find.

• Animal proteins contain potassium, phosphorus, sulfur, zinc, and iron. Dried peas and beans contain iron, potassium, and calcium.
• Fats, oils, and sugars contain almost no minerals.

Minerals in health promotion

The recommended dietary intake to meet the requirements of adults varies for each mineral. (See *Mineral requirements, deficiencies, and toxicities.*)

Calcium and sodium are the minerals that cause the most health concerns. Most Americans consume less than optimal amounts of calcium, increasing their risk of osteoporosis, and more sodium than they need, placing them at risk for hypertension.

Calcium

Calcium is an important mineral throughout life. Adequate calcium intake may play a role in preventing hypertension and colon cancer and can slow the rate of bone loss. (See *Calcium consequence.*)

The latest recommendations for calcium intake are set at levels associated with maximum retention by the body. Many Americans don't consume the recommended amount of calcium. They may take in enough to meet their requirement but fall short of the recommendation. Calcium supplements are appropriate for people who can't or won't eat adequate calcium from foods alone.

People who take calcium supplements should:
• do so only in moderation (calcium is best absorbed when taken in amounts of 500 mg or less.; if higher doses are needed, doses should be spread out throughout the day)
• know the kind of calcium they're taking and how it should be taken (calcium carbonate is best absorbed with food, and calcium citrate is best absorbed on an empty stomach)
• avoid taking it with iron (calcium can interfere with iron absorption)
• drink fluids (constipation is a common adverse effect of calcium supplements; drinking adequate amounts of fluids can reduce the risk)
• remember that supplements should add to what's already consumed (calcium supplements shouldn't be taken to replace dietary consumption of calcium).

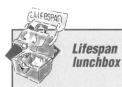

Lifespan lunchbox

Calcium consequence

Adequate calcium intake is important in all stages of life. During the first few decades of life, attaining maximum bone density is a safeguard against the inevitable net bone loss that occurs with aging. After age 30, adequate calcium alone can't stop net bone loss, but it can slow the rate.

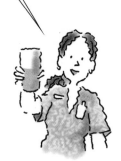

Drink up! Drinking adequate amounts of fluid can decrease the risk of constipation for patients taking calcium supplements.

Mineral requirements, deficiencies, and toxicities

This table lists the daily requirements of common minerals as well as the signs and symptoms of deficiency and toxicity for each.

Minerals	Adult requirements	Signs and symptoms of deficiency	Signs and symptoms of toxicity
Major minerals			
Calcium*	1,000 mg (ages 19 to 50) 1,200 mg (age > 50)	Arm and leg numbness, brittle fingernails, heart palpitations, insomnia, muscle cramps, osteoporosis	Renal calculi, impaired absorption of iron
Chloride*	2.3 g (ages 19 to 50) 2 g (ages 51 to 70) 1.8 g (age > 70)	Disturbance in acid-base balance	None
Magnesium†	*Men:* 400 mg (ages 19 to 30) 420 mg (age > 30) *Women:* 310 mg (ages 19 to 30) 320 mg (age > 30)	Confusion, disorientation, nervousness, irritability, rapid pulse, tremors, muscle control loss, neuromuscular dysfunction	Cardiac rhythm disturbances, hypotension, respiratory failure
Phosphorus†	700 mg	Appetite loss, fatigue, irregular breathing, nervous disorders, muscle weakness	None
Potassium*	2,000 mg	Muscle weakness, paralysis, anorexia, confusion, weak reflexes, slow, irregular heartbeat	Cardiac disturbances, paralysis
Sodium*	500 mg	Appetite loss, intestinal gas, muscle atrophy, vomiting, weight loss	Edema and elevated blood pressure
Sulfur	No recommended intake	None	None
Trace minerals			
Chromium*	50 to 200 mcg	Glucose intolerance (in diabetic patients)	None
Cobalt	Unknown	Indigestion, diarrhea or constipation, weight loss, fatigue, poor memory	None
Copper†	1.5 to 3 mg	General weakness, impaired respiration, skin sores, bone disease	Vomiting, diarrhea

*Adequate intake   †Recommended dietary allowance

(continued)

Mineral requirements, deficiencies, and toxicities *(continued)*

Minerals	Adult requirements	Signs and symptoms of deficiency	Signs and symptoms of toxicity
Trace minerals (continued)			
Fluoride*	*Men:* 4 mg *Women:* 3 mg	Dental caries	Mottling and pitting of permanent teeth, increased bone density and calcification
Iodine[†]	150 mcg	Cold hands and feet, dry hair, irritability, nervousness, obesity, simple goiter	Enlarged thyroid gland
Iron[†]	*Men:* 8 mg *Women:* 18 mg (ages 19 to 50) 8 mg (age > 50)	Brittle nails, constipation, respiratory problems, tongue soreness or inflammation, anemia, pallor, weakness, cold sensitivity, fatigue	Abdominal cramps and pains, nausea, vomiting, hemosiderosis, hemochromatosis
Manganese*	*Men:* 2.3 mg *Women:* 1.8 mg	Ataxia, dizziness, hearing disturbance or loss	Severe neuromuscular disturbances
Molybdenum[†]	45 mcg	None	Headache, dizziness, heartburn, weakness, nausea, vomiting, diarrhea
Selenium[†]	55 mcg	None	Nausea, vomiting, abdominal pain, hair and nail changes, nerve damage, fatigue
Zinc[†]	*Men:* 15 mg *Women:* 12 mg	Delayed sexual maturity, fatigue, smell and taste loss, poor appetite, prolonged wound healing, slowed growth, skin disorders	Anemia, impaired calcium absorption, fever, muscle pain, dizziness

*Adequate intake   [†]Recommended dietary allowance

Sodium

The *Dietary Guidelines for Americans 2005* suggest limiting sodium intake by choosing and preparing foods with less salt. Americans are advised to limit their intake of sodium to less than 2,300 mg/day. The average daily intake from food alone (not count-

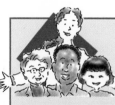

Bridging the gap

Salt sensitivity in blacks

Because blacks tend to be sensitive to salt, have low intake of potassium, and be at increased risk for hypertension, they may benefit from a sodium intake restriction to no more than 1,500 mg/day. Also encourage these patients to consume 4,700 mg of potassium each day through food sources because salt sensitivity might be reduced by increasing potassium intake.

ing salt added at the table) is more than 4,000 mg for men and almost 3,000 mg for women. (See *Salt sensitivity in blacks*.)

High sodium intake is linked to high blood pressure, which can lead to stroke or heart attack. In order to help your patient limit his sodium intake, recommend these actions:
• Reduce sodium intake gradually in order to reduce the desire for salt.
• Read Nutrition Facts labels to avoid or limit foods that contain too much sodium.
• Compare the labels of different brands of similar items to identify the product with the lowest sodium content.
• Avoid processed foods.
• Be aware that high-sodium foods may not taste salty.
• Taste food before adding additional salt.
• Experiment with herbs, spices, and vinegars as alternatives to salt.

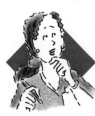

Quick quiz

1. Which water-soluble vitamin requires intrinsic factor to be absorbed?
    A.   Vitamin B_{12}
    B.   Vitamin B_2
    C.   Folate
    D.   Biotin

Answer: A. Vitamin B_{12} requires the gastric protein intrinsic factor, the ingredient for absorption in the small intestine.

2. In which organ does the digestion of vitamins occur?
   A.   Stomach
   B.   Large intestine
   C.   Small intestine
   D.   Liver

Answer: C. Digestion of vitamins occurs in the small intestine.

3. The number of major minerals is:
   A.   4.
   B.   6.
   C.   7.
   D.   10.

Answer: C. There are seven major minerals: calcium, chloride, magnesium, phosphorus, potassium, sodium, and sulfur.

4. Which mineral helps maintain osmotic balance?
   A.   Phosphorus
   B.   Thiamine
   C.   Potassium
   D.   Niacin

Answer: C. Potassium is a mineral that's needed to help regulate fluid distribution and osmotic pressure.

Scoring

☆☆☆   If you answered all four questions correctly, great job! You've certainly been fortified with all of your essential vitamins and minerals.

☆☆   If you answered three questions correctly, keep up the good work! It looks like traces of this chapter settled in your body.

☆   If you answered fewer than three questions correctly, don't worry! Maybe the information on water-soluble vitamins will make more sense after the next chapter — Fluids.

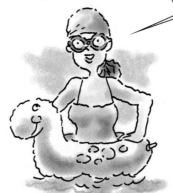

Grab your goggles and then wade through the next chapter on fluids.

7

Fluids

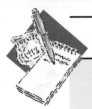

Just the facts

This chapter presents the basics of fluids and fluid balance and explains their importance in body functioning. In this chapter, you'll learn:

♦ the importance of water in the body

♦ the way fluids move in the body

♦ factors that regulate fluid balance.

A look at fluids

A continual supply of water is one of our most basic nutritional needs. Without water, a person can survive no longer than a week. Ensuring balanced distribution of fluids to all body cells is an essential physiologic function.

A salute to solutes

Water makes up 50% to 80% of a person's total body weight. Body water contains solutes, or dissolved substances, that are necessary for physiologic functioning. Solutes include electrolytes, glucose, amino acids, and other nutrients.

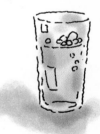

Fluid compartments

The body holds fluids in two basic areas, or compartments—inside the cells and outside the cells. Fluid inside cells is called *intracellular fluid* (ICF); fluid outside cells is *extracellular fluid* (ECF). ICF and ECF are separated by capillary walls and cell membranes.

ECF consists of interstitial fluid, which surrounds the cells, and intravascular fluid or plasma (the liquid portion of blood). In an adult, interstitial fluid accounts for about 75% of ECF. Plasma accounts for the other 25%.

To maintain proper fluid balance, fluid distribution between ICF and ECF must stay relatively constant. In an adult, the total amount of ICF averages 40% of body weight, or about 28 L. The total amount of ECF averages 20% of body weight, or about 14 L.

Where's the water?

Skeletal muscle cells hold much of the body's water. Fat cells contain little water. That's why women, who normally have a higher ratio of fat to skeletal muscle than men, typically have a lower relative water content. Likewise, an obese person may have a relative water content level as low as 45%. In an obese person, accumulated body fat increases weight without boosting the body's water content. Age also affects the proportion of water in the body. (See *Body water differences*.)

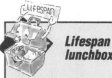

Lifespan lunchbox

Body water differences

Age affects the proportion of water in the body. Specifically, infants' bodies are 75% water, compared with 50% to 65% of adults' bodies. Preterm infants' bodies can be as much as 80% water by weight. Infants reach the adult proportion of water to weight between ages 9 and 12 months.

Functions of fluid

Fluid has many functions within the body. It:
• gives structure and shape to cells
• helps form the structure of large molecules, such as protein and glycogen
• serves as a lubricant (for example, within the eyes and joints)
• helps regulate body temperature (for instance, fluid absorbs the heat produced during a fever; blood then carries the excess heat to the skin, where it dissipates)
• acts as a solvent for minerals, vitamins, glucose, amino acids, and other small molecules
• aids nutrient digestion and absorption
• transports nutrients to cells
• carries waste products away from cells through urine, feces, and expiration
• serves as a medium for all biochemical reactions in the body
• participates in chemical reactions, including the breakdown of proteins to amino acids and the synthesis of hormones and enzymes.

Keeping the joints lubricated is just one of the many functions fluid serves in the body.

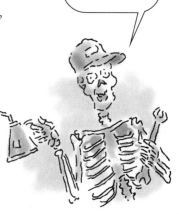

Water absorption and storage

A small amount of water can be absorbed into the bloodstream from the stomach. Over the course of 1 hour, roughly 1 L of water can be absorbed from the small intestine. Water moves through the intestinal membrane by diffusion (a process we'll discuss later).

The body doesn't really store water. Instead, water moves continually from one compartment to another, and the body often reuses it to perform different tasks. However, if a person's adaptive mechanisms are disrupted, water may be retained. Excessive fluid may accumulate between cells, causing a condition called *edema*. This occurs in heart failure, hypothyroidism, and certain kidney conditions. Less commonly, the opposite occurs, with excessive fluid being dispersed throughout the body — a condition called *water intoxication*.

How fluids move in cells

Just as the heart beats constantly, fluids and solutes move constantly within the body. This movement allows the body to maintain homeostasis — the constant state of balance it seeks.

Solutes within the various compartments move through the membranes separating those compartments. The membranes are semipermeable, meaning they allow some solutes to pass through but not others. Solutes move through cell membranes by diffusion or active transport. Fluid moves by osmosis.

Diffusion

In diffusion, solutes move from an area of higher concentration to an area of lower concentration. Eventually, this movement results in equal distribution of solutes within the two areas. Diffusion is a form of passive transport. It requires no energy; it just happens. Like fish traveling downstream, the solutes simply go with the flow. (See *Diffusion: The power of passivity*.)

Active transport

In active transport, proteins within a semipermeable membrane move solutes from an area of lower concentration to an area of higher concentration. Think of active transport as swimming upstream. When a fish swims upstream, it has to expend energy. The energy a cell expends to move a solute against the concentration gradient comes from adenosine triphosphate (ATP), a substance stored in all cells. (See *Active transport: Swimming upstream*, page 94.)

Diffusion: The power of passivity

In diffusion, solutes move from areas of higher concentration to areas of lower concentration until their concentration is equal in both areas.

Area of lower concentration

Area of higher concentration

Semipermeable membrane

Solutes shifting into area of lower concentration

In active transport, solutes move from an area of lower concentration to an area of higher concentration.

Pump it up

Sodium and potassium move in and out of cells in a form of active transport fueled by ATP called the *sodium-potassium pump*. Other solutes that require active transport to cross cell membranes include calcium ions, hydrogen ions, amino acids, and certain sugars.

Pin-up

An engulfing process called *pinocytosis* is a type of active transport used by larger particles, such as proteins and fats. In this process, tiny cavities called *vacuoles* take droplets of fluid containing dissolved substances into the cell. The engulfed fluid is then used in the cell. (See *Pinocytosis: When cells gulp up fluid.*)

Osmosis

Osmosis refers to passive movement of fluid across a membrane from an area of lower solute concentration and comparatively more fluid into an area of higher solute concentration and comparatively less fluid. Osmosis stops when enough fluid has moved through the membrane to equalize the solute concentration on both sides of the membrane. (See *Understanding osmosis*, page 96.)

How fluids move in the vascular system

In the vascular system, only capillaries have walls thin enough for solutes to pass through. Movement of fluids and solutes through capillary walls plays a key role in fluid balance.

May the force be with you

Fluid movement through capillaries—a process called *capillary filtration*—results from blood pushing against the capillary walls. That pressure, called *hydrostatic* (fluid-pushing) *pressure*, forces fluids and solutes through the capillary wall.

When hydrostatic pressure inside the capillary exceeds pressure in the surrounding interstitial space, fluids and solutes inside the capillary are forced out into the interstitial space. When pressure outside the capillary exceeds pressure within it, fluids and solutes move back into the capillary.

Active transport: Swimming upstream

During active transport, energy from a molecule called *adenosine triphosphate (ATP)* moves solutes from an area of lower concentration to an area of higher concentration.

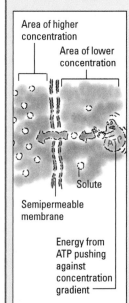

Area of higher concentration

Area of lower concentration

Solute

Semipermeable membrane

Energy from ATP pushing against concentration gradient

Pinocytosis: When cells gulp up fluid

The illustrations below show the steps of pinocytosis, in which solutes encased in the microbody of a cell enter the cell's main body and are exposed to the cell enzymes for metabolism.

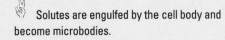 Large solutes attach to the cell membrane.

Solutes are engulfed by the cell body and become microbodies.

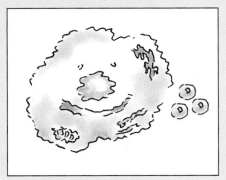

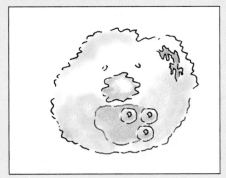

Microbodies are carried across the cell membrane and into the cell.

Once inside the cell, the microbodies open and solutes are metabolized by cells.

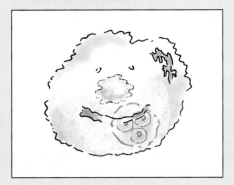

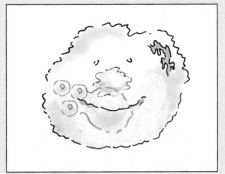

Fluid reabsorption

A process called *reabsorption* prevents too much fluid from leaving the capillaries — no matter how much hydrostatic pressure exists within them. When fluid filters through a capillary, the protein albumin remains behind in the diminishing volume of water. Because it's a large molecule, albumin normally can't pass through capillary membranes. As the albumin concentration inside a capil-

Understanding osmosis

In osmosis, fluid moves passively from areas with more fluid (and a lower solute concentration) to areas with less fluid (and a higher solute concentration). Remember that in osmosis, fluid moves, whereas in diffusion, solutes move.

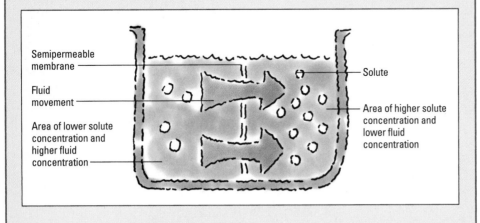

Semipermeable membrane

Fluid movement

Area of lower solute concentration and higher fluid concentration

Solute

Area of higher solute concentration and lower fluid concentration

lary rises, fluid starts to move back into the capillaries through osmosis.

H₂O attraction

Albumin acts as a water magnet. The osmotic, or pulling, force of albumin in the intravascular space is called *plasma colloid osmotic pressure*. In capillaries, this pressure averages about 25 mm Hg.

As long as capillary blood pressure (hydrostatic pressure) exceeds the plasma colloid osmotic pressure, water and solutes can leave the capillaries and enter the interstitial fluid. When capillary blood pressure falls below the plasma colloid osmotic pressure, water and diffusible solutes return to the capillaries.

Normally, blood pressure in a capillary exceeds plasma colloid osmotic pressure in the arteriole and falls below it in the venule end. As a result, capillary filtration occurs along the first half of the vessel; reabsorption, along the second half. As long as capillary blood pressure and plasma albumin levels remain normal, the amount of water that moves into the vessel equals the amount that moves out. When albumin levels in the blood are low, the patient develops edema.

When capillary blood pressure and plasma albumin levels remain normal, the amounts of water moving into and out of a vessel are equal.

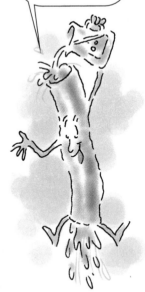

Fluid gains and losses

In a healthy body, fluid gains match fluid losses to maintain proper physiologic functioning. The skin, lungs, kidneys—in fact, nearly all of the major organs—work together to maintain the balance of body fluids. To maintain fluid balance, the amount of fluid gained throughout the day must equal the amount lost. (See *How the body gains and loses fluid.*)

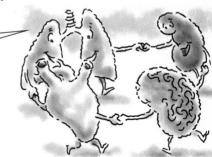

Nearly all of us major body systems work together to maintain the balance of body fluids.

How the body gains and loses fluid

Each day the body takes in fluid from the GI tract (in foods and liquids as well as from metabolism) and loses fluid through the skin, lungs, intestines (feces), and urinary tract (urine). This illustration shows the primary sites involved in fluid gains and losses as well as the average amount of normal daily fluid intake and output.

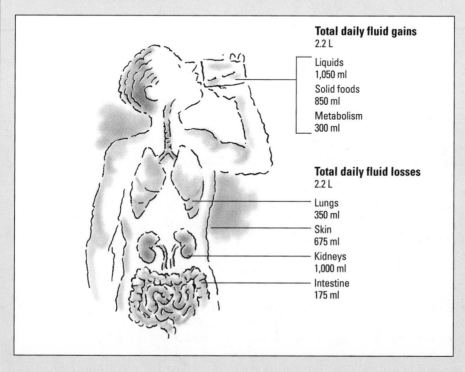

Total daily fluid gains
2.2 L

Liquids
1,050 ml
Solid foods
850 ml
Metabolism
300 ml

Total daily fluid losses
2.2 L

Lungs
350 ml
Skin
675 ml
Kidneys
1,000 ml
Intestine
175 ml

Gains

Fluid gains come mostly from drinking water and other beverages. The body also gains fluid from solid foods and the metabolism of carbohydrates, proteins, and fats.

Losses

The body loses fluid through sensible and insensible means.

Sense and sensibility

Fluid losses from urination, defecation, wounds, and other means are termed *sensible* because they can be measured. Urination accounts for the largest sensible fluid loss.

A certain amount of water must be present in urine to transport out of the body the products of metabolism that the body doesn't need. This amount is called *obligatory* water loss because it must occur daily for health. The kidneys may also put out additional water each day, depending on activities and needs. This *optional* water loss varies with climate and physical activities.

Typically, an adult loses 150 to 200 ml/day of fluid through defecation. In severe diarrhea, these fluid losses may exceed 5,000 ml/day.

Don't count on it

Fluid losses from the skin (through perspiration) and lungs (through expiration) are called *insensible* because they can't be measured — or, to a large extent, even seen. Losses from fluid evaporation through the skin are fairly constant but depend on the body surface area. For instance, an infant has a greater body surface area than an adult, relative to their respective weights. As a result, infants typically lose more water through their skin than adults. Changes in humidity also affect the amount of fluid lost through the skin.

Likewise, respiratory rate and depth affect the amount of fluid lost through the lungs. Tachypnea causes more water to be lost; bradypnea, less. Fever increases insensible fluid losses through both the skin and lungs.

Thirst

Thirst, the conscious desire for water, is the primary regulator of fluid intake. Thirst occurs as a result of even small fluid losses. Losing body fluids or eating salty foods leads to an increase in the osmolarity (osmotic pressure) of ECF. This increase causes the

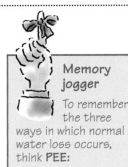

Memory jogger

To remember the three ways in which normal water loss occurs, think **PEE:**

Perspiration — through the skin

Exhalation — from the lungs

Elimination — through urine and feces

mucous membranes of the mouth to become dry, in turn stimulating the thirst center in the hypothalamus.

The brain then directs motor neurons to satisfy thirst, causing the person to drink enough fluid to restore ECF levels to normal. The ingested fluid is absorbed from the intestine into the bloodstream, where it moves freely between fluid compartments. This movement leads to a rise in the amount of fluid in the body and a drop in the concentration of solutes, thus balancing fluid levels throughout the body.

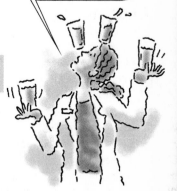

Liquids are the only water sources that meet the body's fluid needs, so advise your adult patient to drink 8 to 12 glasses of water per day!

Sources of fluid

Liquids are the only water sources that meet the body's fluid needs. However, solid foods and metabolic water also contribute to total fluid intake. Solid foods supply about 700 to 1,000 ml of water daily in an average diet. By weight, solid foods range from 0% water (vegetable oil) to 95% water (lettuce). The metabolism of carbohydrates, fats, and proteins yields roughly 250 ml of water daily.

Fluids in health promotion

Many people don't drink enough fluids, which puts them at risk for chronic mild dehydration. Physical effects of dehydration include:
• increased risk of kidney stones
• reduced physical performance, such as difficulty concentrating, headache, irritability, sleepiness, dizziness, and loss of balance.

Under normal circumstances, water is the best fluid to consume. Tap water is available virtually everywhere at no cost; bottled water costs relatively little and may taste better than tap water. What's more, water has no calories, fat, caffeine, or cholesterol. Other good beverage choices are low-fat milk and 100% fruit juices, both of which contain essential nutrients.

Although carbonated drinks provide fluid, they also deliver empty calories along with a high sugar content (unless they're diet drinks). Caffeinated beverages and alcohol actually increase fluid loss by causing frequent urination. (See *Promoting fluid intake*, page 100.)

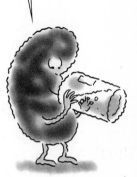

Not everybody must get stoned! Tell your patients to drink up because dehydration increases the risk of kidney stones.

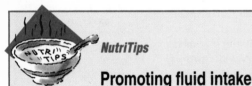

NutriTips

Promoting fluid intake

To help ensure adequate fluid intake, provide the following suggestions to patients:
• Keep bottled water at your desk so you can take sips throughout the day.
• Choose liquids that taste good. If you prefer cold water, refrigerate the water bottle or a glass.
• Consider installing a water filter, or buy bottled water.
• Drink before you get thirsty. If you wait until you're thirsty, you'll need to drink even more fluid.
• Drink a glass of water before each meal. If you're dieting, water helps inhibit your appetite so you eat less.
• Include water as part of your meal. That way, drinking water won't seem like an extra chore that calls for planning.
• Try sparkling water with a touch of lime or lemon. Seltzer is calorie-free and full of bubbles!
• Eat plenty of fruits and vegetables, which are high in water content. Six ounces of fruit juice equals one serving from the fruit group.
• Pack bottled water with your lunch to help you stay away from high-calorie soft drinks.
• Avoid alcohol and caffeinated beverages, which lead to fluid loss from frequent urination.
• Drink low-fat milk. It provides essential nutrients, such as fluids, vitamin D, calcium, and protein.
• Drink extra fluids before, during, and after exercise. Drink at least 16 oz (473 ml) of fluid up to 2 hours before a competitive event; at least 4 to 8 oz (118 to 236 ml) of water or a sports drink 5 to 10 minutes before a workout. During strenuous exercise, drink 8 to 10 oz (236 to 296 ml) every 15 to 20 minutes.

When possible, suggest that your patient wet his whistle with water! Drinking alcoholic beverages, such as wine, and caffeinated beverages, such as coffee and tea, can actually increase fluid loss by causing frequent urination.

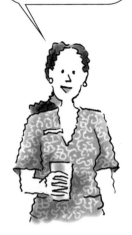

Water requirement

To maintain fluid balance, a person's daily fluid intake should equal fluid output. On average, an adult loses about 1,450 to 2,800 ml of water daily from sensible and insensible losses. Roughly speaking, an adult needs 1 to 1.5 ml of water per calorie consumed. So someone who consumes 2,000 calories daily needs a total fluid intake of 2,000 to 3,000 ml. Of this intake, at least 60% should be consumed as water, with the remainder obtained from foods and metabolism. (See *Fluid balance in infants.*)

A bit more, a tad less

Despite these guidelines, actual water requirements vary greatly among individuals—and in the same individual as circumstances change. For instance, the body's water requirement increases with:
• high ambient temperature—As the temperature of the surrounding environment rises, the body loses water to help maintain

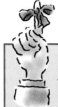

Memory jogger

Remember that individuals may need a **TADD** more or less water, depending on these four factors:

Temperature

Activity

Disease

Diet.

a normal temperature. This loss necessitates increased water intake.

• increased activity level—Strenuous physical activity causes a person to lose more water through sweating and to need more water for the increased metabolic work involved in the physical activity. As a result, the water requirement rises.

• functional losses—Any disease process that interferes with normal functioning of the body can affect fluid requirements. For instance, prolonged diarrhea or vomiting may cause loss of large amounts of water, increasing the fluid need.

• special diets—If you eat a high-fiber diet, your water requirement increases because fiber absorbs water in the GI tract. A high-sodium or high-protein diet also increases the need for fluid.

Fluid imbalances

Most of the time, the body adequately compensates for minor fluid imbalances. If it can't, however, any of several problems may result. These include dehydration (fluid volume deficit), hypervolemia (fluid volume excess), and water intoxication.

Dehydration

The body loses water all the time. A person responds to the thirst reflex by drinking fluids and eating foods that contain water. However, if water isn't adequately replaced, the body's cells can lose water. This loss causes dehydration, or fluid volume deficit. Dehydration refers to a fluid loss of 1% or more of body weight.

Signs and symptoms of dehydration include:
• dizziness
• irritability
• delirium
• extreme thirst
• dry skin and mucous membranes
• poor skin turgor
• increased heart rate
• falling blood pressure
• decreased urine output
• seizures and coma (in severe dehydration).

Laboratory values may include a serum sodium level above 145 mEq/L (145 mmol/L) and serum osmolality above 303 mOsm/kg (303 mmol/kg).

Treatment of dehydration involves determining its cause (such as diarrhea and decreased fluid intake) and replacing lost fluids—orally or I.V. Most patients receive hypotonic, low-sodium fluids,

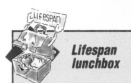

Lifespan lunchbox

Fluid balance in infants

Infants need 1.5 ml of water per calorie, or 1,500 ml of water per day, because of their large body water content (about 70% to 75% of total weight). Also, a relatively large amount of their total body water is located outside the cells, so body water is more easily lost than in adults.

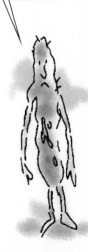

Don't hang me out to dry! Cells like me can become dehydrated if fluid balance isn't maintained.

such as dextrose 5% in water. (See *Dehydration in elderly patients.*)

Hypervolemia

Hypervolemia refers to an excess of isotonic fluid (water and sodium) in the ECF. The body has mechanisms to compensate for hypervolemia. If these fail, however, signs and symptoms develop.

Hypervolemia can occur if a person consumes more fluid than needed, if fluid output is impaired, or if too much sodium is retained. Conditions that may lead to hypervolemia include kidney failure, cirrhosis, heart failure, and steroid therapy.

Depending on the severity of hypervolemia, signs and symptoms may include:
* edema
* distended neck and hand veins
* heart failure
* initially, rising blood pressure and cardiac output; later, falling values.

Laboratory tests may reveal a normal serum sodium level and serum osmolality less than 280 mOsm/kg (280 mmol/kg).

Treatment involves determining the cause and treating the underlying condition. Typically, patients require fluid and sodium restrictions and diuretic therapy.

Water intoxication

Water intoxication occurs when excess fluid moves from the ECF to the ICF. Excessive low-sodium fluid in the ECF is hypotonic to cells; cells are hypertonic to the fluid. As a result, fluids shift into the cells, which have comparatively less fluid and more solutes. That fluid shift occurs to balance the concentrations of fluid between the two spaces.

Water intoxication may occur in a patient with the syndrome of inappropriate antidiuretic hormone, which can result from central nervous system or pulmonary disorders, head trauma, tumors, or the use of certain drugs. Other causes of water intoxication include:
* rapid infusion of hypotonic solutions
* psychogenic polydipsia (a psychological disturbance in which a person drinks large amounts of fluid that aren't needed).

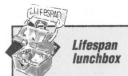

Lifespan lunchbox

Dehydration in elderly patients

Institutionalized elderly patients are at particularly high risk for dehydration because of their diminished thirst perception and physical, cognitive, speech, mobility, and visual impairments.

Poor skin turgor may be an unreliable sign of hydration in older people because of the reduction in the amount of subcutaneous tissue that occurs with age. Check turgor by pinching the subcutaneous tissue at the forehead or over the xiphoid process and watching for a quick return to baseline.

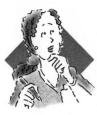

Quick quiz

1. Fluid gains come mostly from:
   A.   solid foods.
   B.   carbohydrates.
   C.   proteins.
   D.   drinking water.

Answer: D. Fluid gains come mostly from drinking water and other beverages.

2. Which type of fluid transport requires no energy?
   A.   Active transport
   B.   Diffusion
   C.   Pinocytosis
   D.   Sodium-potassium pump

Answer: B. Diffusion is a form of passive transport because no energy is required.

3. Dehydration may cause:
   A.   euphoria.
   B.   delirium.
   C.   high blood pressure.
   D.   anuria.

Answer: B. Delirium is a possible sign of dehydration.

4. Which of the following mechanisms is the primary regulator of fluid intake?
   A.   Serum potassium level
   B.   Ratio of fat to skeletal muscle
   C.   Thirst
   D.   Active transport

Answer: C. Thirst is the primary regulator of fluid intake. Even a small fluid loss makes you thirsty and causes the osmotic pressure of ECF to rise. As a result, the mucous membranes of the mouth become dry, which stimulates thirst.

5. Which of the following factors is a source of insensible fluid loss?
   A.   Skin
   B.   Kidneys
   C.   GI tract
   D.   Wounds

Answer: A. Fluid losses from the skin and lungs are called *insensible losses* because they can't be measured or seen. Fluid losses from urination, defecation, and wounds are called *sensible losses* because they can be measured.

Scoring

☆☆☆   If you answered all five questions correctly, celebrate! The information in this chapter diffused quite easily into your system.

☆☆   If you answered four questions correctly, way to go! You must have learned by osmosis.

☆   If you answered fewer than four questions correctly, hang in there. Give the chapter another read, and maybe you'll absorb more of the information.

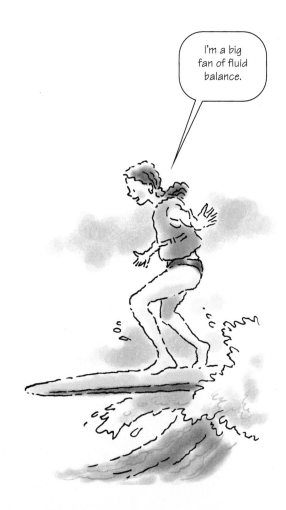

I'm a big fan of fluid balance.

Part II Assessment

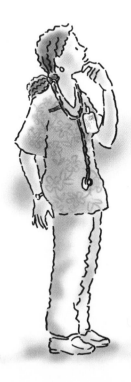

Assessing nutritional status

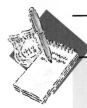

Just the facts

Assessing nutritional status is an important part of patient care. In this chapter, you'll learn:

♦ clinical uses of nutritional screening guidelines

♦ components of a comprehensive nutritional assessment

♦ physical findings that pertain to nutritional status

♦ laboratory studies used to detect poor nutrition.

Evaluating nutritional status

A healthy, balanced diet should be the goal for every individual. This goal is met when nutrient supply, or intake, meets the demand, or requirement. An imbalance occurs when there's overnutrition (supply exceeds demand) or undernutrition (demand exceeds supply).

Seeking status symbols

A person's nutritional status is evaluated by examining information about the patient from several sources. A nutritional screening, along with the patient's medical history, physical examination findings, and laboratory results, can be used to detect potential imbalances. The sources used depend on the patient and setting. A comprehensive nutritional assessment may then be conducted to set goals and determine interventions to correct actual or potential imbalances.

Enacting a plan

Based on the information gathered in the comprehensive nutritional assessment, the patient may require restrictions in diet, such as a reduction in calories, fat, saturated fat, cholesterol, sodium, or other nutrients. Other diet plans involve

> Nutritional screening is an effective way to evaluate nutritional status.

> I just don't get the point of this!

SECURITY ID REQUIRED

therapeutic correction of imbalances, such as by increasing or decreasing certain minerals or vitamins.

Nutritional screening

Nutritional screening also examines certain variables to determine the risk of nutritional problems in specific populations. A screening may target pregnant women, the elderly, or those with certain disorders (such as cardiac disorders) to detect deficiencies or potential imbalances. A dietitian, diet technician, or other qualified health care professional may perform the screening on an individual who may or may not be in the target population. Routine screening occurs during the initial history and physical assessment.

Making value judgments

The most commonly examined values are:
• height and weight history
• unintentional weight loss (more than 5% in 30 days or 10% in 180 days)
• laboratory values
• skin integrity
• appetite
• diet
• present illness or diagnosis
• medical history
• functional status
• advanced age (age 80 and older).

Wellness screen

Wellness screens have been developed by the Nutritional Screening Initiative, a project of the American Academy of Family Physicians, the American Dietetic Association, and the National Council on the Aging. This screening tool also assesses body mass index (BMI), which evaluates height in relationship to weight as well as eating habits, living environment, and functional status. (See *How to use a wellness screen.*)

Risk assessment

When the screening is complete, a level of risk of nutritional problems is assigned. Those individuals at higher risk should be given a comprehensive nutritional assessment, whereas those at lower to moderate risk should be periodically reevaluated.

How to use a wellness screen

A wellness screen is a handy assessment tool for evaluating nutritional status. It provides useful information about the patient's body mass index (BMI), eating habits, living environment, and functional status. A checkmark next to any statement indicates that the patient is at risk and requires further assessment. If indicated, contact appropriate resources who can provide additional help.

Patient's name: _Robert Harrison_ **Date:** _4/30/06_

Body mass index

The BMI measures total body fat based on height and weight. To calculate your patient's BMI, first obtain his height to the nearest inch and his weight to the nearest pound. Then consult the grid on page 117 or use this formula:

([weight ÷ height] ÷ height) × 703.

BMI values are:
< 18.5 = underweight
18.5 to 24.9 = normal
25.0 to 29.9 = overweight
≥ 30 = obese.

Height (in): _71_
Weight (lb): _220_
BMI: _31_

Check if the patient:
☐ lost or gained 10 lb or more in the past 6 months.
☐ has a BMI less than 18.5.
☑ has a BMI greater than 24.9.

Eating habits

Check if the patient:
☐ doesn't have enough food to eat each day.
☐ usually eats alone.
☐ doesn't eat anything on one or more days each month.
☐ has a poor appetite.
☐ is on a special diet.
☑ eats vegetables two or fewer times per day.
☑ drinks milk or eats milk products once or less per day.
☐ eats fruit or drinks fruit juice once or less per day.
☐ eats breads, cereals, pasta, rice, or other grains five or fewer times per day.
☐ has difficulty chewing or swallowing.
☑ has more than one alcoholic drink per day (if a woman) or more than two drinks per day (if a man).
☐ has pain in the mouth, teeth, or gums.

Living environment

Check if the patient:
☐ lives on an income of less than $6,000 per year (per individual in the household).
☑ lives alone.
☐ is housebound.
☐ is concerned about home security.
☐ lives in a home with inadequate heating or cooling.
☐ doesn't have a stove or refrigerator.
☐ can't or won't spend money on food (less than $25 per person each week).

Functional status

Check if the patient needs help with:
☐ bathing.
☐ dressing.
☐ grooming.
☐ toileting.
☐ eating.
☐ walking or moving about.
☐ traveling (outside the home).
☑ preparing food.
☑ shopping for food or other necessities.

How many vegetables do you eat each day?

Er...Do french fries and corn chips count?

Comprehensive nutritional assessment

When the nutritional screening has identified a person at risk, a comprehensive nutritional assessment is conducted to examine additional factors and better determine the degree of malnutrition. Using this assessment, a baseline nutritional status is determined and effective nutritional care is planned. Because of the extensive training required and the need for accuracy, a registered dietitian is usually responsible for conducting this assessment.

> I sentence those at high risk for poor nutrition to a comprehensive nutritional assessment.

Crunching the numbers

The comprehensive nutritional assessment is commonly performed on moderate- to high-risk patients with some degree of protein-calorie malnutrition. Major parameters examined include:
• medical history
• physical examination findings
• laboratory test results.

Multiple criteria must be examined to provide an accurate evaluation of the individual's nutritional status. No single criterion can be used to evaluate an individual, and it may not be necessary to gather all possible information for every patient. The decision to consider information is left to the dietitian's discretion.

Medical history

A medical history is usually gathered from the patient's medical record or through an interview with the patient.

Current and past health history

Current and past health history is important as it relates to nutritional status and as it affects nutrient supply or demand. Findings that may affect nutritional status negatively include:
• chewing and swallowing problems resulting from ill-fitting dentures, missing teeth, or mechanical problems, such as obstruction, inflammation, or edema
• neurologic problems, such as dysphagia, Parkinson's disease, stroke, or traumatic brain injury
• anorexia or loss of appetite
• cognitive impairments
• paralysis or physical disabilities that may impair the ability to feed oneself.

Excessive nutrient intake

Conditions may also be found in the patient's history that may result in excessive nutrient intake. Examples of these conditions include bulimia nervosa and obesity.

GI disorders

Other problems can also impair digestion and absorption, resulting in altered nutritional status. Check the patient's health history for inflammatory, obstructive, or functional disorders of the GI tract, such as:
• lactose intolerance
• cystic fibrosis
• pancreatic disorders
• inflammatory bowel diseases
• minimal function in the small intestine due to a disorder, such as Crohn's disease or surgical excision (short-gut syndrome)
• radiation enteritis
• liver disorders.

Altered metabolism

Nutrition may also be affected by conditions known to accelerate metabolism. These conditions include:
• pregnancy
• fever
• sepsis
• thermal injuries
• pressure ulcers
• cancer
• acquired immunodeficiency syndrome
• major surgery
• trauma
• burns.

  Some conditions, such as diabetes mellitus, hormonal imbalances, and starvation, alter nutrient metabolism. In addition, diarrhea and malabsorption syndromes, such as celiac disease, cause increased nutrient excretion. Other conditions, such as renal insufficiency, impair nutrient excretion.

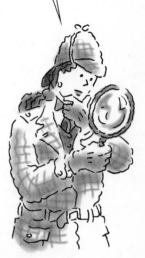

Knowing if a health problem exists helps to detect potential nutritional problems.

Detection is the key

In the history, it's important to identify an existing condition that might affect nutritional status. The condition's impact on nutritional status depends on its severity and how long the patient has been afflicted. (See *Tips for detecting nutritional problems*, page 112.)

Tips for detecting nutritional problems

Nutritional problems may stem from physical conditions, drugs, diet, or lifestyle factors. The lists below will help you determine if your patient is at risk for a nutritional problem.

Physical condition
• Chronic illnesses (diabetes or neurologic, cardiac, or thyroid problems)
• Family history of diabetes or heart disease
• Draining wounds or fistulas
• Obesity or a weight gain of 10% above normal body weight
• Unplanned weight loss of 10% below normal body weight
• History of or recent GI disturbances
• Anorexia or bulimia
• Depression or anxiety
• Severe trauma
• Recent chemotherapy or radiation therapy
• Physical limitation (paresis or paralysis)
• Recent major surgery
• Pregnancy, especially teen or multiple birth

Drugs and diet
• Fad diets
• Steroid, diuretic, or antacid use
• Mouth, tooth, or denture problems
• Excessive alcohol intake
• Strict vegetarian diet
• Liquid diet or nothing by mouth for more than 3 days
• Polypharmacy

Lifestyle
• Lack of support from family and friends
• Financial problems
• Isolation or homebound status

Intake information

Intake information helps you assess what and how much your patient eats. This information can help identify problems in nutritional status and behaviors that need improvement.

Survey says...

Observing what the individual eats provides an objective measurement of the kinds and amount of foods consumed. Of course, close observation is rarely possible. A screening, commonly a questionnaire geared to nutritional problems, can help fill this information gap. Open-ended questions are more useful than closed, "yes-or-no" questions for obtaining accurate information. Important areas for questioning include:
• number of meals and snacks eaten in a 24-hour period
• unusual food habits
• time of day most of the calories are consumed
• skipped meals
• meals eaten away from home
• number of fruits and vegetables eaten daily
• number of servings (and types) of grains eaten daily
• how often red meat, poultry, and fish are eaten, including type and amount

• how often meatless meals are consumed
• number of hours of television watched daily
• types and amount of dairy products consumed daily
• how often desserts and sweets are eaten
• types and amount of beverages (including alcohol) consumed
• food allergies or intolerances
• dietary supplements and why they're taken
• medications, including over-the-counter products and herbal supplements.

Diet history tools

More formal tools for taking a diet history have been developed. The 24-hour food recall and the food frequency record are tools that examine what, how much, and how often a person typically eats to determine nutritional status.

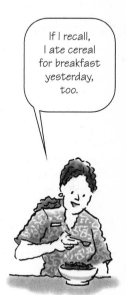

If I recall, I ate cereal for breakfast yesterday, too.

24-hour food recall

A quick and easy method of evaluating an individual's intake is through the 24-hour food recall. In order to complete this tool, the person must be able to recount all the types and amounts of foods and beverages consumed during a 24-hour period.

Working around the clock

The time period may be the past 24 hours or a typical 24-hour period. To help the person identify portion sizes, food models or pictures of typical portions can be used. Specific details may be necessary in some recall situations, such as food preparation (for example, frying versus dry roasting meat). Open-ended questions also reveal more information than typical "yes-or-no" questions. Once obtained, the recall information is then evaluated to see if nutritional needs are being met.

Food frequency record

The food frequency record is a checklist of particular foods that helps determine what's consumed and how often. The checklist may list the foods in one column, and the person marks off how often he eats the foods in other columns. The choices may include how often the food is consumed (such as per day, per week, or per month) or if the food is eaten frequently, seldom, or never. The checklist typically doesn't include the serving size, and it may only include specific foods or nutrients suspected of being deficient or excessive in the diet.

Getting into groups

Another method of gathering information for the food frequency record is to use a questionnaire that lists food items organized by food groups. In this document, the patient records the type of food consumed and how often.

Two are better than one

Either checklist provides a more complete dietary picture when used in conjunction with the 24-hour recall. When deficiencies or excesses are identified, goals may be developed to address nutritional and educational needs.

Psychosocial factors

Other factors could be uncovered during the history that may influence the patient's nutritional habits, including:
- illiteracy
- language barriers
- knowledge of nutrition and food safety
- cultural or religious influences
- social isolation
- limited or low income
- inadequate cooking resources, such as major appliances or kitchen access
- limited access to transportation
- physical inactivity or illness
- use of tobacco or recreational drugs
- limited community resources. (See *Understanding cultural and economic influences.*)

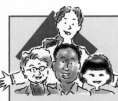

Bridging the gap

Understanding cultural and economic influences

What your patient eats may depend on various cultural and economic influences. Understanding these influences will give you more insight into the patient's nutritional status. Consider these points:
- Socioeconomic status may affect the patient's ability to purchase healthful foods in quantities needed to maintain proper health. Low socioeconomic status can lead to nutritional problems, especially for small children as well as pregnant women, who may experience complications of labor or may give birth to infants with low birth weight.
- Work schedule affects the amount and type of food a patient eats, especially if he works full-time at night.
- Religion can restrict food choices. For example, many Jews and Muslims don't eat pork products, and many Catholics avoid meat on Ash Wednesday and Fridays during Lent.

Teach according to each patient's needs

You should incorporate the patient's individual psychosocial factors into his teaching plan, as appropriate. For example, if you identify that your patient can't read or doesn't read well, giving him a picture guide on which foods are appropriate and which should be avoided may be more helpful to the patient than written words alone.

Physical findings

Physical examinations help determine your patient's health status and identify illness. Physical factors discovered during the comprehensive nutritional assessment may be related to an alteration in nutritional status and malnutrition. However, such findings as height and weight reflect chronic changes in nutritional status rather than acute processes.

Height

Measure height using a fixed measuring stick with the individual standing as straight as possible, without shoes, against a wall. Adaptations may be needed if the patient can't stand or cooperate. (See *Overcoming height measurement problems* and *Growth spurts and diminishing height*.)

Weight

Measure weight using a beam-balance scale or a bed scale if the person is bedridden. The information gathered is more helpful if weight is measured on the same scale at the same time of day (typically before breakfast and after voiding), in the same amount of clothing, and without shoes. (See *Nutrition and infant growth rate*, page 116.)

Lifespan lunchbox

Growth spurts and diminishing height

When measuring height, note the growth of children as well as diminishing height in older adults. Growth of children may be noted on standardized charts, such as those developed by the American Academy of Pediatrics, to assess growth patterns for possible abnormalities. Diminishing height in older adults may be related to osteoporotic changes and should be investigated.

Overcoming height measurement problems

A patient confined to a wheelchair or one who can't stand straight because of scoliosis poses a challenge in measuring accurate height. An approximate measurement of height can be obtained by measuring "wingspan."

Winging it
Have the patient hold his arms straight out from the sides of his body. Children may be told to hold their arms out "like bird wings." Measure from the tip of one middle finger to the tip of the other. That distance is the patient's approximate height.

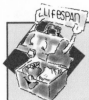

Lifespan lunchbox

Nutrition and infant growth rate

The rate of growth in infants is an indicator of nutritional status. Infants who are breast-fed have satisfactory but slower rates of growth than infants who are formula-fed. However, by age 12 to 16 months, breast-fed infants weight approximately the same as infants who are formula-fed. Undernourished or sick infants with slow growth rates typically reach normal weight percentiles by age 2 years.

Body mass index

BMI measures weight in relationship to height. It can be calculated using conventional pounds and inches or the metric system (using kilograms and centimeters). (See *Calculating BMI*.) BMI can also be estimated without doing any calculations. (See *Determining BMI*.)

Using BMI to evaluate body weight requires little skill. The major disadvantage of using BMI is that it works on the assumption that excess weight is a result of excess fat. It doesn't account for such other reasons as edema and large muscle mass.

> When weighing your patient, remember: same scale, same time of day, same amount of clothing, and no shoes!

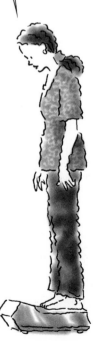

Calculating BMI

Use one of the formulas below to calculate your patient's BMI.

$$BMI = \left(\frac{\text{weight in pounds}}{\text{height in inches} \times \text{height in inches}} \right) \times 703$$

OR

$$BMI = \left(\frac{\text{weight in kilograms}}{\text{height in centimeters} \times \text{height in centimeters}} \right) \times 10{,}000$$

OR

$$BMI = \left(\frac{\text{weight in kilograms}}{\text{height in meters} \times \text{height in meters}} \right)$$

Determining BMI

Body mass index (BMI) measures weight in relation to height. The BMI ranges shown here are for adults. They aren't exact ranges for healthy or unhealthy weights; however, they show that health risks increase at higher levels of overweight and obesity. To use the graph below, find your patient's weight along the bottom and then go straight up until you come to the line that matches his height. The shaded area indicates whether your patient is healthy, overweight, or obese.

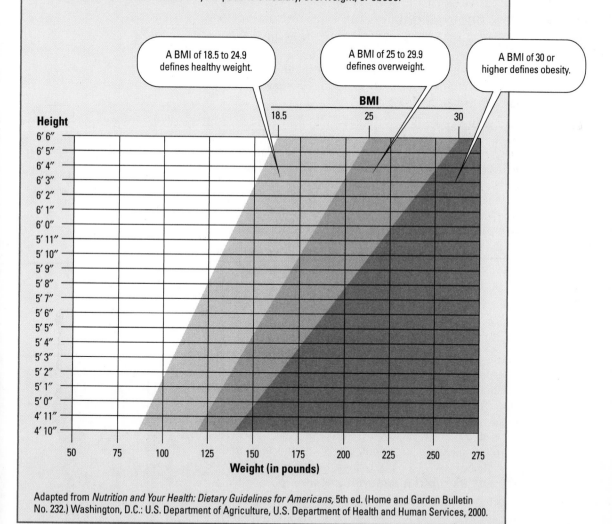

A BMI of 18.5 to 24.9 defines healthy weight.

A BMI of 25 to 29.9 defines overweight.

A BMI of 30 or higher defines obesity.

Adapted from *Nutrition and Your Health: Dietary Guidelines for Americans,* 5th ed. (Home and Garden Bulletin No. 232.) Washington, D.C.: U.S. Department of Agriculture, U.S. Department of Health and Human Services, 2000.

Interpretation station

BMI is interpreted as follows:
• An underweight person has a BMI of less than 18.5.

- A person whose weight is normal for his height has a BMI of 18.5 to 24.9.
- An overweight person has a BMI of 25.0 to 29.9.
- A person in obesity class 1 has a BMI of 30.0 to 34.9; in obesity class 2, a BMI of 35.0 to 39.9; and morbid obesity, 40.0 or greater.

All measures other than normal place the patient at a higher health risk, and nutritional needs should be assessed accordingly.

Ideal body weight

Ideal body weight (IBW), also helpful in assessing nutritional status, is a reference standard for clinical use. For men, this measurement is 106 lb for a height of 5′, plus an additional 6 lb for each inch over 5′. For women, IBW is 100 lb for a height of 5′, plus 5 lb for each inch over 5′.

Measuring up to the ideal

IBW range can be 10% higher or lower depending on body size. The percentage of IBW is obtained by dividing the patient's true weight by the IBW and then multiplying that number by 100. This percentage can be used to determine the patient's weight status and accompanying health risk:

- An obese person is greater than 120% of IBW.
- An overweight person is 110% to 120% of IBW.
- A person whose weight is normal is 90% to 110% of IBW.
- A mildly underweight person is 80% to 90% of IBW.
- A moderately underweight person is 70% to 79% of IBW.
- A severely underweight person is less than 70% of IBW.

Body composition measurements

Measurements of body composition include the triceps skinfold measurement, the midarm circumference, and the midarm muscle circumference. These measurements provide quantitative information about body composition made up of fat or muscle tissue. Measurements may be compared with reference standards or may be used to evaluate changes. If measurements are less than 90% of the reference value, nutritional intervention is indicated.

Triceps skinfold measurements

Triceps skinfold measures subcutaneous fat stores and is an index of total body fat. To measure the skinfold, the individual's arm hangs freely and a fold of skin located slightly above midpoint is grasped between the thumb and forefinger. As the skin is pulled away from underlying muscle, calipers are applied and the measurement is read to the nearest millimeter. (See *Taking anthropometric arm measurements.*)

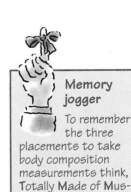

Memory jogger

To remember the three placements to take body composition measurements think, Totally Made of Muscle, Man:

Triceps skinfold

Midarm circumference

Midarm Muscle circumference.

Taking anthropometric arm measurements

Follow the steps below to determine triceps skinfold thickness, midarm circumference, and midarm muscle circumference.

Triceps skinfold thickness

1. Find the midpoint circumference of the arm by placing the tape measure halfway between the axilla and the elbow. Grasp the patient's skin with your thumb and forefinger, about ⅜" (1 cm) above the midpoint, as illustrated below.

2. Place calipers at the midpoint and squeeze for 3 seconds.

3. Record the measurement to the nearest millimeter.

4. Take two more readings and use the average.

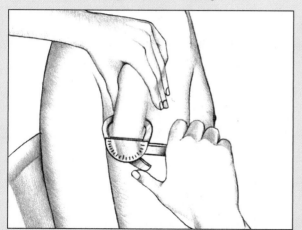

Midarm circumference and midarm muscle circumference

1. Measure the midarm circumference at the midpoint, as illustrated below. Record the measurement in centimeters.

2. Calculate the midarm muscle circumference by multiplying the triceps skinfold thickness (measured in millimeters) by 3.14.

3. Subtract this number from the midarm circumference.

Recording the measurements

Record all three measurements as a percentage of the standard measurements (see chart below), using this formula:

$$\frac{\text{Actual measurement}}{\text{Standard measurement}} \times 100\%$$

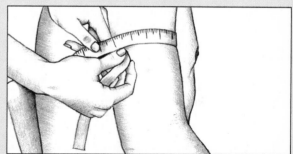

After taking and recording the measurements above, consult the chart at right to determine your patient's caloric status. A measurement less than 90% of the standard indicates caloric deprivation. A measurement over 90% indicates adequate or more than adequate energy reserves.

Measurement	Standard	90%
Triceps skinfold thickness	Men: 12.5 mm Women: 16.5 mm	Men: 11.3 mm Women: 14.9 mm
Midarm circumference	Men: 29.3 cm Women: 28.5 cm	Men: 26.4 cm Women: 25.7 cm
Midarm muscle circumference	Men: 25.3 cm Women: 23.3 cm	Men: 22.8 cm Women: 20.9 cm

Take three

Three readings of the skinfold measurements are taken. These readings may be from the same site or other appropriate sites (bicep, thigh, calf, subscapular, or suprailiac skinfolds). The readings are then added together and divided by 3 to record the average. For men, 11.3 mm is 90% of standard; for women, 14.9 mm.

Midarm circumference

Midarm circumference measures muscle mass and subcutaneous fat. To obtain this value, ask the patient to flex the forearm of his nondominant arm 90 degrees. Then place the arm in a dependent position, place a measuring tape around the midupper arm between the top of the acromion process of the scapula and olecranon process of the ulna, and measure from the midpoint. Hold the tape firmly — but not too tightly — and record to the nearest millimeter.

Midarm muscle circumference

Midarm muscle circumference provides an index of muscle mass and indicates somatic protein stores. Calculate this value by multiplying the triceps skinfold measurement by 3.14 and then multiplying that value by the midarm circumference measurement. Record the value in centimeters. This value is minimally affected by edema and provides a quick estimation.

Appearance

Physical examination of the individual may reveal signs of malnutrition related to a nutritional deficiency. However, signs may also be due to other conditions or disorders and can't be considered indicative, but only suggestive of a nutritional deficiency. In addition, remember that physical signs and symptoms may vary among populations because of genetic and environmental differences. (See *Evaluating nutritional disorders*.)

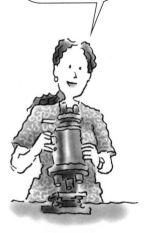

Lab values can detect nutritional problems before physical signs and symptoms appear.

Laboratory data

Laboratory tests can detect nutritional problems in early stages before physical signs and symptoms appear. Most of the routine tests assess protein-calorie information, with serum albumin used most commonly to screen for nutritional problems. Tests are done to help determine adequacy of protein stores. Some tests measure by-products of protein catabolism (such as creatinine) and others measure products of protein anabolism (such as albumin level, transferrin level, hemoglobin level, hematocrit, prealbumin, retinol binding protein, and total lymphocyte count).

Evaluating nutritional disorders

This chart can help you interpret your nutritional assessment findings. Body systems are listed below with signs or symptoms and the implications for each.

Body system or region	Sign or symptom	Implications
General	• Weakness and fatigue • Weight loss	• Anemia or electrolyte imbalance • Decreased calorie intake, increased calorie use, or inadequate nutrient intake or absorption
Skin, hair, and nails	• Dry, flaky skin • Dry skin with poor turgor • Rough, scaly skin with bumps • Petechiae or ecchymoses • Sore that won't heal • Thinning, dry hair • Spoon-shaped, brittle, or ridged nails	• Vitamin A, vitamin B-complex, or linoleic acid deficiency • Dehydration • Vitamin A deficiency • Vitamin C or K deficiency • Protein, vitamin C, or zinc deficiency • Protein deficiency • Iron deficiency
Eyes	• Night blindness; corneal swelling, softening, or dryness; Bitot's spots (gray triangular patches on the conjunctiva) • Red conjunctiva	• Vitamin A deficiency • Riboflavin deficiency
Throat and mouth	• Cracks at the corner of the mouth • Magenta tongue • Beefy, red tongue • Soft, spongy, bleeding gums • Swollen neck (goiter)	• Riboflavin or niacin deficiency • Riboflavin deficiency • Vitamin B_{12} deficiency • Vitamin C deficiency • Iodine deficiency
Cardiovascular	• Edema • Tachycardia, hypotension	• Protein deficiency • Fluid volume deficit
GI	• Ascites	• Protein deficiency
Musculoskeletal	• Bone pain and bow leg • Muscle wasting	• Vitamin D or calcium deficiency • Protein, carbohydrate, and fat deficiency
Neurologic	• Altered mental status • Paresthesia	• Dehydration and thiamine or vitamin B_{12} deficiency • Vitamin B_{12}, pyridoxine, or thiamine deficiency

Albumin

The serum albumin level test assesses protein levels in the body. Albumin makes up more than 50% of total proteins in blood and affects the cardiovascular system because it helps maintain osmotic pressure. Keep in mind that albumin production requires functioning liver cells and an adequate supply of amino acids, the building blocks of proteins.

Bum albumin levels

The serum albumin level is decreased with serious protein deficiency and loss of blood protein due to burns, malnutrition, liver or renal disease, heart failure, major surgery, infections, or cancer.

Creatinine height index

The creatinine height index involves a 24-hour urine collection to measure urinary excretion of creatinine. It helps define body protein mass and evaluate protein depletion. Test results are interpreted using a formula that compares results with ideal height standards.

Creatin' creatinine confusion

Creatinine values decrease with age because of a normal decrease in lean muscle mass. The test is of limited value because results are greatly altered by age, amount of exercise, stress, menstruation, and the presence of severe illness. Increased values may indicate decreased protein stores.

Transferrin

Transferrin is a "carrier" protein that transports iron. The molecule is synthesized mainly in the liver. Transferrin levels decrease along with protein levels and indicate depletion of protein stores. The serum transferrin level reflects the patient's current protein status more accurately than albumin because of its shorter half-life. A normal transferrin value is greater than 200 mg/dl (SI, 2 g/L).

Trackin' transferrin

Decreased transferrin values may also indicate inadequate protein production due to liver damage, protein loss from renal disease, acute or chronic infection, or cancer. Elevated levels may indicate severe iron deficiency.

Hemoglobin

Hemoglobin (Hb) is the main component of red blood cells (RBCs), which transport oxygen. Its formation requires an adequate supply of protein in the form of amino acids. Hb values help assess the blood's oxygen-carrying capacity and are useful in diagnosing anemia, protein deficiency, and hydration status.

Globin trekker

Decreased Hb suggests iron deficiency anemia, protein deficiency, excessive blood loss, or overhydration. Increased Hb suggests dehydration or polycythemia. Normal Hb values vary with age and type of blood sample tested. The following values reflect normal Hb concentrations (in grams per deciliter):
- neonates — 17 to 22 g/dl (SI, 170 to 220 g/L)
- 1 week — 14.5 to 24.5 g/dl (SI, 145 to 245 g/L)
- 1 month — 12.5 to 20.5 g/dl (SI, 125 to 205 g/L)
- 3 months — 10.7 to 17.3 g/dl (SI, 107 to 173 g/L)
- 10 years — 10.3 to 14.9 g/dl (SI, 103 to 149 g/L)
- adult males — 14 to 17.4 g/dl (SI, 140 to 174 g/L)
- females — 12 to 16 g/dl (SI, 120 to 160 g/L).

Hematocrit

The hematocrit (HCT) level reflects the proportion of blood occupied by the RBCs. This test helps diagnose anemia and dehydration.

Don't omit hematocrit

Decreased values suggest iron deficiency anemia or excessive fluid intake or blood loss. Increased values suggest severe dehydration or polycythemia. Normal HCT values reflect age, sex, sample type, and the laboratory performing the test. The following ranges represent normal HCT values for different age-groups:
- neonates — 55% to 68% (SI, 0.55 to 0.68)
- 1 week — 44% to 64% (SI, 0.44 to 0.64)
- 1 month — 39% to 59% (SI, 0.39 to 0.59)
- 3 months — 35% to 49% (SI, 0.35 to 0.49)
- 10 years — 32% to 42% (SI, 0.32 to 0.42)
- adult males — 42% to 52% (SI, 0.42 to 0.52)
- adult females — 36% to 48% (SI, 0.36 to 0.48).

Prealbumin

The prealbumin test is also more sensitive than albumin because of its short half-life (2 days). It isn't as affected by liver disease and hydration status as albumin; however, it's also more expensive to perform. A normal prealbumin value is 19 to 38 mg/dl (SI, 190 to 380 mg/L).

Retinol binding protein

Measurement of retinol binding protein can help you detect an acute change in a patient's nutritional status. This protein responds quickly to nutritional repletion due to a small body pool and short half-life (10 to 12 hours). A normal retinol binding protein value is 2.6 to 7.7 mg/dl (SI, 1.43 to 2.86 mmol/L).

Total lymphocyte count

A lymphocyte (leukocyte) is a white blood cell (WBC), the main cell responsible for fighting infection. Leukocytes are responsible for destroying organisms as well as for phagocytosis, which promotes cellular repair. Normal WBC counts range from 4,000 to 10,000 cells/mm³ (SI, 4 to 10 × 10⁹ L). This test is useful for diagnosing the severity of a disease.

There are five types of leukocytes:

neutrophils, which fight pyogenic infections

eosinophils, which fight allergic disorders and parasitic infections

basophils, which fight parasitic infections

lymphocytes, which fight viral infections

monocytes, which fight severe infections.

The WBC differential will provide specific information about which type of WBC is being affected and is a diagnostically useful test.

Malnutrition decreases the total number of lymphocytes, impairing the body's ability to fight infection. The total lymphocyte count is used in evaluating the health of the immune system and assists in evaluation of protein stores. The total lymphocyte count may also be affected by many medical conditions, so the value is limited.

Totaling it up

Decreased lymphocyte values may indicate malnutrition when no other cause is apparent and may point to infection, leukemia, or tissue necrosis.

Other measures of poor nutrition

In addition to the patient's medical history, physical findings, and laboratory test results, you can use other criteria to detect nutritional deficiencies, including immunocompetence and bone integrity.

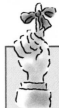

Memory jogger

To remember the five types of leukocytes (WBCs), think Must Examine Low Blood Numbers:

Monocytes

Eosinophils

Lymphocytes

Basophils

Neutrophils.

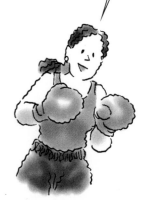

Malnutrition takes the fight out of the immune system by decreasing the number of lymphocytes.

Cutaneous hypersensitivity reactions

Immunocompetence may be evaluated by placing small quantities of recall antigens (*Candida*, mumps, or purified protein derivative of tuberculin) under the skin. Normally, a positive reaction occurs in 24 to 48 hours with a red area of 5 mm or more. However, in the individual with malnutrition, a delayed reaction, a reaction to only one antigen, or no reaction at all (anergy) may occur. (See *Delayed hypersensitivity reactions.*)

X-rays

X-rays can be used to determine bone integrity and, especially in older women, to detect possible osteoporosis. A bone mineral density test is a specialized X-ray that detects the amount of change in a bone. (Bones with higher mineral density allow fewer X-rays to pass through.) The beam detects the intensity and shows the physician how dense the bones are. A bone scan, another type of X-ray, takes a picture of the bone and identifies fractures, tumors, or inflammation. It's also sensitive enough to recognize structural changes. X-rays may also be used to evaluate the GI tract for integrity and diagnose disorders that may cause malnutrition. The specific X-rays performed will be influenced by the patient's symptoms and diagnosis. Multiple tests may be necessary before a definitive diagnosis is made.

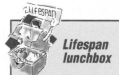

Lifespan lunchbox

Delayed hypersensitivity reactions

Age can cause delayed cutaneous hypersensitivity reactions, making the test less helpful for determining protein status. Elderly patients may have altered laboratory values because of:
• hydration status
• chronic diseases
• organ function changes
• drug regimen.

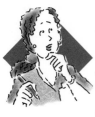

Quick quiz

1. You should measure a patient's midarm circumference whenever you:
    A.   conduct a basic nutritional assessment.
    B.   want to confirm an abnormal protein level.
    C.   want to obtain information about body composition.
    D.   determine a person's weight.

Answer: C. Midarm circumference is one of three measurements used to provide information about the percentage of fat or muscle tissue in the body.

2. To identify individuals at moderate or high risk for nutritional problems, you can obtain information quickly by using which of the following tools?
    A.   Comprehensive nutritional assessment
    B.   Laboratory data
    C.   Physical examination
    D.   Nutritional screening

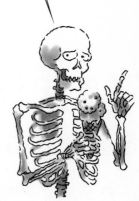

I have lots of integrity. Must be all this calciummmm...

Answer: D. Screening uses a minimal amount of information to identify people at risk. Those identified as being at risk will need a comprehensive nutritional assessment.

3.   Which of the following measures helps classify a person as underweight, normal, or obese?
- A.   Body mass index
- B.   Triceps skinfold
- C.   Midarm circumference
- D.   Midarm muscle circumference

Answer: A. Body mass index uses the patient's height and weight to obtain a value that's useful for determining nutritional status.

4.   The serum albumin test assesses:
- A.   protein levels in the body.
- B.   the ratio of protein to albumin.
- C.   how well the liver metabolizes proteins.
- D.   amino acid levels.

Answer: A. The serum albumin test assesses protein levels in the body.

Scoring

☆☆☆   If you answered all four questions correctly, wow! You've achieved star status in nutritional assessment!

☆☆   If you answered three questions correctly, you've been screened for great things! Your evaluation shows no imbalances when it comes to comprehension!

☆   If you answered fewer than three questions correctly, don't worry! If you're still feeling starved for information, go back and review this chapter!

Nutrition across the lifespan

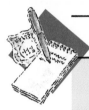

Just the facts

This chapter discusses the ways in which nutritional needs and considerations change throughout life. In this chapter, you'll learn:

♦ stages of growth and development throughout life

♦ nutritional needs unique to each stage of life

♦ nutritional problems common in each stage of life.

A look at nutrition across the lifespan

Nutrition plays a major role throughout each stage of the life cycle. From pregnancy and infancy to the older adult years, each stage of life has specific nutrition requirements to keep the body functioning at its best.

Nutrition during pregnancy

Maternal diet and nutritional status directly impact the course of pregnancy and the fetus. Malnutrition that occurs in the early months of pregnancy can affect the embryo's ability to survive; poor nutrition during the latter half of pregnancy can affect fetal growth.

Physiologic changes

Pregnancy produces various physiologic changes that influence the mother's nutritional needs and how nutrients are used in her body. These changes include alterations in metabolism, GI function, and weight.

Nutrient metabolism

A pregnant woman's nutrient metabolism changes to adjust to the growing fetus:

• Carbohydrate and fat metabolism are altered during pregnancy to provide glucose to the fetus. Maternal fat stores increase during the first half of pregnancy as fat becomes the primary maternal fuel source. During the second half of pregnancy, these stores are used by the mother's body for energy, allowing glucose to be used as an energy source for the fetus.

• Protein metabolism is increased for growth of maternal and fetal tissues.

GI function

Nausea and vomiting are common symptoms of pregnancy in the first trimester. These GI alterations may be related to hypoglycemia (low blood glucose level), decreased gastric motility, relaxation of the cardiac sphincter, or anxiety.

Smoothing things out

During pregnancy, production of the hormone progesterone is increased, causing relaxation of smooth-muscle cells. This action helps the uterus expand to accommodate the growing fetus and slows GI motility, allowing for increased nutrient absorption.

Feeling the burn

As pregnancy progresses, the displacement of the stomach and the intestines caused by the enlarging uterus may contribute to heartburn and constipation. Some women also experience taste and odor changes and some become thirsty frequently.

Weight gain

Growth of the fetus, the placenta, maternal blood volume, maternal fat stores, and tissues all contribute to weight gain during pregnancy. The amount of weight a woman gains, especially during the second and third trimesters, is an important indicator of fetal growth. A woman should gain 2 to 4 lb during the first trimester and 1 lb per week (3 to 4 lb per month) during the second and third trimesters.

Fluid factors

A woman's body gains a large amount of water during pregnancy — total body water can increase by 7 to 10 L (1.8 to 2.6 gal). This fluid weight gain (edema) accounts for a large percentage of weight gain at term. Up to 75% of women experience edema. Minor edema may be considered normal as long as the mother doesn't have other

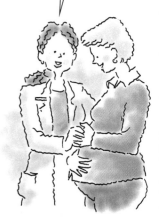

An expectant mother's body undergoes many changes that influence her nutrition needs.

Pregnancy weight gain recommendations

Here are recommendations for weight gain during pregnancy, based on body mass index (BMI).

Prepregnancy weight status	Recommended gain
Underweight (BMI less than 18.5)	28 to 40 lb (12.7 to 18.1 kg)
Normal weight (BMI 18.5 to 24.9)	25 to 35 lb (11.3 to 15.9 kg)
Overweight (BMI 25 to 29.9)	15 to 25 lb (6.8 to 11.3 kg)
Obese (BMI 30 or more)	At least 15 lb (6.8 kg)
Twin pregnancy	35 to 45 lb (15.9 to 20.4 kg)

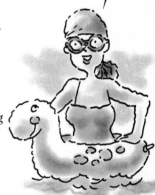

The weight a woman gains during pregnancy is primarily water — up to 7 to 10 liters!

complications, such as hypertension and proteinuria. In addition, blood and plasma volume increase significantly during pregnancy.

Tipping the scales toward a healthy infant

The amount of weight gained during the second and third trimesters can be a valuable indicator of fetal development. Inadequate weight gain during pregnancy increases the risk of having a low-birth-weight (LBW) infant — a baby weighing less than 2,500 g (5.5 lb). LBW babies tend to be malnourished, especially if born full-term, and have a higher incidence of postnatal complications and mortality.

Putting on pounds for pregnancy

Current weight gain recommendations are influenced by prepregnancy weight status. The higher a woman's weight is before pregnancy, the lower the amount of weight she needs to gain during pregnancy to produce a healthy-sized baby. However, young adolescents should be encouraged to achieve gains at the upper ends of the ranges to accommodate for their own growth during pregnancy. (See *Pregnancy weight gain recommendations.*)

Bad influences

It's important to remember, however, that other factors also influence birth weight; adequate maternal weight gain doesn't ensure the delivery of a healthy-birth-weight infant. These factors include:
- smoking
- alcohol intake

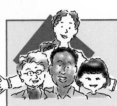

Bridging the gap

Cultural practices during pregnancy

When assessing the nutritional status of pregnant women, be sure to ask about cultural food preferences, restrictions, and taboos because these practices can impact your nursing care. For example, consider these cultural differences:
• In the Haitian culture, pregnant women avoid spices that may irritate the fetus. They also eat red fruits because they believe that these fruits enhance fetal blood.
• Pregnant Filipino women may avoid prunes because they believe these fruits cause a baby to be wrinkled. They may also avoid squid because it's thought to cause the umbilical cord to twist in the womb.

• maternal health status. (See *Cultural practices during pregnancy.*)

Nutrient needs

The requirements for many nutrients increase during pregnancy. Calorie and protein requirements grow to meet the needs of the heart's increased workload, increased energy needs for respiration, growth of maternal tissues, uterine muscles, and the baby's rapid growth. Vitamins and minerals — specifically folate (folic acid), B vitamins, calcium, and iron — also play critical roles in this phase of the life cycle and require specific attention.

Calories

During the first trimester, energy needs are essentially the same as those in a nonpregnant woman. In the second and third trimesters, however, the increased need for energy ranges from 300 to 400 cal/day. An additional 300 cal/day is equal to only two extra cups of low-fat milk and one slice of bread. Because nutrient needs increase more than calorie needs, a pregnant woman's food choices need to be nutrient dense. More calories (2,700 to 3,000 per day) may be needed for active, large, or nutritionally deficient mothers.

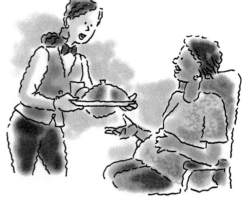

For the second trimester of pregnancy, we're adding 300 calories per day to your menu.

Protein

Recommended protein intake during pregnancy increases by only 10 to 15 g/day, to 60 g/day total. Many nonpregnant women consume more than this already and don't need to increase protein intake. Good sources of protein include milk, eggs, cheese, and meat.

Carbohydrates

A pregnant woman needs at least 100 g/day of carbohydrates to provide enough energy in a usable form for the baby.

Folate

Folate also is critical during the early periconceptional period (from approximately 2 months before pregnancy to 6 weeks' gestation) to ensure healthy embryonic tissue development and prevent spina bifida and neural tube defects. The daily recommended intake of folate is 600 mcg.

The *Dietary Guidelines for Americans 2005* recommend that women of childbearing age who may become pregnant obtain adequate amounts of synthetic folic acid each day from fortified foods or supplements in addition to eating a varied diet rich in folate.

A fortified feast

In recent years, fortification of folic acid in refined grain products, such as breads and cereals, has helped improve the folate status in women of childbearing age. Foods that contain highly usable forms of folate include oranges, orange juice, and pineapple juice.

Calcium

Calcium is needed during pregnancy for the formation of the fetal skeleton and teeth. An additional 300 mg of calcium is recommended for women during pregnancy—for a total of 1,300 mg/day for women ages 14 to 18 and 1,000 mg/day for women ages 19 to 50.

Increasing calcium 1 cup at a time

A diet that includes 3 cups of fortified milk or calcium-fortified soy milk or 2 cups of calcium-fortified orange juice and 1 cup of milk can provide adequate calcium for the increased needs during pregnancy.

Iodine

Adequate iodine intake is essential for the production of thyroxine, the thyroid hormone responsible for controlling the increased metabolic rate that occurs during pregnancy.

Iron

A pregnant woman needs an extra 30 mg/day of iron during the last two trimesters — twice the requirement of a nonpregnant woman. Iron is essential to maintain the increased hemoglobin synthesis necessary for increased maternal blood volume as well as the baby's necessary prenatal iron storage.

Ironing out iron difficulties

Because iron occurs in such small amounts in food, it's standard for a pregnant woman in the United States to take a 30-mg iron supplement daily after 12 weeks of pregnancy. Some of this iron is transferred to the fetus, where it's stored in the liver for use during the first 4 to 6 months of life. The remainder is used to support the mother's blood volume.

The *Dietary Guidelines for Americans 2005* recommend that women of childbearing age who may become pregnant consume foods rich in heme-iron, plant foods high in iron, or iron-fortified foods. These foods should be consumed with foods high in vitamin C to enhance iron absorption.

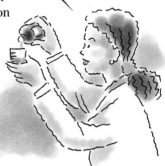

Iron supplements are recommended after the 12th week of pregnancy because foods offer only a small amount of iron.

Developing a healthful diet

A daily diet that supports a healthful pregnancy can be arranged using recommendations of the *Dietary Guidelines for Americans 2005* and MyPyramid food intake patterns. For example, an easy-to-implement core food plan that meets daily pregnancy needs includes:
- milk products (4 cups) — such as milk, yogurt, and cheese (1½ to 2 oz per serving)
- meat and bean group (6- to 8-oz equivalents) — lean meats, eggs, nuts, seeds, and cooked, dry beans
- vegetables (2½ to 3½ cups) — fresh, frozen, canned, or dried vegetables
- dark green or orange vegetables (at least 2 to 3 cups/week)
- fruits (2 cups) — fresh, frozen, canned, or dried fruits and fruit juices, including vitamin C–rich sources
- grains (6- to 10-oz equivalents) — at least half should be whole grains
- oils (6 to 8 tsp) — emphasize those containing omega-3 fatty acids and monounsaturated fats.

Fluid challenge

It's important to drink plenty of fluids during pregnancy—10 cups per day. For many women, thirst will help meet this need without much effort.

Nutrition and breast-feeding

Nutritional needs for a woman who's breast-feeding are only slightly different from those during her pregnancy. Folate and iron needs decrease after giving birth, and energy requirements increase.

Fueling milk production

While breast-feeding, a healthy woman should consume 2,300 to 2,700 cal/day, approximately 500 cal/day more than prepregnancy recommendations. If maternal intake is poor, which can occur when a breast-feeding woman is dieting, the nutrient content of her breast milk may become inadequate and the quantity of milk she produces may decrease.

Water hydrant

Adequate hydration encourages ample milk production, so it's important for new mothers to drink plenty of fluids—2 to 3 qt (2 to 3 L)/day. The mother should also drink one 8-oz glass of fluid each time the infant nurses to ensure she's staying hydrated. Water and such beverages as fruit juices and milk are good choices to maintain adequate hydration.

Keep contaminants out!

Most substances that the mother ingests are secreted into her milk. Therefore, beverages containing alcohol and caffeine should be limited or avoided because they may be harmful to the infant. In addition, the mother should check with her pediatrician before taking any medication. Some researchers believe that components of the maternal food may contribute to colic or the infant's fussiness.

Women who are pregnant or breast-feeding can reduce the risk of mercury poisoning, which can cause brain damage in the fetus and developing child, by avoiding the consumption of shark meat, swordfish, king mackerel, and tilefish. They should also limit their intake of other fish and shellfish.

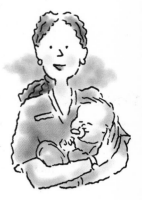

Breast-feeding requires more energy! Therefore, breast-feeding mothers can't afford to cut calories.

Nutritional concerns

Other important nutrition-related considerations during pregnancy include use of artificial sweeteners, alcohol, caffeine, and supplements; smoking; and food-borne illnesses.

Artificial sweeteners

Currently, there's no evidence that consumption of artificial sweeteners, such as aspartame (NutraSweet) or sucralose (Splenda), is harmful during pregnancy. Regardless, many artificially sweetened beverages and foods are low-nutrient foods that serve as poor substitutes for more nutrient-rich foods in the diet.

Alcohol

Prenatal exposure to alcohol is the leading preventable cause of birth defects, mental retardation, and developmental disorders. Alcohol can easily cross the maternal-fetal barrier and the growing fetus hasn't yet developed enzymes to break alcohol down, so it lingers in the fetus's circulation. Be sure to tell your pregnant patient to exclude alcohol-containing beverages from her diet.

Caffeine

Caffeine has long been suspected of causing negative effects in pregnant women. For example, some research suggests that high caffeine consumption during pregnancy can lead to miscarriage. It's also responsible for increasing heart rate, stimulating the central nervous system, and acting as a diuretic.

Some evidence suggests that high caffeine intake may also affect the developing fetus. Caffeine passes through the placenta into fetal circulation, which stimulates fetal activity, leading to increased heart rate and blood pressure.

Coffee break

Because of the high amount of caffeine in coffee, general recommendations limit intake to about 2 cups per day during pregnancy, or no more than 300 mg of caffeine per day.

Smoking

Smoking has negative effects on an unborn child. Babies born to women who smoke during pregnancy commonly have low birth weights.

Supplements

Vitamin and mineral supplements may be recommended for an individual when a nutritional assessment indicates that she's deficient in a particular nutrient. (See *Supplements and pregnancy*.)

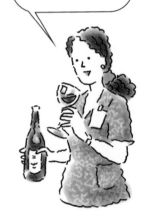

Don't toast too soon! A fetus hasn't developed the enzymes to break down alcohol. That's why it's important for mothers to avoid alcohol during pregnancy.

Herbal helpers?

Herbal supplement use is increasingly more common during pregnancy. However, there's little well-supported research about the safety and effectiveness of this practice.

Food-borne illnesses

Food-borne illnesses, such as listeriosis and *Escherichia coli* infection, can be life-threatening during pregnancy. Pregnant women are more susceptible to food-borne infections because of increased hormone or progesterone levels. To prevent food-borne illnesses, pregnant women should avoid raw fish, oysters, soft cheeses such as Brie, raw or undercooked meat, and unpasteurized milk.

Nutrition during infancy

As humans grow, energy and nutrient requirements change to meet the body's changing needs. Tissue rebuilding and metabolic functioning go on throughout life. However, growth and activity are most rapid during infancy and childhood, resulting in increased nutritional requirements during these stages. The *Dietary Guidelines for Americans 2005* recommendations don't include children under age 2 years.

Growth and development

During infancy, energy, protein, vitamin, and mineral requirements per pound of body weight are higher than at any other time during the lifespan. These high requirements are necessary to support rapid growth and development during this stage of life. An infant's birth weight doubles in the first 4 to 6 months of life and triples within the first year.

Assessing growth

The primary tool for assessing adequacy of nutrition is growth. Most health care professionals chart an infant's growth (weight and length) each visit on a standardized grid provided by the National Center for Health Statistics. As long as the height-to-weight ratio is consistent and the infant's growth follows the curve, nutrition is most likely adequate. In addition, the infant is checked for the development of musculoskeletal milestones at an appropriate age.

Supplements and pregnancy

It's recommended that certain groups of women at high risk for poor dietary intake take a vitamin and mineral supplement. These groups include women who:
• have poor-quality, unchangeable diets
• are pregnant with more than one baby
• smoke cigarettes
• have iron deficiency anemia
• abuse alcohol or use drugs.

Laboratory values followed the first year include serum hematocrit (greater than 29%) and hemoglobin level (greater than 10 g/dl), urine glucose and protein, and the presence of white or red blood cells in the urine.

Physiologic changes

During this time, important physiologic changes can be seen throughout the body, including several major body systems.

GI system

Because an infant's stomach capacity is small — approximately 90 ml at birth — and gastric emptying time is 2.5 to 3 hours, small, frequent feedings are important to meet the infant's energy needs. Digestive enzymes are produced only in small quantities at birth, which is why breast milk and formula are initially the only dietary nutrients babies consume.

Adding to the menu

By age 3 months, secretion of digestive enzymes begins in quantities sufficient to digest some of the starches found in cereal. However, cereals and other solid foods shouldn't be added to an infant's diet until age 6 months, when lipase and bile (enzymes that help to digest fat) are produced. Foods should be introduced to the diet one at a time in order to gauge infant preferences and observe for food allergies and intolerances.

Renal system

The ability of the kidneys to concentrate urine develops rapidly during the first 6 weeks. Before that, however, the infant is highly susceptible to dehydration, especially if he's being fed formula that's overly concentrated.

Neuromuscular system

An important factor in obtaining enough nutrients for small infants is their ability to ingest them. At birth, the infant relies on the sucking reflex and only gradually develops muscle control of the tongue, jaw, head, and neck. Eventually, developing fine motor control allows the infant to chew and drink and to grasp food so that he can feed himself. By age 9 months, the infant can bring the thumb and first finger together to grasp objects, such as small pieces of food, a cup, or a spoon.

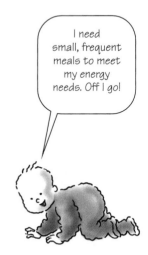

I need small, frequent meals to meet my energy needs. Off I go!

Nutrient needs

Infants' calorie needs range from 80 to 120 cal/kg of body weight. Infants under age 6 months need an average of 108 cal/kg of body weight to supply them with adequate energy; infants ages 6 to 12 months need 98 cal/kg.

Protein needs for infants ages 6 months and younger are 2.2 g/kg of body weight; ages 6 to 12 months, 1.6 g/kg.

Fat-free? No need!

There's no specific recommended amount of fat for infants and restriction isn't recommended. For infants up to age 2, at least 40% of calories consumed should be from fat. Protein and fat requirements are met by human milk or formula.

Fluid figures

Infants need about 2 oz of fluid daily per pound of body weight. Infants typically consume enough breast milk or formula to supply this amount. However, during periods of illness—for example, diarrhea, vomiting, or fever—or exposure to sun, additional fluids may be needed.

ABCs of supplementation

Formula and breast milk provide most of the necessary vitamins and minerals needed by the growing infant. However, supplementation is recommended for certain nutrients:
• Vitamin K is routinely given by injection to all infants at birth to supply the vitamin until the infant's intestinal tract can synthesize it on its own.
• The American Academy of Pediatrics recommends that formula-fed infants be given formula with iron fortification from birth. Because the body's iron stores are generally depleted by age 6 months, it's recommended that oral iron intake be increased for breast-fed infants after this age. Solid foods such as iron-fortified cereals may be used to help meet these iron needs.
• Vitamin D is recommended for some breast-fed infants.
• Fluoride supplementation is recommended for infants ages 6 months to 1 year, unless their food is prepared with fluoridated water.

Nutrient intake

Human milk consumed through breast-feeding is considered optimal for neonates. Even so, not all mothers can or choose to breast-feed. Medical conditions, cultural background, anxiety, drug abuse, and various other factors can prevent a woman from breast-feeding. Rarely, some infants can't take in enough breast

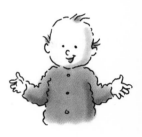

Talk about baby fat! Up to age 2, I'm supposed to consume at least 40% of my daily calories from fat.

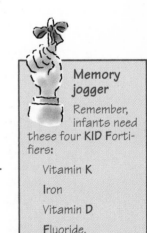

Memory jogger

Remember, infants need these four **KID** Fortifiers:

Vitamin K

Iron

Vitamin D

Fluoride.

milk through breast-feeding to meet nutritional needs. Although breast milk is usually the best food for premature infants, some breast milk may be insufficient in calcium, protein, and essential vitamins. In these cases, bottle-feeding with infant formula is an acceptable alternative or may be used to supplement breast-feeding. (See *Tips for preparing formula*.)

Breast-feeding

Breast-feeding is widely supported in the medical community. The American Academy of Pediatrics and the American Dietetic Association recommend breast-feeding exclusively for the first 4 to 6 months and then in combination with infant foods until age 1. (See *Advantages of breast-feeding*.)

Formula feeding

Formula feedings can provide adequate nutrition in cases where the mother shouldn't or can't breast-feed her infant. Infant formulas are constituted to provide the proper variety and amount of carbohydrates, protein, fats, and micronutrients needed for healthy growth and development. The Food and Drug Administration regulates the composition, labeling, and inspection of infant formula to ensure infant safety.

Women are strongly urged to use commercially prepared formulas rather than homemade formulas made with cow's milk because cow's milk:

- doesn't meet all of an infant's nutritional needs
- can be difficult to digest
- can strain the infant's renal system.

Unlocking the secret formula

Most formulas are based on cow's milk, although preparations based on soy and casein hydrosylate are available for infants who can't tolerate cow's milk–based preparations. There are also special formulas for infants with diseases, such as phenylketonuria and other metabolic diseases. Formula comes in powder form, concentrated liquid, and ready-to-feed forms. Ready-to-feed formulas are convenient and prevent problems based on incorrect dilution and preparation but are more expensive. Special care should be used so that formula isn't improperly mixed and stored, which can be hazardous to the infant.

Introducing solid foods

Introducing solid foods to an infant's diet depends on such factors as nutritional need for iron, physiologic capability to digest starch, and physical ability to chew and swallow. Breast-milk or iron-

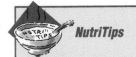

NutriTips

Tips for preparing formula

Here are a few tips for properly preparing infant formula:

- Wash your hands before preparing formula.
- Boil water for 1 to 2 minutes, and then let it cool. (The American Academy of Pediatrics recommends boiling water before use because of contamination of water supplies.)
- Wash utensils in warm, soapy water and rinse them well to ensure that they're safe to use. Also, keep separate utensils for preparation.
- Avoid using microwave ovens because they fail to sanitize utensils and cause uneven heating, which increases the risk of burns.
- Discard a prepared bottle of formula after it has been offered to the infant or has sat at room temperature for more than 1 hour.
- Cover and store opened cans of liquid formula in the refrigerator; discard after 48 hours.

Advantages of breast-feeding

It's a well-known fact that breast-feeding is best for an infant. Here are five reasons why.

 Passive immunity

Human milk provides passive immunity to the infant. Colostrum is the first fluid secreted from the breast (occurs almost immediately) and provides immune factor and protein to the neonate. Many components of breast milk protect against infection — it contains antibodies (especially immunoglobulin A) and white blood cells that protect the infant from some forms of infection. Breast-fed babies also experience fewer allergies and intolerances.

 Easily digestible

Breast milk provides essential nutrients in an easily digestible form for the neonate. It contains lipase, which breaks down dietary fat, making it easily available to the infant's system.

 Brain booster

The lipids in breast milk are high in linoleic acid and cholesterol, which are needed for brain development. Breast milk also contains docosahexaenoic acid (an omega-3 fatty acid that's important for brain and eye development).

 Low protein content

Cow's milk contains proportionally higher concentrations of electrolytes and protein than are needed by human infants. It must be cleared by the immature kidneys and thus isn't recommended until after a baby is at least 12 months old.

 Convenience and price

Breast-feeding saves the time and money that must be spent to buy and prepare formula.

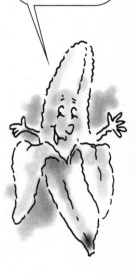

Pleased to meetcha! It's okay to introduce solid finger foods such as bananas to infants between ages 7 and 9 months.

fortified formula satisfies all of an infant's nutritional requirements until age 6 months. Signs that an infant is ready to try solid foods and eat from a spoon include the ability to sit with some support and move the head to participate in the feeding process as well as reaching and grabbing for food. (See *Solid foods and infant age*, page 140.)

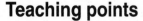

Teaching points

Be sure to stress these points about feeding and nutrition to the parents of an infant:

• Be observant for behaviors that indicate feeding preferences. Turning the head away, biting, and chewing followed by swallowing all indicate preferences and satiety. If the infant rejects a food initially, don't force him to eat it. Offer the food again later.

• Keep the baby in the upright feeding position.

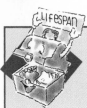

Lifespan lunchbox

Solid foods and infant age

This table gives an overview of solid foods that are appropriate for a developing infant.

Age	Type of food	Rationale
6 months	Rice cereal mixed with formula or breast milk; strained vegetables and fruits	Less likely than wheat to cause an allergic reaction (offer vegetables first because they may be more readily accepted)
7 to 9 months	Finger foods (bananas, crackers); pureed and mashed foods	Promote self-feeding
10 to 12 months	Ground meats, cheese, yogurt, pudding; mashed egg yolk (avoid whites until age 1); bite-size cooked food	Provide important source of iron, add variety to the diet, and decrease the risk of choking (although the infant chews well, be careful to avoid foods likely to cause choking)
12+ months	Foods from the adult table	Add variety to the diet (chop or mash according to the infant's ability to chew foods)

• Let the baby decide how much to eat. Don't try to make him eat more to finish the serving or portion.

• Initially, offer iron-fortified rice cereal. Avoid wheat-based cereals until age 9 months because of the increased risk of allergic reaction.

• Introduce new foods one at a time, waiting 5 to 7 days between foods, to assess for allergy or intolerance.

• Avoid foods that are choking hazards, such as cut-up hot dogs, whole grapes, and nuts, until the infant develops adequate chewing and swallowing skills.

• Diluted juice may be introduced when the infant is able to drink from a cup (usually around age 9 months). Only 100% fruit juice with no added sugar should be used. Limit juice to 4 oz per day for infants ages 6 to 12 months and to 6 oz per day for children ages 1 to 4 years.

• If a history of food allergies is present, delay offering eggs (especially whites), wheat-based products, and citrus fruits.

• Avoid honey and corn syrup. These products may contain the harmful bacteria *Clostridium botulinum,* which can lead to botulism. Botulism can be fatal in children younger than age 1 year.

Nutritional concerns

Some nutritional concerns for the infant include iron deficiency anemia, dental health, colic, diarrhea, constipation, and food allergies.

Iron deficiency anemia

When older infants consume few solid foods rich in iron, they're at risk for developing iron deficiency anemia. By age 6 months, the iron stores in the liver are depleted and the infant must rely on ingestion and absorption to provide the iron necessary for tissue building.

Initially, iron-fortified cereals are recommended. Later, red-meat products can be consumed as tolerated (usually pureed) to meet iron requirements. Iron supplements are available for infants who are diagnosed with iron deficiency anemia.

Dental health

Fluoride and dental caries are two potential nutrition-related problems that can compromise dental health. Fluoride is incorporated into forming teeth, including those in early stages of development. Most infants who live in areas where fluoridated water is available don't require an additional source of fluoride. The American Academy of Pediatrics recommends fluoride supplementation only if the family's water supply doesn't contain fluoride. Bottled water isn't recommended

The bottle can let a baby down

Dental caries are a potential problem if an infant is put to bed with a bottle. An infant can fall asleep with formula in his mouth, which leads to the development of caries. Fruit juices can also contribute to dental caries.

Colic

Repeated crying episodes that don't respond to feeding, holding, or diaper changes are characteristic of infants with colic. The infant is generally unhappy and fussy and cries a lot. About 10% to 20% of infants suffer from colic, which is thought to be due to swallowing air (for bottle-fed babies, when nipple holes are too large or too small) or to a reaction to gas-producing foods. (See *Tips for reducing colic.*)

Diarrhea

Noninfectious diarrhea, which may result from overfeeding and food intolerances, can put an infant at risk for dehydration. Be-

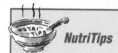
NutriTips

Tips for reducing colic

Colic usually resolves by about age 3 months and isn't associated with later dysfunction or disease. Here are several ways to reduce the discomfort caused by colic:
• Change the diet for mothers who are breastfeeding. Avoid onions, cow's milk, chocolate, broccoli, cauliflower, and brussels sprouts.
• Change the routine. Try different positions during feeding. Also try using warm water, diluting formula, holding, rocking, and using a pacifier.

cause an infant's body is 75% water, fluid loss due to diarrhea can quickly cause dehydration. A careful diet history commonly uncovers the cause of diarrhea.

Although it isn't uncommon, diarrhea can be dangerous and parents should notify the infant's health care provider if diarrhea persists beyond 12 hours or if it's accompanied by fever or vomiting.

Battling dehydration

If an infant develops diarrhea, special electrolyte-replacement formulas, such as Pedialyte, may be recommended to help with rehydration in the short term. Babies who are breast-fed should continue to feed from the breast. Formula is commonly withheld temporarily. The infant should receive 120 ml of the electrolyte solution plus the amount lost in each stool. After about 12 hours, if diarrhea has stopped, half-strength formula can be offered.

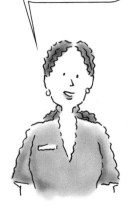

Diarrhea puts infants at high risk for dehydration.

Constipation

Constipation is rare in breast-fed infants. However, it's occasionally a problem for formula-fed infants. In many cases, it's a result of inadequate carbohydrate intake or consumption of overly concentrated formula. The parents should be instructed to adjust the dilution of the formula and, for older infants, add fiber to the diet by feeding fresh fruits and vegetables as indicated.

Food allergies

Foods that commonly pose allergy risks include milk, eggs, and wheat. It's important to introduce solid foods to the diet slowly to assess for allergy or intolerance. If a reaction occurs after the introduction of a food, the response should be noted for further evaluation. If a similar reaction occurs the second time the food is consumed, the food should be eliminated from the diet. It's important to notify the pediatrician of suspected allergies.

Nutritional considerations for premature infants

Babies who are born prematurely (gestational age less than 37 weeks) require special nutritional care. Each premature infant has different needs, depending on his weight and length of gestation. Breast milk is especially beneficial in easing digestion for premature infants.

Other nutritional concerns in premature infants include:
• increased caloric and nutrient requirements
• lack of enzymes that enable digestion and absorption
• neuromuscular immaturity

- small gastric capacity
- risk of dehydration due to immature kidney function and proportionally high body-surface area
- risk of hypoglycemia due to immature liver function, hypothermia, or respiratory distress syndrome
- vitamin E deficiency due to inability to digest and absorb fats.

Tired out

Many immature infants also have a hard time feeding long enough and efficiently enough to take in adequate amounts of breast milk. For this reason, breast milk can be pumped, saved, and fed to the infant through a nasogastric tube or bottle.

Rapid response

Breast milk is commonly supplemented with such nutrients as calcium, phosphorus, sodium, and protein, which are necessary to supplement a premature infant's rapid growth.

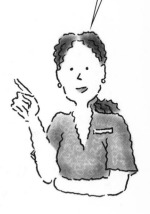

Breast milk can help ease digestion in premature infants.

Nutrition during childhood

As children grow, energy and nutrient needs continue to change to meet the body's changing needs.

Growth and development during childhood

Childhood growth and development can be divided into three stages:
- toddler (ages 1 to 3)
- preschool age (ages 3 to 5)
- school age (ages 5 to 10).

Obtaining adequate energy and nutrient requirements during each of these stages is essential to achieving full growth and development potential.

Sprouting up

Growth during childhood is steady but not as great as during infancy or adolescence. Toddlers gain about 0.5 lb (0.2 kg) and grow ⅜″ (1 cm) in height per month, whereas preschool children gain approximately 4 to 5 lb (1.8 kg to 2.3 kg) and grow approximately 2″ (5.1 cm) in height per year (or about ⅛″ [0.4 cm] per month). By the time a child reaches school age, his weight should be about double what it was at age 1. This decreased growth rate is commonly associated with a reduced appetite and food intake in toddlers and preschool children.

Eating behaviors

Eating behaviors vary with each stage of childhood development.

Toddler

During the toddler years, exploration and a sense of individuality begin to develop. The toddler may demonstrate a change in appetite and may be easily distracted from eating. Because of these changes, it's best to offer a toddler various foods and smaller portions. In addition, a toddler shouldn't be forced to eat foods. It's also a good idea to keep nutritious foods, such as fruits, available to serve as snacks.

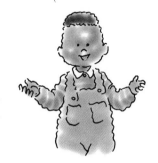

Sometimes I can be easily distracted from eating. Mom says I'm showing my individuality.

Preschool age

During the preschool-age period, parents and caregivers still have a fair amount of control over a child's food intake. Nutritional concerns focus on offering a proper selection and amount of nutrients needed by the growing child.

A preschool-age child responds best to regular mealtimes. Three meals per day aren't enough for this age-group, and snacks are recommended as part of a regular eating pattern. Research indicates that snacks typically provide 20% of a child's total caloric intake and, therefore, can be a good way to provide protein, calories, and nutrients to a young child. At this age, it's good to begin involving a child in meal-related activities, such as food selection and preparation.

School age

The school-age child is more independent of adults. Meeting the nutritional needs of this age-group must be balanced with the child's need for decision making and peer acceptance. A school-age child spends much of the day at school, away from parents and, in many cases, only marginally supervised at lunchtime. In addition, peers' behaviors are an increasing influence, as is exposure to different types of food and eating behaviors. A child at this age begins to make independent choices about what to eat. (See *Tips for ensuring childhood health*.)

Nutrient needs

Preschool children need approximately 1,000 to 1,600 calories/day. School-age children need between 1,200 and 2,200 calories per day, depending on specific age and activity level (sedentary, moderately active, or active). Protein requirements vary by age-group. (See *Energy and protein requirements for infants and children*, page 146.)

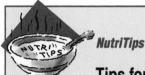

NutriTips

Tips for ensuring childhood health

To help ensure that children take in a balanced diet and maintain a healthy lifestyle, recommend these tips to parents and caregivers:

• Schedule regular mealtimes and allow the child to participate in planning, preparation, and serving as well as clean up.

• Maintain variety because it's normal for a child to prefer certain foods for a while and then suddenly refuse to eat them.

• Have nutritional snacks readily available, especially when the child gets home from school. Carrot and celery sticks and yogurt in cups or squeeze tubes are good possibilities.

• Prepare mildly flavored single-food dishes, which children tend to prefer. Many children don't like casseroles.

• Have the child get up early enough to be able to eat breakfast unhurriedly. Breakfast is an important meal.

• Encourage physical activity. Sports are increasingly an important and beneficial part of a young child's life. Also, keep in mind that physical activity other than sports is valuable as well and should be encouraged. Walks, bike rides, and other forms of loosely organized activities can be beneficial.

• Eat with a child to model good eating habits.

• Avoid using food as a reward or bribe.

• Turn off the television during meals.

Supplemental information

Research confirms that most normal, healthy children in the United States don't require supplementation of vitamins and minerals in their diet.

Nutritional concerns

Some things to consider when planning nutritional care for a child include caffeine consumption, irregular eating habits, overeating and obesity, and lead poisoning.

Caffeine

Children may ingest caffeine in such products as tea, chocolate, and soft drinks. Therefore, it's important to monitor the caffeine content of certain beverages. For example, 8 oz of hot chocolate or 12 oz of a soft drink contain 50 mg of caffeine.

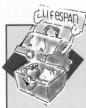

Lifespan lunchbox

Energy and protein requirements for infants and children

This table lists the recommended dietary allowances for energy and protein needs of infants and children.

Age	Estimated energy requirement (kcal/day)*	Protein (g/day)
First 6 months	438 to 645	9.1
7 to 12 months	608 to 844	11
1 to 3 years	768 to 1,184	13
4 to 8 years	1,133 to 2,225	19
9 to 13 years	1,415 to 3.308	34

* Actual energy requirement depends on activity level and gender.

The facts about caffeine

Some people believe that because caffeine is a stimulant, its consumption leads to hyperactivity. However, research has disproven this assumption. Even so, although most children don't require caffeine restriction, parents should be aware of how much caffeine a child ingests daily.

Irregular eating habits

Be aware of patterns of irregular eating, such as food jags, skipped meals, and overeating, when preparing nutritional care for a child. Some irregular eating habits are a major concern for this age-group.

Bag the jag?

Children commonly go on food jags where they eat one particular food in preference to most others. As long as they're getting adequate amounts of nutrients, food jags aren't problematic and parents should be reassured.

Physiologic anorexia may be logical

At times, some children will display a lack of interest in food, especially as growth rate fluctuates. This "physiologic anorexia" isn't a cause for concern, as long as intake doesn't drop off too sharply and the child is behaving normally otherwise.

Don't let 'em skip out on you

Skipping meals, especially breakfast, is common in older children. The maintenance of a regular pattern for meals and snacks (within reason) is very important to help children eat regularly. Getting children up early enough before school so that they wake up fully and become hungry will help in getting them to eat breakfast.

Overeating and obesity

Overweight and obesity are growing problems in children from industrialized cultures. Obesity is defined as being 20% or more above the mean weight for children of the same height. The cause of the increase in childhood obesity rates is thought to be sedentary lifestyle and consumption of high-fat, starchy food in greater proportion than proteins and complex carbohydrates.

According to the *Dietary Guidelines for Americans 2005*, the incidence of weight problems among children and adolescents is significantly increasing, with as much as 16% of this population being overweight.

Sticks and stones break bones but names hurt, too

Although the major health concern is in overweight children going on to become overweight adults with ill-health effects, obese children also undergo psychosocial stress. They're the target of teasing and disapproval, due to conceptions among adults that obesity is related to weakness and laziness, and the fact that these perceptions are passed on to children.

Not merely baby fat

The severity of childhood obesity is affected by the age of onset and the presence of factors such as parental obesity. If obesity develops after age 3, the likelihood of lasting into adulthood is greater; the same is true if the obesity is severe or if one or more parents is obese. Studies show that obese children's intake isn't significantly higher than that of nonobese children. Experts currently believe that lack of physical activity is the reason for the weight gain.

Setting a schedule for success

Prevention and treatment are based on the establishment of regular meal and snack times, having nutritious snacks readily available, and encouraging (especially through role modeling) regular

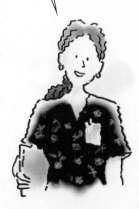

The risk of growing into an obese adult increases if a child's obesity develops after age 3.

physical activity. The *Dietary Guidelines for Americans 2005* recommend that children shouldn't be placed on weight reduction diets without first consulting with a professional.

According to the *Guidelines*, the goal for overweight children and adolescents is to reduce the rate of weight gain while allowing for normal growth and development. The guidelines recommend that children and adolescents consume fewer calories and increase physical activity to control their weight. They should participate in at least 60 minutes of physical activity on most, if not every day of the week. The total fat intake for children should be limited to 30% to 35% of calories in children 2 to 3 years old and between 25% to 35% in children and adolescents 4 to 18 years old. The majority of fats should come from polyunsaturated and monounsaturated fats.

Lead poisoning

Children under age 6 are susceptible to lead toxicity because they have a higher rate of intestinal absorption, their neurologic tissues are still developing, and they tend to put things in their mouths, increasing the risk of exposure. Lead poisoning can cause stunting of growth as well as cognitive deficits and other neurologic problems. Lead toxicity occurs more readily (and is, therefore, more common in children with iron deficiency).

Nutrition during adolescence

Nutritional requirements during adolescence are more individualized than during other periods of life. They depend on the timing and duration of the growth spurt, which can vary from person to person and is different for males and females.

Protein needs vary with the degree of growth and development, and requirements based on developmental age are more accurate than those based on chronological age.

Growth and development during adolescence

During adolescence, increases in lean body mass, skeletal mass, and body fat that occur during puberty influence energy and nutrient needs. The growth rate is different for boys and girls and each growth rate is individualized.

Girls get a head start...

In girls, the growth spurt usually begins between ages 10 and 11, peaks at age 12, and ceases at age 15. Girls have lower caloric needs during this time because of more fat deposition (particularly to the abdomen and pelvic girdle).

...But boys bone up

In boys, the growth spurt usually begins between ages 12 and 13, peaks at age 14, and stops at age 19. Because boys experience an increase in muscle mass, bone, and lean body tissue, they have higher caloric needs during this stage.

My growth spurt usually peaks around age 12.

Mine usually peaks later — around age 14.

Nutrient needs

Sedentary adolescent boys require 1,800 to 2,400 cal/day, whereas those who are moderately active require 2,000 to 2,800 cal/day. Adolescent girls who are sedentary require 1,600 to 1,800 cal/day, while those who are moderately active require 2,000 cal/day. Adolescent boys who participate in sports may need up to 3,200 cal/day while athletic adolescent girls may need up to 2,400 cal/day. Active adolescents may need additional niacin, thiamin, and riboflavin. Three servings of dairy products per day are recommended to help adolescents meet their calcium requirements of 1,300 mg/day.

Zinc again!

Zinc is important during adolescence for its role in sexual maturation. Males who are deficient in zinc experience growth failure and delayed sexual development. Generally, boys and girls consume adequate amounts of iron and zinc in their diets unless they follow strict vegetarian diets.

Focus on folate

Because of folate's role in deoxyribonucleic acid, ribonucleic acid, and protein synthesis, poor folate status can be an issue for adolescent females who become pregnant. Inadequate intake of folate before pregnancy can increase the incidence of spina bifida and neural tube defects. Studies show that many adolescents have inadequate folate levels. However, this number may be reduced by the fortification mandates requiring that grains and cereals be enriched with folate.

More to watch for

According to the *Dietary Guidelines for Americans 2005*, dietary intakes of calcium, potassium, fiber, magnesium, and vitamin E may be of concern for children and adolescents.

Developing a healthful diet

Many adolescents in the United States eat low-nutrient, high-calorie, high-sugar, high-fat foods. Usually, these diets fall short of meeting the requirements recommended by the *Dietary Guidelines for Americans 2005*. Many adolescents, especially adolescent girls, also don't consume adequate amounts of vitamins and minerals.

Snack attack

Usually, adolescents get one-fourth to one-third of all their energy and major nutrients from snacks. In addition, soft drinks are a favorite beverage among adolescents. These drinks contain large amounts of calories in the form of sugar, which is filling and may interfere with intake of more nutritious foods. Soft drinks also commonly replace milk as the drink of choice and may hinder an adolescent from getting adequate amounts of calcium.

Although snacking seems like a nutritional problem, it can become a healthy part of the adolescent diet. Snacking habits can be slightly altered to allow the adolescent independence in choices and to help establish a healthful lifelong eating pattern. These habits can be achieved by using Food Guide recommendations to plan snacks. One good tip for improving snacking behavior is to have nutritious foods already prepared and available. Good examples include fortified cereals, fresh fruit, cut up vegetables, and high-fiber, multigrain snack bars.

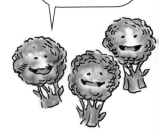

We're a cut above the rest! If you keep us around in precut pieces, we make a pretty good snack!

Nutritional concerns

Some common nutritional concerns for adolescents include dieting and eating disorders, calcium deficiency, tobacco and alcohol use, hormonal contraceptive use, and special diets.

Dieting and eating disorders

Because of preoccupations with appearance and peer acceptance, adolescents are notorious for fad dieting. Meals are skipped, food intake is severely restricted, or whole food groups may be cut out of the diet. Dieting behaviors should be monitored because they may lead to more serious eating disorders. Dieting behaviors should be of particular concern in an adolescent who isn't overweight.

Adolescent preoccupations with eating can range from mild body shape dissatisfaction to serious eating disorders, such as anorexia nervosa and bulimia nervosa. Symptoms of eating disorders should be further investigated because inadequate nutritional intake can adversely affect growth, development, and health outcomes. Keep in mind that you should be supportive and understanding of an adolescent's feelings while promoting adequate nutritional intake.

Calcium deficiency

Inadequate calcium intake is a common concern, especially for teenage girls, because lack of calcium during this critical time can greatly affect the development of osteoporosis later in life. It's common for teens to stop drinking milk, so suggest yogurt, cheese, and calcium-fortified orange juice to help an adolescent continue to meet her calcium requirements.

Getting enough calcium during my teen years can help me avoid osteoporosis later in life.

Tobacco and alcohol use

The use of tobacco, alcohol, and other drugs can also impact an adolescent's nutritional health. It's important to discuss these issues with adolescents, making them aware of the adverse affects associated with these substances.

Tobacco troubles

Tobacco, which may be consumed by an adolescent who's trying to lose weight, has been associated with a range of health problems, most of which don't manifest during adolescence.

Drinking away needed nutrients

Alcohol consumption can interfere not only with the ingestion of required nutrients but also with their digestion and absorption.

Hormonal contraceptive use

It's common for adolescent girls to begin taking hormonal contraceptives—some as a form of birth control and some to decrease or regulate bleeding associated with menstruation. Hormonal contraceptives may also help with iron deficiency problems. Use of progestin-based contraceptives may be a concern for weight-conscious teens because these forms have been reported to increase appetite.

Special diets

Some adolescents, such as athletes and vegetarians, choose to follow special diets that can affect their nutritional requirements.

Athletes

An athlete's dietary intake should follow the *Dietary Guidelines for Americans 2005*, although the athlete's increased energy needs may require him to consume the upper limit of the recommendations. Depending on the duration and intensity of his sport, an athlete may require 500 to 1,500 extra calories per day to meet his energy needs. If an athlete loses much weight, caloric intake is most likely inadequate to support growth and development and should be increased. Protein should supply 15% to 20% of total calories.

Keep an eye on iron

Iron loss during exercise puts an athlete at higher risk for developing iron deficiency anemia. Iron status should be monitored in athletes, especially vegetarians and females who have begun menstruating.

Vegetarians

Lacto-ovo vegetarians generally aren't at great risk for inadequate intake of protein, calcium, phosphorus, zinc, and other nutrients obtained from meat. However, strict vegetarians or vegans are at a risk for deficiencies if their diets aren't well planned.

Nutrition and the adult

Because growth and maturation are complete by early adulthood— approximately age 19—nutritional considerations for the adult focus more on maintaining a healthy body weight and physical fitness, avoiding excess weight gain, and continuing to build strength. General calorie requirements for adults are established by the recommended dietary allowances and depend on activity levels.

According to the *Dietary Guidelines for Americans 2005*, for adults ages 19 to 50 years of age, a sedentary man requires 2,200 to 2,600 cal/day; a moderately active man, 2,400 to 2,800 cal/day; and an active man, 2,800 to 3,000 cal/day. A sedentary woman in this age range requires 1,800 to 2,000 cal/day; a moderately active woman, 2,000 to 2,200 cal/day; and an active woman, 2,200 to 2,400 cal/day.

Fighting illnesses before they begin

Between ages 40 and 60, such chronic illnesses as heart disease, hypertension, and diabetes commonly begin to develop. Establishing healthful food and exercise habits, such as reducing total fat intake, eating fruits and vegetables, and maintaining a balance of food intake and physical activity to stabilize weight, can modify risk factors for developing chronic illness in later years.

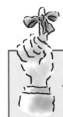

Memory jogger

The U.S. Department of Agriculture's **ABCs** of good nutrition can help adults establish healthful eating and exercise habits. They encourage Americans to:

Aim for fitness every day

Build a health base (using the Food Guide recommendations)

Choose sensibly.

Nutrition and the older adult

Life expectancy in the United States has increased dramatically over the last century. In the early 1900s, fewer than one-half of all Americans lived past age 65. Today, more than 80% of Americans are expected to do so.

Pills and ills

Older adults have special nutritional needs because their tissues and organ systems are aging. In addition, many older adults take medications for chronic illness. More than 80% of adults over age 65 suffer from arthritis, hypertension, heart disease, diabetes, or a combination of these diseases. Nutritional health can help older adults maintain active and pleasurable lives, protect them from disease, lessen the severity of disease, and hasten recovery.

Development and change

Older adults experience an array of changes that can affect their nutritional health. Some changes are directly related to the body whereas others are associated with external influences.

Physiologic changes

Even after a person reaches adulthood at age 20, the body continues to change. These changes may include gradual loss of lean body mass and gain of adipose tissue. Some changes can be offset, however, through strength training and aerobic exercise.

GI system changes

Several GI problems that affect nutritional status can arise for older adults:
• Loss of dentition, periodontal disease, and jawbone deterioration can cause problems with chewing.
• Saliva production is decreased, commonly as an adverse effect of medications, and may cause difficulty swallowing.
• Secretion of gastric digestive enzymes falls off, making it more difficult to digest certain foods. Poor lactase secretion, for example, makes it difficult to digest milk products.
• Absorption of nutrients decreases as blood supply to the intestine decreases and gastric mucosa degenerates.
• Intestinal motility slows, and constipation can become a problem.

Metabolic changes

As adipose tissue replaces lean body mass, the metabolic rate slows. Glucose metabolism can be problematic in older adults, manifesting as glucose intolerance.

Central nervous system (CNS) changes

Common CNS problems that can prevent an older adult from eating a balanced diet include tremors, slowed reaction time, short-term memory loss, cognitive deterioration (from such diseases as Alzheimer's disease), and depression.

Renal system changes

As blood flow decreases and new renal tissue fails to generate, the ability to clear nitrogenous and other waste products from the body is impaired. In addition, loss of sphincter tone can contribute to urinary incontinence in many older adults. Males may also experience prostate dysfunction.

Sensory changes

All sense organs lose some function as people age, and some people are more severely affected than others:
- Hearing loss begins to develop at about age 30.
- Loss of visual acuity, especially in low-light settings, begins at approximately age 40.
- Sense of smell or olfactory function decreases.
- Taste changes due to olfactory function loss, visual acuity loss, and loss of taste buds and saliva. Sweet and salty tastes are the first to be lost, followed by bitter and sour.
- The sense of thirst is less acute, leaving older adults at risk for dehydration. Dehydration can manifest in older adults as confusion or lethargy.

Economic and social changes

The focus on physiologic function during nutritional assessment may lead to other factors—such as economic and social changes—being overlooked.

Spare changes

Many older adults live on fixed incomes, and approximately 20% of adults older than age 65 live in poverty. Economic hardships can limit a person's ability to eat a well-balanced diet. In many cases, meat and dairy products are cut out of the diet because of their cost. However, these foods are important to the health of older adults because they provide protein and various other nutrients, such as iron, B vitamins, and zinc.

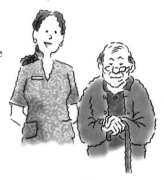

A multitude of physiologic changes can affect the nutritional intake of older adults.

Isolating the problem

Some older adults experience social isolation due to lack of mobility, loss of sensory acuity, and other functional limitations. In addition, coping with the loss of friends and lack of interest in eating can also add to isolation, leading to poor eating habits and severely affecting nutritional intake. This situation is compounded in institutionalized elderly patients, who experience inadequate diets due to quality of food, food preferences, illnesses, and taste alterations.

Nutrient needs

The *Dietary Guidelines for Americans 2005* include recommendations for the older adult. Calorie requirements diminish and nutrient requirements may stay the same or increase with age.

Calories

Calorie needs diminish as the human body ages and lean muscle mass decreases. Exact calorie requirements in an older adult depend on degree of mobility, illness, overall health, and level of fitness.

According to the *Dietary Guidelines for Americans 2005*, for adults 51 years of age and older, a sedentary man requires 2,000 to 2,200 cal/day; a moderately active man requires 2,200 to 2,400 cal/day; and an active man requires 2,400 to 2,800 cal/day. A sedentary woman in this age range requires 1,600 cal/day; a moderately active woman requires 1,800 cal day; and an active woman requires 2,000 to 2,200 cal/day.

Protein

Currently, the recommendation for daily protein intake for an older adult is the same as that for other adults: 0.6 g/kg of body weight or 63 g/day for males and 50 g/day for females. Impaired GI tract function and medications, however, can lead to decreased absorption of amino acids and micronutrients, leading to increased intake requirements. Some studies suggest that 0.7 to 1.1 g/kg/day may be necessary to maintain nitrogen balance.

Iron

Although the physiologic requirement for iron is lessened in older adults, decreased absorption of iron due to antacid interference, decreased stomach acid secretion, blood loss from disease (such as GI ulcers), or medications (such as aspirin), and the inability to ingest adequate amounts of iron-rich foods put some older adults at risk for iron deficiency. Leading sources of iron in the American diet include ready-to-eat cereals and beef.

Calcium

The RDA of calcium is 1,200 mg for adults ages 51 and older. Low calcium intake has been linked to colon cancer and hypertension. In many cases in this population, the dietary reference intake (DRI) for calcium isn't achieved and supplements are recommended.

Magnesium

Magnesium is needed for bone and tooth formation, nerve activity, glucose utilization, and synthesis of fat and proteins. A high percentage of adults ages 70 and older don't meet the DRI for magnesium (420 mg/day for men, 320 mg/day for women). Magnesium can be an issue for older adults, not only because of low intake from food but also because of malabsorption due to GI disorders, chronic alcoholism, and diabetes. Signs of deficiency include personality changes (such as irritability and aggressiveness), vertigo, muscle spasms, weakness, and seizures.

Maxing out magnesium levels

Magnesium is also overconsumed by some elderly patients. Many medications used by older adults, such as magnesium-based antacids and cathartics, may lead to magnesium overdose. Signs of magnesium toxicity include diarrhea, dehydration, and impaired nerve activity.

Vitamin D

Vitamin D levels are also subject to age-associated changes. The skin's decreased ability to synthesize vitamin D in older adults may be compounded by their limited exposure to sunlight due to use of sunscreen or limited mobility. In addition, medications commonly used by older adults may also interfere with vitamin D metabolism. Fortified foods such as milk are the main sources of vitamin D; however, older adults tend to consume less milk and other vitamin D sources, such as fortified cereals, eggs, liver, salmon, and tuna. The *Dietary Guidelines for Americans 2005* recommend that older adults consume additional vitamin D from vitamin D–fortified foods or supplements.

B vitamins

As the body gets older, it uses vitamin B_{12} less efficiently. Vitamin B_{12} deficiency can occur due to lack of intrinsic factor secretion, which is required for vitamin B_{12} absorption. Another cause is inadequate secretion of gastric acid, which can impair the ability to break down foods and make B_{12} available for absorption. If gastric

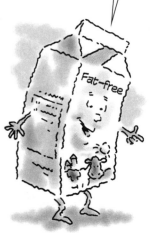

Low calcium intake has been linked to colon cancer and hypertension.

acid secretion is a problem, supplements of B_{12} in its synthetic, nonprotein-bound form, can help prevent deficiency. B_{12} is better absorbed in synthetic form and can be found in fortified foods, such as cereals and soy products. The *Dietary Guidelines for Americans 2005* recommend that older adults ingest vitamin B_{12} in its crystalline form, such as fortified foods or supplements.

Risk factors for poor nutrition

Researchers estimate that as many as two-thirds of older adults are at risk for nutritional deficits. The populations at the greatest risk are those with limited education, those who live alone, and those with limited incomes.

Older adults who have limited mobility due to chronic disease are at increased risk for malnutrition as well, especially those in institutions. Only 3% to 6% of the elderly population suffers from malnutrition. However, the risk is much higher after admittance to a health care facility.

Teaching points

Because of the high prevalence of eating disorders among this age-group, it's important to stress these points to your elderly patient:

• Concentrate on variety and pleasure. If calories are a concern, try to moderate portion size rather than cutting foods out altogether. Follow the *Dietary Guidelines for Americans 2005*, paying special attention to protein intake.

• Choose high-fiber foods. Whole grain breads and cereals and dried peas and beans are good choices. Fresh fruits and vegetables are also high in fiber and should be encouraged. Be aware, however, that many older adults can't tolerate or chew raw fruits and vegetables. In this case, cooked fruits and vegetables can be substituted but shouldn't be overcooked.

• Drink six to eight 8-oz glasses of water per day. This recommendation can exacerbate incontinence, however, so try to schedule intake at appropriate times.

• Take supplements as recommended. Dietary nutrient supplements such as Ensure can be useful for older persons whose diets fall short of meeting recommended levels. General recommendations are to take vitamin and mineral supplements that contain no more than 100% of RDAs. There's no conclusive, scientific evidence that herbal supplements have beneficial effects on the health of older adults.

Nutritional assessment for the older adult

It's important to accurately assess the nutritional status of the older adult to reduce the risk of disease and promote health. The Mini Nutritional Assessment is an easy tool that both screens and assesses for malnutrition in the older adult. (See *Mini Nutritional Assessment.*) Here are some additional guidelines:

• Physical assessment of height and weight can be challenging in older adults, especially those who are bedridden or obese.

• An adequate diet history can also be difficult to obtain unless family and friends are available to give additional information.

• A thorough diet history is important for understanding social and economic limitations (such as access to a food market), in addition to cognitive ones.

• The patient should be asked specifically about a 10-lb (4.5-kg) weight gain or loss in the previous 6 months.

• Ongoing height and weight measurements are important for noting trends. Dentition should be assessed regularly as well.

• Blood tests for hemoglobin, hematocrit, serum lipids, and glucose are important. An especially valuable parameter for assessment of protein status is serum albumin, which should be 3.5% or higher. Urinalysis for glucose, ketones, protein, and occult blood is important to assess kidney function and glucose metabolism.

Nutritional concerns

The consequences of poor nutrition are especially severe for older adults. Primary nutritional concerns for elderly patients include dehydration and decreased immunity.

Dehydration

Dehydration can cause lethargy and confusion, which are commonly overlooked as effects of the "normal" aging process.

Decreased immunity

Inadequate protein intake can make older adults more susceptible to infectious diseases and exacerbations of chronic diseases as well as pressure ulcers and other wounds.

> Don't mistake the lethargy and confusion that can result from dehydration with "normal" aging in the older adult.

Mini Nutritional Assessment

The Mini Nutritional Assessment can help you screen your older adult patients for malnutrition. The form has two parts: screening and assessment. If the patient scores 11 points or less on the screening portion, the second part of the tool is completed to provide a more detailed assessment.

Last name: *Brown*   First name: *Jennifer*   Sex: *F*   Date: *6/10/06*

Age: *76*   Weight (kg): *65*   Height (cm): *160*   I.D. number: *123456*

SCREENING

A Has food intake declined over the past 3 months due to loss of appetite, digestive problems, chewing, or swallowing difficulties?
0 = severe loss of appetite
1 = moderate loss of appetite
2 = no loss of appetite ☑

B Weight loss during the last 3 months
0 = weight loss greater than 3 kg (6.6 lbs)
1 = does not know
2 = weight loss between 1 and 3 kg (2.2 and 6.6 lbs)
3 = no weight loss ☑

C Mobility
0 = bed or chair bound
1 = able to get out of bed or chair but does not go out
2 = goes out ☑

D Has suffered psychological stress or acute disease in the past 3 months
0 = yes
2 = no ☑

E Neuropsychological problems
0 = severe dementia or depression
1 = mild dementia
2 = no psychological problems ☑

F Body Mass Index (BMI) (weight in kg)/(height in m2)
0 = BMI less than 19
1 = BMI 19 to less than 21
2 = BMI 21 to less than 23
3 = BMI 23 or greater ☑

Screening score subtotal (max. 14 points) ☐ ☐
12 points or greater = Normal (not at risk, no need to complete assessment)
11 points or below = Possible malnutrition (continue assessment)

ASSESSMENT

G Lives independently (not in a nursing home or hospital)
0 = no   1 = yes ☐

H Takes more than 3 prescription drugs per day
0 = yes   1 = no ☐

I Pressure sores or skin ulcers
0 = yes   1 = no ☐

J How many full meals does the patient eat daily?
0 = 1 meal
1 = 2 meals
2 = 3 meals ☐

K Selected consumption markers for protein intake
• At least one serving of dairy products (milk, cheese, yogurt) per day?
Yes ☐   No ☐
• Two or more servings of legumes or eggs per week?
Yes ☐   No ☐
• Meat, fish, or poultry every day?
Yes ☐   No ☐
0.0 = 0 or 1 yes
0.5 = 2 yes
1.0 = 3 yes ☐.☐

L Consumes two or more servings of fruits or vegetables per day?
0 = no   1 = yes ☐

M How much fluid (water, juice, coffee, tea, milk…) is consumed per day?
0.0 = less than 3 cups
0.5 = 3 to 5 cups
1.0 = more than 5 cups ☐.☐

N Mode of feeding
0 = unable to eat without assistance
1 = self-fed with some difficulty
2 = self-fed without any problem ☐

O Self view of nutritional status
0 = views self as being malnourished
1 = is uncertain of nutritional state
2 = views self as having no nutritional problem ☐

P In comparison with other people of the same age, how does the patient consider his or her health status?
0.0 = not as good
0.5 = does not know
1.0 = as good
2.0 = better ☐.☐

Q Mid-arm circumference (MAC) in cm
0.0 = MAC less than 21
0.5 = MAC 21 to 22
1.0 = MAC 22 or greater ☐.☐

R Calf circumference (CC) in cm
0 = CC less than 31
1 = CC 31 or greater ☐

Assessment score subtotal (max. 16 points) ☐ ☐.☐

Screening score subtotal ☐ ☐
Assessment score subtotal ☐ ☐.☐
Total score (max. 30 points) ☐ ☐.☐

Malnutrition indicator score
17 to 23.5 points = at risk of malnutrition ☐
Less than 17 points = malnourished ☐

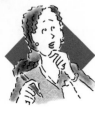

Quick quiz

1. What vitamin is essential in a pregnant woman's diet to prevent neural tube defects?

A. Vitamin E
B. Folic acid
C. Vitamin C
D. Iodine

Answer: B. Folic acid ensures healthy embryonic development.

2. Infants have trouble with cow's milk–based formulas because:

A. cow's milk has inadequate amounts of lactose.
B. cow's milk has small amounts of protein.
C. infants can't digest milk protein from cows.
D. the taste of the formula is sour.

Answer: C. Cow's milk protein is hard for an infant to digest because the intestinal tract isn't mature.

3. What vitamin is absorbed less efficiently by older adults?

A. Vitamin B_{12}
B. Vitamin E
C. Vitamin A
D. Vitamin C

Answer: A. Older adults have decreased secretion of intrinsic factor, which is necessary for vitamin B_{12} to be absorbed in the intestinal tract.

Scoring

☆☆☆   If you answered all three questions correctly, take center stage! You should receive a lifespan achievement award!

☆☆   If you answered two questions correctly, you've hardly been upstaged. In fact, you're developing nicely into your role of nutrition-know-it-all!

☆   If you answered fewer than two questions correctly, don't get stage fright! Look over the chapter again and you're sure to become a star of stages of nutrition!

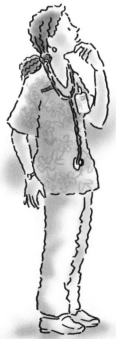

Part III Clinical nutrition

Feeding patients

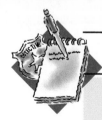

Just the facts

Knowing how to feed patients is an important part of their nutritional care. In this chapter, you'll learn:

♦ purposes, advantages, and disadvantages of oral supplemental feedings, enteral nutrition, and parenteral nutrition

♦ tubes used for enteral feedings

♦ components of oral supplements and enteral and parenteral nutrition formulas

♦ enteral and parenteral nutrition therapy monitoring

♦ complications of enteral and parenteral nutrition therapy.

A look at patient feeding methods

Ideally, a patient meets his nutritional needs by chewing and swallowing — in other words, through normal oral intake. However, ensuring adequate nutritional intake is more difficult if your patient is unconscious or acutely ill, can't chew or swallow, is too weak or confused to eat, or needs extra nutrients to speed healing.

A patient who can't or won't consume an adequate oral diet needs an alternative feeding method. Depending on his condition, he may require oral supplemental feedings, enteral nutrition therapy (tube feedings), or parenteral nutrition therapy.

It's okay to be choosy

When choosing the optimal feeding method, one principle holds sway: If the gut works, use it. Whenever possible, a patient should eat orally and independently. If he can't take in enough nutrients to maintain adequate nutrition, first consider giving oral supplements. If he's unable or unwilling to take oral supplements, provide enteral nutrition. Consider parenteral nutrition as a last resort — to be used only when oral supplements and enteral feedings are out of the question.

Oral supplemental feedings

Oral supplemental feedings (primarily beverages) may be given between or with meals if your patient can't meet his nutritional requirements through normal oral intake. They're also used extensively to wean patients from enteral or parenteral nutrition therapy.

Oral supplements come in several categories — clear supplements, milk-based drinks, prepared liquid supplements, specially prepared foods, and modular products. Commercially available formulas differ in calories, protein source, osmolality, lactose content, and cost. Most formulas provide 1 cal/ml. The choice of supplement depends on such factors as the condition of the patient's GI tract, the degree of digestion required, and the patient's nutritional needs.

Taster's choice

Such oral supplements as Boost and Ensure are easy to consume and well accepted by most patients. Because they leave the stomach quickly, they serve as good between-meal snacks. Each brand tastes different. A patient who doesn't like one brand may accept another.

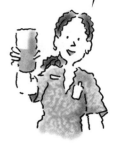

Oral supplemental feedings — most of which come in liquid form — can help your patient meet his nutritional needs.

Clear liquid supplements

Clear liquid supplements are useful for patients on clear liquid diets. They come as a powder to be mixed with water or in ready-to-use form. They provide protein, calories, or both; have little residue; and are extremely low in fat. However, some patients find them unpalatable, even though they come in various flavors.

Milk-based supplements

Milk-based supplements may be made from scratch, prepared with powdered commercial mixes, or bought as commercially prepared products. They provide significant proteins and calories, have an acceptable taste, and are relatively cheap. However, they aren't appropriate for patients who need complete nutritional support or who have lactose intolerance.

Commercially prepared liquid supplements

Commercially prepared liquid supplements vary in composition, taste, and cost. Besides convenience, they offer consistent quality and a range of flavor choices. Standard commercial supplements are low in residue and contain no lactose. Typically, they provide 1 to 1.2 cal/ml, with 14% to 16% of total calories coming from protein. Examples include Boost, Ensure, and Resource Standard. Depending on the brand, one serving (8 oz) of a commercially prepared supplement provides about 240 to 250 calories and 8.8 to 10 g of protein.

Commercial supplements should be used only after the patient's nutritional requirements have been thoroughly evaluated.

Variations from the form

Many commercial supplements come in variations of the standard formula, including high-protein, high-calorie, light, and added-fiber versions. Ensure and Boost offer high-protein, high-calorie, and added-fiber supplements. Ensure also offers a light version, which contains less fat and fewer calories than standard supplements.

Commercial supplements should be used only after the patient's nutritional requirements have been thoroughly evaluated.

Commercially prepared supplemental foods

As an alternative to liquid supplements, manufacturers have introduced puddings, bars, and other food products that provide a concentrated source of calories and protein. A 5-oz serving of Boost Pudding, for instance, provides 240 calories and 7 g of protein.

Modular supplements

Modular supplements boost nutrient intake without increasing intake volume. They contain a single nutrient — either carbohydrate (for example, hydrolyzed cornstarch), protein (such as whey protein), or fat (such as medium-chain triglycerides) — for use in a special situation. For instance, a patient with chronic renal failure who needs to gain calories without increasing protein intake may receive carbohydrate-fortified mashed potatoes.

Modular supplements may be added to foods, other types of oral supplements, or tube (enteral) feedings. They're sold under such brand names as:
• Moducal, Polycose, Sumacal (carbohydrate modules)
• ProMod, Propac, Casec (protein modules)
• Microlipid (a fat module).

Be aware, however, that modular supplements are subject to calculation errors, may lead to nutrient imbalances if added to tube feedings, and may become contaminated by bacteria. Also, they cost more than standard formulas.

Elemental formulas

Elemental formulas are available in liquid or powder form and contain partially digested nutrients that are useful for the patient with impaired digestion or absorption. These formulas contain little lactose and residue and can be ingested or given through a tube. Examples include Vital, Criticare HN, and Vivonex.

Elemental formulas are expensive and should be used only for patients with limited GI function or metabolic disorders. Also, they're less palatable than commercially prepared supplements, so some patients may reject them.

Disease-specific supplements

Specialized formulas are tailored for patients with certain diseases or disorders. A specialized formula may have:
• decreased carbohydrate content for patients with respiratory disease
• increased branched chain amino acids for patients with liver disease
• decreased protein content for patients with kidney disease
• added fiber for patients with constipation.

Also, lactose-free formulas are made for patients with lactase deficiency. Elemental formulas based on free amino acids and monosaccharides are suitable for patients with malabsorption.

Special considerations

Here are some additional points about oral supplemental feedings that are important to remember:
• An intact (polymeric), rather than a predigested nutrient, formula should be used if the patient has a functioning GI tract and needs all of the essential nutrients in a specific volume. Intact formulas are made from whole complete proteins or protein isolates. Because they contain complex protein, carbohydrate, and fat molecules, they require normal digestion and absorption. Dozens of commercially prepared intact formulas are available.
• A complete nutritional supplement should always be used if the formula is the patient's sole nutritional source. Complete supplements include Ensure, Sustacal, Resource, and Meritene.
• Patients with water restrictions, such as those with syndrome of inappropriate antidiuretic hormone, can receive increased calories with formulas that provide 1.5 to 2 cal/ml.
• Nutrient-dense formulas are hyperosmolar and may cause diarrhea.

• Oral supplements should be given between meals and at least 1 hour before the next meal.
• To minimize taste fatigue, serve oral supplements cold and offer various flavors. Most commercial brands come in vanilla and chocolate. Some brands also offer strawberry, coffee, eggnog, and butterscotch flavors.

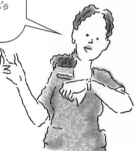

Keep your eye on the clock. Be sure to give oral supplements at least 1 hour before the patient's next meal.

Enteral nutrition

Enteral nutrition (also called tube feeding) delivers a liquid formula through a tube placed in the patient's stomach (gastric feeding) or intestine (duodenal or jejunal feeding). Enteral nutrition therapy preserves the health of the GI mucosa and stimulates lymphoid tissue in the GI tract. It's less likely than parenteral nutrition to cause infection or fluid and electrolyte imbalance, and it's cheaper.

For patients with normal digestion, nutrients in tube feedings should be provided intact rather than predigested. Because intact nutrients force the body to produce all the secretions and enzymes needed for digestion, they preserve normal functioning of the gut.

Gastric enteral nutrition typically is indicated for:
• patients who can't eat normally because of dysphagia or oral or esophageal obstruction or injury
• patients who are unconscious or intubated
• patients who are recovering from GI tract surgery and can't ingest food orally.

Duodenal or jejunal enteral feedings decrease the risk of aspiration because the formula bypasses the pylorus. (See *Indications for enteral nutrition.*)

Feeding tubes

The type and placement of a feeding tube for enteral nutrition depends on:
• anticipated duration of enteral feedings
• condition of the patient's GI tract
• patient's overall condition
• patient's aspiration risk.

Location explanation

A feeding tube is identified by where it enters the body and where its tip is placed. A tube may be placed:
• through the mouth, with its tip resting in the stomach (orogastric tube), jejunum (orojejunal tube), or duodenum (oroduodenal tube)

Indications for enteral nutrition

Enteral nutrition may be used for a patient with:
• dysphagia (difficulty swallowing)
• coma
• delirium
• dementia
• mechanical ventilation.

Enteral nutrition may also be used for a patient in a hypermetabolic state, which may result from burns, sepsis, multiple trauma, and cancer. For a patient in this state, nutritional needs can't be met with oral diet alone.

• through the nose, with its tip resting in the stomach (nasogastric [NG] tube), jejunum (nasojejunal [NJ] tube), or duodenum (nasoduodenal tube)
• through a surgical opening, with its tip resting in the stomach (gastrostomy tube) or small intestine (jejunostomy tube).

Surgical solutions

A percutaneous endoscopic gastrostomy (PEG) tube is placed through the abdomen into the stomach without the need for laparotomy or general anesthesia. It's held in place with a button.

For jejunal access, a percutaneous endoscopic jejunostomy (PEJ) tube may be placed. This tube commonly has two ports—a gastric port used to decompress gastric secretions and a jejunal port used for feedings. (For indications and contraindications for PEG and PEJ tubes, see *Percutaneous feeding tubes*.)

Tube selection

Follow these guidelines for proper tube selection:
• NG tubes typically are used in patients who have satisfactory stomach emptying and are expected to need enteral feedings for at least 30 days, or if the duration of enteral feedings hasn't been determined.
• NJ tubes may be used for patients with impaired stomach emptying, pancreatitis, or a high risk of aspiration.
• Nasoduodenal tubes are used for patients with impaired stomach emptying or a high risk of aspiration.
• Orogastric, oroduodenal, and orojejunal tubes are used in critically ill patients to minimize the risk of sinusitis.

Other tube features

Feeding tubes are classified by length, diameter, and presence or absence of a weighted tip. The outer diameter is measured in French sizes. Each French size unit equals 0.33 mm. Although a tube with a smaller diameter promotes patient comfort, it's more likely to clog. PEG tubes, with their larger diameters, are less likely to clog. Small-diameter feeding tubes need to be flushed often to prevent clogging.

Enteral feeding formulas

In enteral feeding formulas, osmolality (the number of particles in solution, expressed as milliosmols per kilogram [mOsm/kg]) is determined by the concentration of sugars, amino acids, and electrolytes. Isotonic formulas have roughly the same osmolality as blood—about 300 mOsm/kg.

Percutaneous feeding tubes

A percutaneous endoscopic gastrostomy (PEG) or jejunostomy (PEJ) tube is used to deliver enteral nutrition to a patient who:
• needs long-term tube feedings (more than 4 weeks)
• requires gastric decompression
• has a swallowing dysfunction
• has mental status problems that prevent oral intake
• has a tracheoesophageal fistula.

These tubes are contraindicated for patients with:
• GI obstructions
• hemodynamic instability
• coagulation disorders
• no stomach
• scarring from previous abdominal surgery.

Most patients tolerate formulas that are isotonic or mildly hypertonic (with a slightly higher osmolality than blood). Formulas that are more hypertonic are poorly tolerated—especially when delivered at full strength into the intestine. The high osmolality draws water into the intestine to dilute the particle concentration, causing nausea, abdominal cramping, and diarrhea.

Content with the contents

Formula residue consists of fiber (carbohydrates not digested in the GI tract), undigested food, intestinal secretions, bacterial cell bodies, and cells shed from the intestinal lining. Enteral formulas vary in their residue content. Most standard intact formulas are low in residue, although some have added fiber.

Fiber may help normalize bowel function in patients with diarrhea or constipation. With long-term tube feedings, adding fiber to the formula may help maintain GI integrity. However, formulas that contain fiber may cause gas and bloating in some patients. They're usually inappropriate as initial feedings in patients who have been on bowel rest, have certain GI disorders, or have undergone GI surgery.

Types of enteral feeding formulas

More than 80 types of enteral feeding formulas are available. They range from inexpensive standard formulas to costly disease-specific ones. Enteral feedings can also be made from table food—a cheaper alternative to commercial formulas. Careful formula selection can prevent unneeded expense for the patient and health care system.

Standard formulas

Standard formulas provide about 1 cal/ml and have a moderate protein content.

Calorie-dense formulas

Calorie-dense formulas range from 1.2 to 2 cal/ml. Those used for patients with renal failure are low in potassium, phosphorus, and magnesium; they also require less volume. Other calorie-dense formulas are simply high in calories.

Fiber-containing formulas

Fiber-containing formulas usually provide 10 to 15 g of fiber per 1,000 calories. The fiber source may be mostly insoluble fiber or a mixture of soluble and insoluble fiber. These formulas help to prevent constipation and solidify loose stools. To prevent fecal impaction, the patient must be adequately hydrated.

High-protein formulas

High-protein formulas are given to patients with high protein needs — for example, those with major wounds, critical illnesses, or burns; those recovering from surgery or trauma; and overweight or elderly patients who have high protein needs relative to their calorie needs.

Elemental formulas

Elemental (hydrolyzed) formulas contain partially digested nutrients, including proteins in the form of amino acids, or amino acids along with peptides. Used for patients with impaired digestion or absorption, these formulas provide 1 to 1.5 cal/ml, with 8% to 17% of total calories coming from protein. Stress formulas — elemental formulas high in branched-chain amino acids — may be used for energy during stress.

Disease-specific formulas

Disease-specific formulas are tailored to meet the nutritional needs of patients with specific medical problems.
• Diabetic formulas contain fiber and relatively low amounts of carbohydrates. Useful for patients with hard-to-control blood glucose levels, they're effective among patients in long-term care facilities. However, their effectiveness in acute-care patients hasn't been established.
• Renal formulas are dense in calories; low in potassium, magnesium, and phosphorus; moderately low in protein; and low in fat-soluble vitamins. The renal formulas currently available are so low in protein that they must be supplemented with protein powder to meet the patient's protein needs. Renal formulas are used primarily for patients with renal failure who aren't on dialysis.
• Pulmonary formulas are dense in calories, high in fat, and relatively low in carbohydrates.
• Immune-enhancing formulas may contain extra arginine, omega-3 fatty acids, nucleic acids, and glutamine. They're sometimes used in health care facilities in an attempt to reduce infectious complications. However, experts haven't determined which patient populations benefit from these formulas.

Modular formulas

Modular formulas are used when the patient's nutritional needs can't be met with other available formulas. They provide supplemental proteins, carbohydrates, lipids, and fiber. A modular formula can be added to a tube feeding or infused through the tube between feedings.

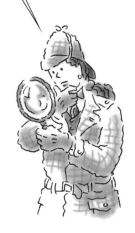

It's elemental, my dear Watson. Because elemental formulas contain partially digested nutrients, they aid digestion and absorption.

Administering enteral nutrition

Enteral feedings may be given continuously or on a cyclic or nocturnal schedule.

Never a dull moment

Recommended when the formula is delivered directly into the patient's small intestine, *continuous* feedings are administered 24 hours per day by gravity drip or infusion pump. The rate is increased gradually to allow the patient's GI tract to adjust to the formula. To prevent clogging, the tube should be flushed every 4 to 6 hours. To prevent contamination, the formula bag should hang no longer than 4 hours, unless it's packaged in a sterilized delivery system.

Nighttime is the right time

A *nocturnal* schedule usually delivers a feeding over 8 to 14 hours. The feeding may be infused over a longer period to allow gradual transition to nocturnal feedings — for instance, if the patient can't tolerate rapid increases in the hourly feeding rate.

Nocturnal feedings give the patient increased daytime mobility. They're also used during the transition to an oral diet to supply part of the patient's caloric needs. As oral intake improves, the volume of tube feedings can be reduced until the patient's oral intake is sufficient to discontinue tube feedings. Also, if the patient's caloric needs can't be met during the daytime alone, the patient may benefit from extra calories delivered during night time feedings, such as in the patient with cystic fibrosis.

Gastric feedings

Generally, gastric feedings can be given via syringe, infusion pump, or intermittent gravity drip.

Bolus feedings

Bolus feedings provide a 4- to 6-hour volume of solution within a few minutes. They're given by syringe into tubing that leads to the stomach. Bolus feedings may cause abdominal discomfort, cramping, and nausea. However, some home care patients prefer this method, especially if they work or go to school. To prevent contamination or clogging, the tube should be flushed with water after each bolus feeding.

Intermittent feedings

Intermittent feedings usually are given by gravity drip or syringe over 15 to 30 minutes, depending on patient tolerance. Jejunal or

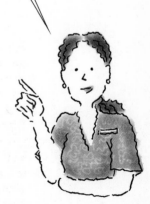

The adverse effects of bolus feedings aren't bogus! Bolus feedings may cause abdominal discomfort, cramping, and nausea.

duodenal feedings are given by infusion pump because of the gastric emptying rate.

Typically, the patient receives four to six feedings daily of up to 500 ml per feeding. The infusion rate and volume per feeding are based on patient tolerance and the doctor's orders. Flush the feeding tube with warm water before and after each feeding to prevent clogging.

Initiating feedings

Tube placement must be verified, usually by examining X-rays and confirming bowel sounds, before feeding begins. To check tube placement, remove the cap or plug from the feeding tube, and attach a syringe. Gently aspirate gastric secretions. Examine the aspirate and place a small amount on the pH test strip. Proper placement of the tube is likely if the aspirate has a typical gastric fluid appearance (grassy-green, clear and colorless with mucous shreds or brown) and the pH is 5 or less. To help prevent aspiration during feedings, elevate the patient's head at least 30 degrees during feedings and for at least 30 minutes afterward.

Tube feedings don't need to be diluted. Give additional fluids as flushes to maintain tube patency.

When giving an isotonic formula, start at full strength, infusing at a rate of 50 ml/hour. Increase the rate by 25 ml/hour every 12 to 24 hours, until the desired rate is achieved. Use a much slower infusion rate if the patient is malnourished, under severe stress, or receiving intestinal feedings. After patient tolerance is established, increase the rate gradually.

Flushing the tube

To help ensure patency, flush the feeding tube with 20 to 30 ml of warm water at least every 4 hours, before and after administering medications through the tube, before and after bolus and intermittent feedings, and after checking gastric residual volumes. Pancreatic enzyme solution may also be used to flush feeding tubes, especially in patients at risk for clogged feeding tubes, such as patients receiving high-viscosity formulas and those with small feeding tubes.

Monitoring tolerance

When monitoring your patient's tolerance of enteral feedings, evaluate the factors listed here.

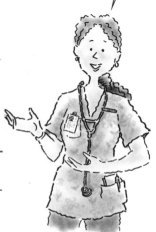

When administering enteral nutrition to your patients, be aware of indications of low tolerance, including high gastric residual content, diarrhea, nausea, vomiting, and abdominal distention.

High gastric residual content

If your patient is receiving gastric feedings, assess gastric empty-ing by aspirating and measuring residual gastric contents. Reinstill any aspirate obtained. Be aware, however, that experts disagree on what constitutes a high gastric residual content. Research sug-gests that in patients with residual volumes under 500 ml, tube feedings shouldn't be held unless the patient is prone to aspira-tion, such as the sedated patient. Each patient's clinical situation and risks should be evaluated when determining whether to hold a tube feeding. Interventions such as elevating the head of the bed, assessing the abdomen for distention, and providing duode-nal or jejunal feedings may reduce the risk of aspiration.

Diarrhea

If your patient develops diarrhea (more than three liquid stools per day), perform a thorough assessment to determine the cause. Review the patient's medications for those with laxative effects —including elixirs sweetened with sorbitol, antibiotics, laxatives, magnesium, and electrolyte supplements.

It isn't *difficile*, or is it?

If medications are ruled out as the cause of diarrhea, check the patient's stool for *Clostridium difficile*. If the stool tests positive for this organism, avoid giving antidiarrheal medications (such as paregoric, Lomotil, and Imodium), which slow intestinal peristal-sis and prolong intestinal transit time. Instead, provide a pectin- or fiber-containing medication, such as Kaopectate or Metamucil, as ordered.

Regardless if *C. difficile* is confirmed, add fiber to the tube feeding — either by changing to a fiber-containing for-mula or mixing a modular fiber supplement with water and infusing it through the feeding tube several times daily.

Since administering cold tube feedings may lead to diar-rhea, check the temperature of the tube feeding. Allow the feeding solution to warm to room temperature before admin-istration. Avoid giving cold feedings straight from the refriger-ator. Reducing the flow rate or volume of the feeding may also help resolve diarrhea. If the patient is receiving a milk-based formula, try switching to one that's lactose-free. Be sure to practice good hand washing when preparing feedings and handling tube feeding equipment. If these measures don't relieve diarrhea, con-sult the doctor about a prescription for antidiarrheal medication.

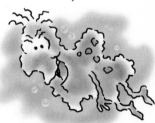

I don't mean to be difficile. It's just who I am.

Nausea

A patient who experiences nausea during tube feedings may need to switch to a formula with a higher caloric density to reduce feeding volume. If this doesn't help, consider giving a prokinetic agent such as Reglan. Prokinetic agents increase upper GI tract motility and relax the pyloric sphincter and duodenal bulb, thus shortening GI transit time.

Vomiting

If the patient vomits during a tube feeding, stop the feeding immediately. Then perform a thorough assessment to evaluate:
• adequacy of gastric emptying (check gastric residual contents)
• proper tube tip location
• possible bowel obstruction, ileus, or constipation.

You may also need to reduce the infusion rate, adjust the formula, or switch formulas — for example, from one that contains fiber to one that doesn't.

Emptying promises

If your patient has impaired gastric emptying, the doctor may order a prokinetic agent. If the problem persists, the patient may need to have a feeding tube placed in the small bowel, antiemetic medications, or further evaluation to determine the cause of vomiting. If the patient has diabetic gastroparesis, a normal blood glucose level must be maintained.

Abdominal distention

Check for abdominal distention during every shift, measuring from one iliac crest to the other. An increase greater than 8 cm from the baseline measurement is cause for concern.

Changing the equipment

For patients in hospitals or long-term-care settings, tubing and formula bags should be changed every 12 to 24 hours or according to facility policy and procedure. For the home care patient, tubing and bags can be changed less frequently — for example, every 24 hours.

Safe keeping

Make sure the formula container is labeled with the date and time of feeding, product name, patient's name, and nurse's name. To avoid contamination, use sanitary technique when mixing and administering tube feedings. Discard unused refrigerated tube feedings after 24 hours. In an open system, hang only 4 to 8 hours of tube feeding at a time. Change a closed system (one that uses ready-to-hang containers) every 24 to 48 hours, according to the manufacturer's guidelines.

Complications

Enteral nutrition can lead to various complications, including aspiration, GI problems, and metabolic imbalances.

Aspiration pneumonia

One of the most serious complications of tube feedings, aspiration pneumonia can occur whether the patient receives feedings in the stomach or intestine. To help prevent aspiration, elevate the head of the bed at least 30 degrees during feedings and for about 30 minutes afterward. Discontinue feedings at least 30 minutes before treatments that require the patient's head to be lowered. If an endotracheal tube is in place, keep the cuff inflated during feedings.

GI problems

Enteral feedings can lead to such GI problems as diarrhea, abdominal cramps, bloating, or gas. To help prevent these problems, warm the formula to room temperature before administration. Also, consider changing to a lactose-free formula with lower osmolality and fat content.

Metabolic problems

Enteral feedings can lead to fluid imbalances, such as dehydration or overhydration. Assess the patient's fluid and electrolyte status and serum glucose levels before feedings begin and throughout enteral nutrition therapy.

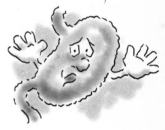

Oh no! Enteral feedings can cause me to become crampy and bloated.

Clogged feeding tube

Causes of a clogged feeding tube include:
• failure to flush the tube adequately after medication delivery
• withholding of tube feedings
• use of calorie-dense formulas (which may coagulate when delivered slowly or by gravity)
• use of a small-diameter feeding tube
• use of gravity drip (the roller clamp may allow residual formula to cling to the wall of the tube, creating buildup)
• delivery of bulk-forming agents (such as Metamucil), antacids, or medications that weren't crushed properly or didn't dissolve completely before delivery
• gastric residual (gastric acid mixes with formula in the tube and causes coagulation)

• stopping or slowing the feeding (which lowers gastric pH, reducing gastric acid dilution of the formula and possibly causing backflow of excess formula into the tube).

To help prevent clogging, flush the tube with warm water after giving medication, whenever a tube feeding is withheld, and at least every 4 hours.

The logistics of unclogging

Flushing the tube with warm water usually dislodges a clog. If that doesn't work, an enzyme mixture can be prescribed to declog the tube. Research doesn't support the use of cola or cranberry juice to unclog feeding tubes. Pancreatic enzyme solution may be used to keep tubes patent in patients at risk for clogged tubes.

Home enteral nutrition

If your patient will receive enteral nutrition at home, teach him and his family how to use an infusion control device to maintain accuracy. Provide instructions on proper use and care of the syringe or bag and tubing, care of the tube and insertion site, and formula mixing.

Instruct the patient to discard any formula not used within 24 hours. If the formula bag must hang for more than 8 hours, advise the patient to use a gavage or pump administration set with an ice pouch to decrease bacterial growth. Tell him to use a new bag daily. Teach family members which signs and symptoms to report to the doctor or home care nurse as well as measures to take in an emergency.

Parenteral nutrition

Parenteral nutrition is the administration of predigested nutrients directly into the bloodstream through an I.V. line. Used for patients who can't receive nutrients through the GI tract, parenteral nutrition enables body cells to function despite the patient's inability to eat or metabolize food. (See *Indications for parenteral nutrition*.)

The patient's diagnosis, history, and prognosis determine the need for parenteral nutrition. Generally, parenteral nutrition isn't indicated for patients with a normally functioning GI tract or for well-nourished patients whose GI tracts will resume normal function within 10 days. Also, it may be inappropriate for patients with a poor prognosis or when the risks outweigh the benefits.

Indications for parenteral nutrition

Generally, parenteral nutrition is prescribed for a patient who can't absorb nutrients through the GI tract for more than 10 days. Common conditions that make parenteral nutrition necessary include:
• GI trauma
• pancreatitis
• short-gut syndrome
• ileus
• inflammatory bowel disease
• intractable vomiting and diarrhea
• GI tract cancer
• GI hemorrhage
• GI obstruction
• paralytic ileus
• short-bowel syndrome
• GI fistula (high output [more than 500 ml/day] enterocutaneous fistula)
• severe malabsorption
• severe radiation enteritis
• critical illness in a patient who's hemodynamically unstable or has impaired GI tract blood flow.

To use or not to use...

In many health care facilities, nutrition support specialists participate in the decision to use — or not use — parenteral nutrition. These specialists may be registered dietitians, doctors, nurses, or pharmacists certified in nutrition support by the American Society of Parenteral and Enteral Nutrition. If the patient is extremely ill, the decision to use parenteral nutrition may hinge on his and his family members' wishes.

Drawbacks

Like any invasive procedure, parenteral nutrition poses certain risks, including catheter-related infection, hyperglycemia (high blood glucose level), and hypokalemia (low blood potassium level). Such complications can be minimized with careful monitoring of the catheter site, infusion rate, and laboratory test results.

Another disadvantage of parenteral nutrition is the need for vascular access. If poor vasculature rules out peripheral access, central access may be necessary, perhaps requiring surgical intervention.

Show me the money

Parenteral nutrition is also expensive — about 10 times as expensive as enteral nutrition for the solutions alone. Therefore, it's used only when necessary.

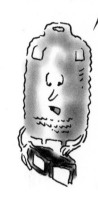

In addition to putting your patient at risk for catheter infection, hyperglycemia, and hypokalemia, parenteral nutrition can lead to empty wallet syndrome. Parenteral solutions cost 10 times more than enteral ones.

Types of parenteral nutrition

Parenteral nutrition may be given through a central or peripheral I.V. line. The administration routes depend on what level of parenteral nutrition is required.

Total parenteral nutrition

A patient who needs parenteral nutrition for more than 5 days usually requires total parenteral nutrition (TPN). TPN provides total caloric needs. It's delivered through a central line, typically placed in the subclavian vein with its tip resting in the superior vena cava. This large central vein can tolerate the concentrated, hypertonic solutions that supply full nutritional support. Alternatives are the internal jugular and femoral veins.

Indications for TPN include:
- debilitating illness lasting longer than 2 weeks
- deficient or absent oral intake for more than 7 days
- loss of at least 10% of pre-illness weight
- serum albumin level below 3.5 g/dl
- poor tolerance of long-term enteral feedings

• chronic vomiting or diarrhea
• continued weight loss despite adequate oral intake
• GI disorders that prevent or severely reduce absorption, such as bowel obstruction, Crohn's disease, ulcerative colitis, short-bowel syndrome, and bowel fistulas
• inflammatory GI disorders, such as wound infection, fistulas, and abscesses.

Peripheral parenteral nutrition

Peripheral parenteral nutrition (PPN, also called partial parenteral nutrition) delivers nutrients through a short catheter inserted into a peripheral vein. It meets basic caloric needs without the risks involved with central venous access. PPN may be used for:
• patients who don't need to gain weight but require nutritional support for up to 3 weeks
• patients who can't absorb enteral feedings
• patients who are receiving oral or enteral feedings and need to supplement low-calorie intake.

Generally, PPN provides fewer nonprotein calories than TPN because it uses lower dextrose concentrations. PPN must infuse a much larger fluid volume to deliver the same number of calories as TPN. Therefore, most patients who require parenteral nutrition therapy receive TPN rather than PPN. (See *Nutrition by many other names…*)

Catheters used for parenteral nutrition

The type of catheter used depends mainly on how long the patient is expected to require parenteral nutrition and whether he'll receive a central or peripheral infusion. PPN is administered through a peripheral vein. TPN is administered using one of the methods listed here.

For short-term use

For short-term TPN, a stiff, triple-lumen catheter typically is used. Generally, the I.V. line is inserted percutaneously into the jugular or subclavian vein — usually at the bedside, with a nurse assisting. Strict sterile technique is essential to prevent infection. The catheter tip rests in the vena cava or right atrial area.

For long-term use

A longer silicone central catheter, such as a Hickman or Groshong catheter, is used for long-term TPN. The catheter is tunneled to allow separation of the vein entry site from the skin exit site, thus lowering the infection risk. The catheter tip rests in the vena cava.

Nutrition by many other names…

Parenteral nutrition is known by various names. Some of them are rarely used. Others refer to particular types of therapy.
• Total parenteral nutrition (TPN) — delivers total caloric needs through a central vein
• Total nutrient admixture (TNA), or 3-in-1 solution — contains 1 day's nutrients; combines a lipid emulsion with other parenteral solution components
• Hyperalimentation (HAL) — rarely used term for total parenteral nutrition
• Central parenteral nutrition (CPN) — parenteral nutrition administered through a central vein
• Peripheral parenteral nutrition (PPN) — delivers basic caloric needs through a peripheral vein.

Take your PICC

A peripherally inserted central catheter (PICC) may be used if the patient will need parenteral nutrition for several weeks to several months. PICCs are associated with fewer insertion complications and infections than lines inserted directly into a central vein.

Inserted via the basilic, median antecubital, cubital, or cephalic vein, the PICC is threaded to the superior vena cava or subclavian vein or to a noncentral site such as the axillary vein. In most states, trained nurses are permitted to place PICCs.

Parenteral nutrition solutions

The type of parenteral solution that should be administered depends on the patient's condition and metabolic needs and whether it will be given through a peripheral or central line. The solution usually contains protein, carbohydrates, electrolytes, vitamins, and trace minerals. A lipid emulsion provides the necessary fat.

Parenteral solutions may contain the following elements, each offering a particular benefit:

• dextrose—In parenteral nutrition solutions, most of the calories that can help maintain nitrogen balance come from dextrose. The number of nonprotein calories needed to maintain nitrogen balance depends on the severity of the patient's illness. Dextrose provides 3.4 cal/g.

• amino acids—Amino acids supply enough protein to replace essential amino acids, maintain protein stores, and prevent protein loss from muscle tissue. Commercial amino acid solutions range in concentration from 3% to 15%.

• fats—A concentrated energy source, fats prevent or correct fatty acid deficiencies. They're available in several concentrations and can provide 30% to 50% of daily calories. Lipids can be infused separately (as a lipid emulsion) or mixed in with the carbohydrate and protein.

• electrolytes and minerals—The amount of electrolytes and minerals added to the solution is based on evaluation of the patient's serum chemistry profile and metabolic needs.

• vitamins—To ensure normal body functions and optimal nutrient use, the patient needs daily vitamins. A commercially available mixture of fat- and water-soluble vitamins, biotin, and folic acid may be added to the solution. Parenteral nutrition formulas should contain vitamins A, D, C, E, K, and B_{12}; thiamin; riboflavin; pyridoxine; niacin; pantothenic acid; folic acid; and biotin.

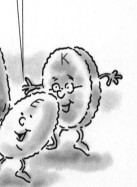

Parenteral nutrition formulas should contain all four of us—and some of our buddies, too!

• trace elements — Trace elements promote normal metabolism. Most commercial solutions contain zinc, copper, chromium, selenium, and manganese. Some peripheral nutrition formulas also contain sodium, potassium, chloride, acetate, phosphorus, magnesium, and calcium.

• water — The amount of water added to a parenteral nutrition solution depends on the patient's fluid requirements and electrolyte balance.

• other components — Depending on the patient's condition, the doctor may order such additives as insulin or heparin. Iron isn't routinely included because of the risk of anaphylactic reactions. However, iron dextran may be added after a test dose is given to determine patient tolerance. Medications other than insulin or heparin also aren't generally added because of the risk of incompatibilities between the nutrients and medications.

TPN solutions

TPN solutions are hypertonic, with an osmolarity of 1,800 to 2,600 mOsm/L. Electrolytes, minerals, vitamins, micronutrients, and water are added to the base solution to satisfy daily requirements. Lipids may be given as a separate solution or as an admixture with dextrose and amino acids. (See *ABCs of TPN*.)

Total nutrient admixture

Daily allotments of TPN solution, including lipids and other parenteral solution components, commonly are given in a single 3-L bag, called a total nutrient admixture (TNA), or 3-in-1 solution. TNA is faster to administer because it requires only one infusion pump (which permits the patient to ambulate). Lipid is available at 10% (1.1 cal/ml), 20% (2 cal/ml) or 30% (3 cal/ml). Because egg phospholipid is used to emulsify lipids, patients with severe allergies to egg yolk shouldn't receive I.V. lipids.

Maintaining glucose balance

Glucose balance is extremely important in a patient receiving TPN. Adults use 0.8 to 1 g of glucose per kg of body weight/hour. That means a patient can tolerate a constant I.V. infusion of hyperosmolar (highly concentrated) glucose without the need to add insulin to the solution. As the concentrated glucose solution infuses, a pancreatic beta-cell response causes serum insulin levels to rise.

Slow and steady

To allow the pancreas to establish and maintain the necessary increased insulin production, start with a slow infusion rate and increase the rate gradually as ordered. Abruptly stopping the infusion may cause rebound hypoglycemia.

ABCs of TPN

To determine the appropriate dosage and administration of total parenteral nutrition (TPN), the primary care doctor or consulting doctor collaborates with the pharmacist and dietitian. Basic components of TPN include:

• dextrose
• amino acids
• lipids (may be given separately or mixed in a 3-in-1 solution)
• sterile water
• vitamins
• mineral and trace elements.

PPN solutions

PPN solutions usually consist of dextrose 5% in water to dextrose 10% in water ($D_{10}W$) and 2.75% to 4.25% crystalline amino acids. Alternatively, PPN solutions may be slightly hypertonic, such as $D_{10}W$, with an osmolarity no greater than 600 mOsm/L. Lipid emulsions, electrolytes, trace elements, and vitamins may be given as part of PPN to add calories and other needed nutrients.

Lipid emulsions

Lipid emulsions prevent and treat essential fatty acid deficiency and provide a major source of energy. In an oral diet, lipid or fat intake should provide 20% to 35% of calories. In parenteral nutrition solutions, lipids provide 9 cal/g. I.V. lipid emulsions are oxidized for energy as needed. As a nearly isotonic emulsion, a concentration of 10% or 20% can be infused safely through a peripheral or central vein.

Administering parenteral nutrition

Parenteral nutrition may be given on a continuous or cyclic schedule. With *continuous* delivery, the patient receives the infusion over a 24-hour period. The infusion begins slowly and increases to the optimal rate, as ordered, to help prevent such complications as hyperglycemia from a high dextrose load. Most hospital patients who receive parenteral nutrition are on a continuous delivery schedule.

Night cap

With *nocturnal* therapy, the patient receives the entire 24-hour volume of solution over a shorter period — perhaps 10, 12, 14, or 16 hours. If the patient ambulates during the day or will be discharged soon on parenteral nutrition, changing to a cyclic nighttime schedule allows freer movement during the day. If the patient on a nighttime schedule isn't sleeping well because of increased urination at night, a daytime schedule may be preferable. Home care parenteral nutrition programs have boosted the use of nocturnal therapy.

Administering TPN

TPN solutions must be infused through a central vein, using one of these devices:
- a PICC whose tip lies in a central vein
- a central venous catheter
- an implanted vascular access device.

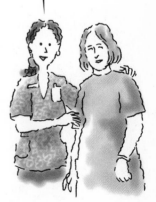

A patient on nocturnal therapy is freer to move about during the day.

Long-term therapy requires:
- a silicone central venous catheter, such as a Hickman, Broviac, or Groshong catheter
- an implanted reservoir, such as an Infuse-A-Port
- an implanted vascular access device.

Solution dilution

Because TPN fluid has about six times the solute concentration of blood, peripheral I.V. administration can cause sclerosis and thrombosis. To ensure adequate dilution, the central venous catheter is inserted into the superior vena cava — a wide-bore, high-flow vein.

Inspecting the infusate

Make careful inspection of the infusate a habit. Check for clouding, floating debris, and color changes. Any of these could indicate contamination, problems with the solution integrity, or a pH change. If you see anything suspicious, notify the pharmacist. Also inform the doctor that there may be a delay in hanging the solution; he may want to order $D_{10}W$ until a new container of TPN solution is available.

Start your infusions!

After removing the TPN solution from the refrigerator, let it warm to room temperature. (Administering chilled solution can cause discomfort, hypothermia, venous spasm, and venous constriction.) Then begin the infusion as ordered. Watch for swelling at the catheter insertion site. This may indicate extravasation of the TPN solution, which can cause tissue damage.

A port of last resort

Remember, never add medication to a TPN solution container. Also avoid using a TPN infusion port for another infusion. To prevent infection, don't use the TPN line to piggyback or infuse blood or blood products, give a bolus injection, administer simultaneous I.V. solutions, measure central venous pressure, or draw blood for laboratory tests. In unavoidable circumstances, the TPN port may be used for electrolyte replacement or insulin drips.

Administering PPN

Because PPN solutions have lower tonicity than TPN solutions, a patient receiving PPN must be able to tolerate infusion of large fluid volumes. Administer the solution through the largest peripheral vein available so the blood can dilute the solution adequately.

Well that isn't so swell

When starting the PPN infusion, watch for swelling at the peripheral insertion site. Swelling may indicate infiltration or extravasation of the solution, which can cause tissue damage.

Withdrawing blood samples

Avoid contaminating a blood sample with parenteral nutrition solution. Each health care facility has its own policy on withdrawing blood from a parenteral nutrition line. Generally, though, you should withhold the feeding formula for a few minutes; then, discard the first several milliliters of blood before filling the laboratory vial. Otherwise, blood glucose level and certain other values may be extremely high.

Complications

Complications of parenteral nutrition therapy may be catheter-related, metabolic, or mechanical in nature. (See *Complications of parenteral nutrition.*)

Catheter-related complications

The most common catheter-related problems are catheter clogging, catheter dislodgment, cracked or broken tubing, pneumothorax and hydrothorax, and sepsis:
- clogged catheter — Suspect a clogged catheter if the infusion flow rate is interrupted or if greater pressure is needed to maintain the infusion at the desired rate.
- catheter dislodgment — The most obvious sign is when the catheter comes out of the vein. You may note that the dressing is wet. With a peripheral catheter, the insertion site may be red or swollen. With a central catheter, swelling may appear around the insertion site. Catheter dislodgment may cause bleeding from the insertion site and an air embolism.
- cracked or broken tubing — If the catheter or vascular access device is damaged, infusate may leak from a cracked part of the insertion site. If the infusion tubing is damaged, the I.V. insertion site remains dry. Both situations pose the risks of bleeding, contamination, and air emboli.
- pneumothorax (air in the pleural cavity) and hydrothorax (fluid in the pleural cavity) — These complications usually result from trauma to the pleurae during insertion of a central venous access device.
- sepsis — The most serious catheter-related complication, sepsis can be fatal. To prevent it, provide meticulous, consistent catheter care.

Complications of parenteral nutrition

- Pneumothorax (air in the chest)
- Hemothorax
- Venous thrombosis (a blood clot)
- Lymphatic injury
- Air embolism (leakage of air into the catheter, obstructing blood flow)
- Catheter embolization (the catheter tip breaks off and obstructs blood flow)
- Phlebitis (vein inflammation)
- Nerve damage at the insertion site
- Infection or sepsis
- Hyperglycemia
- Hypertriglyceridemia
- Electrolyte imbalances, including refeeding syndrome
- Liver dysfunction
- Fluid overload or dehydration

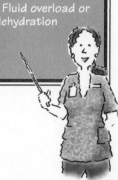

Metabolic complications

During parenteral nutrition therapy, rapid intracellular electrolyte shifts may occur, leading to such complications as:
- high or low blood glucose level
- hyperosmolar hyperglycemic nonketotic syndrome
- high or low blood potassium level
- low blood magnesium, phosphate, and calcium levels
- metabolic acidosis
- liver dysfunction.

Refeeding syndrome

A potentially fatal complication, refeeding syndrome results from rapid and immediate refeeding of a malnourished patient, whose total body stores of potassium, magnesium, and phosphorus are depleted. Accustomed to a state of near starvation, the patient is at risk for metabolic overflow of excess calories and protein. When parenteral nutrition begins and endogenous insulin is released, intravascular potassium, magnesium, and phosphorus move into the cells. Because the body's stores of these electrolytes are already decreased, intravascular levels may become dangerously low. In fact, overaggressive parenteral nutrition has been fatal for some patients. Although refeeding syndrome can occur in patients fed by mouth or enteral nutrition, it's most likely to occur in parenterally fed patients because the I.V. route can infuse larger amounts of nutrition.

To prevent refeeding syndrome, parenteral nutrition therapy shouldn't begin until the patient's electrolyte levels have been normalized. Also, therapy should begin at a low calorie level (25% to 50% of caloric needs), with the calorie level increasing slowly over several days.

Mechanical complications

Mechanical complications of parenteral nutrition therapy can be life-threatening:
- air embolism — Suspect this problem if the patient becomes apprehensive and develops chest pain, tachycardia, hypotension, cyanosis, seizures, loss of consciousness, cardiac arrest, or a churning heart murmur.
- venous thrombosis — This complication causes pain, redness, or swelling at the catheter insertion site; swelling of the arm, neck, or face; malaise; fever; and tachycardia.
- extravasation — Suspect extravasation if swelling and pain occur around the insertion site.
- phlebitis — Pain, tenderness, redness, and warmth at the insertion site and along the vein path may indicate phlebitis.

Monitoring your patient

During parenteral nutrition therapy, monitor the results of routine laboratory tests, including serum electrolyte levels, blood urea nitrogen, and arterial blood gas values. Report abnormal findings to the doctor so that appropriate changes in the nutrition solution can be made. (See *Keeping an eye on lab values*.)

In addition, check glucose levels as ordered, using glucose fingersticks or serum tests. Monitor serum triglyceride levels, which should stay within the normal range during continuous TPN infusion. Typically, alanine aminotransferase, aspartate aminotransferase, alkaline phosphatase, cholesterol, triglyceride, plasma-free fatty acid, and coagulation tests are performed weekly. Also, evaluate the patient for signs and symptoms of nutritional abnormalities, such as fluid and electrolyte imbalances and disturbed glucose metabolism. Some patients may need supplementary insulin throughout TPN therapy. Usually, the pharmacist adds insulin directly to the TPN solution in this case.

Discontinuing therapy

If your patient has been receiving PPN, therapy can be discontinued without weaning because the dextrose concentration is lower than in TPN. With TPN, the patient is weaned while receiving an additional form of nutrition, such as enteral feedings. If the transition to oral or tube feedings will be rapid, parenteral nutrition can be discontinued relatively quickly. Current recommendations are to reduce the TPN rate by 50% for 1 hour, then discontinue TPN and check the patient's blood glucose level 1 hour later.

If the transition to oral or tube feedings is expected to be gradual (for example, if the tube feeding rate will be advanced only by small amounts each day), TPN should be reduced gradually to avoid overfeeding.

Home parenteral nutrition

Patients who require prolonged or indefinite parenteral nutrition may be able to receive the therapy at home. Home parenteral nutrition reduces the need for prolonged hospitalization and allows the patient to resume many of his normal activities.

However, because of the huge expense and potential complications, Medicare and other third-party payers have strict guidelines on reimbursement for home parenteral nutrition.

Meet with the home care patient before discharge to make sure he knows how to perform the administration procedure and how to handle complications. If the patient can't manage the ther-

Keeping an eye on lab values

If your patient is receiving parenteral therapy, monitor:
• serum glucose
• serum sodium
• serum potassium
• serum chloride
• carbon dioxide
• blood urea nitrogen
• serum creatinine
• serum calcium
• serum magnesium
• serum phosphorus
• liver function
• serum triglycerides
• prealbumin
• nitrogen balance
• routine blood glucose every 6 hours
• weight (two to three times per week)
• bone densitometry (with long-term parenteral therapy).

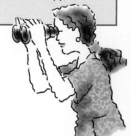

apy himself, a well-trained caregiver must be available to assist with setting up and maintaining the infusion system and changing catheter dressings. The home care patient should be monitored regularly by a clinician with expertise in nutrition support.

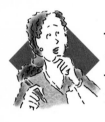

Quick quiz

1. Enteral nutrition is preferred over parenteral because:
    A.   it disturbs the GI mucosa.
    B.   feeding tubes are easier to place than I.V. lines.
    C.   it's more physiologic than parenteral nutrition.
    D.   it costs less.

Answer:　C. Enteral nutrition is a more physiologic way to receive nutrition.

2. A patient receiving gastric feedings should:
    A.   have his head elevated at least 30 degrees during the feedings.
    B.   have his head elevated for 15 minutes after the feeding.
    C.   remain flat in bed.
    D.   lie supine.

Answer:　A. A patient receiving a gastric feeding should have his head elevated at least 30 degrees during feedings and for at least 30 minutes afterward.

3. What's the maximum amount of time that TPN solutions are permitted to hang before the bag must be replaced?
    A.   8 hours
    B.   12 hours
    C.   24 hours
    D.   48 hours

Answer:　C. Don't allow TPN solutions to hang for more than 24 hours.

Scoring

✩✩✩ If you answered all three questions correctly, great job! You've totally taken in the essentials of patient feeding.

✩✩ If you answered two questions correctly, way to go! You obviously used the correct administration route to feed yourself this information.

✩ If you answered fewer than two questions correctly, don't worry! Take a break and then come back and try a different method of intake.

Obesity and eating disorders

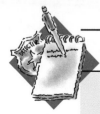

Just the facts

Overeating and eating disorders are among the most common causes of nutritional problems. In this chapter, you'll learn:

♦ definitions for the terms *overweight* and *obesity*

♦ causes of overweight and obesity

♦ treatments for overweight and obesity

♦ signs and symptoms of anorexia nervosa and bulimia

♦ nutritional interventions used to treat eating disorders.

A look at overweight and obesity

Overweight and obesity in the United States have increased markedly over the past two decades. According to the 1999-2000 National Health and Nutrition Examination Survey, 61% of U.S. adults age 20 and older are either overweight or obese—a 5% increase over the estimates obtained in 1994. This study also estimates that 13% of children ages 6 to 11 and 14% of adolescents ages 12 to 19 are overweight. (See *Weight changes in the aging adult*, page 188.)

The high cost of too many calories

Excess weight substantially increases the risk of diabetes, cardiovascular disease, certain types of cancer, and other diseases. Other obesity-related diseases that require identification and appropriate management include gynecologic abnormalities, osteoarthritis, gallbladder disease, and stress incontinence. The risk of death from all causes in obese people is 50% to 100% greater than people with normal weight. In addition, the annual health care cost of obesity is approximately $92.6 billion.

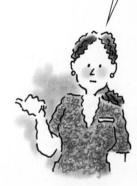

Obesity is a major contributor to preventable deaths and costs more than $90 billion in medical expenses annually.

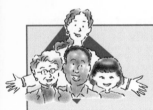

Bridging the gap

Cultural beliefs about weight

Be aware that some cultures and races consider overweight a positive characteristic. Many blacks, for example, believe that carrying extra pounds is important to allow for weight loss during illness. In the Cuban culture, a fat baby is believed to be healthy and attractive. Among Cuban adults, overweight is also considered appealing.

Lifespan lunchbox

Weight changes in the aging adult

As a person ages, the risk for overweight or obesity increases. After age 60, the risk tends to decrease; however, sudden or profound weight changes aren't a normal result of aging.

In addition to the risk of morbidity from obesity-related diseases, obesity can increase the morbidity of other preexisting disorders. Overweight and obese patients with existing coronary artery disease, type 2 diabetes, stroke, and sleep apnea are at high risk for developing disease-related complications that may lead to death.

Obesity is also associated with complications during surgery, pregnancy, and labor and delivery. It's a major contributor to preventable deaths, and it also leads to low self-esteem, negative self-image, hopelessness, and negative social consequences, such as stereotyping, prejudice, social isolation, and discrimination. (See *Cultural beliefs about weight.*)

Causes

The basic cause of obesity is an energy imbalance that results when the number of calories taken in exceeds the number of calories used for energy. A recurring imbalance leads to weight gain over time. This imbalance most commonly results from overeating, inactivity, or both.

The 500 rule

An easy way to put weight gain in perspective is to recall the so-called "500 rule." Because 1 lb of body fat equals 3,500 calories, a person who eats 500 calories more per day than his body requires will gain 1 lb of body fat in 1 week (500 cal/day × 7 days = 3,500 cal).

Other explanations

You may notice that some people who are overweight eat only moderate amounts of food but still gain weight and that some average-weight people overeat but never gain weight. That's because there are other possible influences on fat accumulation in the body:
• A *family history* of obesity increases a person's chance of becoming obese by 25% to 30%. In addition, body fat distribution is

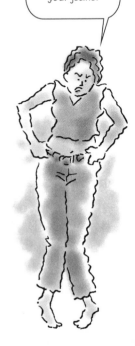

Your genes may play a role in how well you fit into your jeans.

influenced by genetics. Families also share diet and lifestyle habits that may contribute to obesity. (See *Obesity in minorities.*)

• *Environment* also strongly influences obesity. This includes such lifestyle behaviors as eating habits, diet, and level of physical activity. Americans tend to eat high-fat foods and put taste and convenience ahead of nutrition. Also, most Americans don't get enough physical activity. Only 22% of Americans achieve the recommended 30 minutes of physical activity each day.

• *Nutrition* plays an important role in weight gain. Consuming low-fat foods and snacks can decrease the amount of fat in a diet but commonly increases the amount of calories consumed. The high fat content in high-fat foods also contributes to increased calorie consumption.

• *Psychological factors* may also influence eating habits. Many people eat in response to positive emotions, such as excitement, or negative emotions, such as boredom, sadness, and anger.

• Some *illnesses* can lead to obesity or a tendency to gain weight. Examples include hypothyroidism, Cushing's syndrome, depression, and certain neurological problems that can lead to overeating. Also, drugs such as steroids, antipsycotics, and some antidepressants may cause weight gain. A practitioner can tell whether underlying medical conditions are causing weight gain or making weight loss difficult.

• *Sociocultural factors*, such as race, gender, income, education, and ethnicity, may also contribute to overweight and obesity.

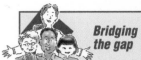

Bridging the gap

Obesity in minorities

The prevalence of overweight and obesity in minorities is different than in whites, especially in minority women. Native-Americans, Hispanics, and blacks have the greatest prevalence of overweight and obesity while Asians have the lowest prevalence in the population as a whole. Approximately 77% of black females and 61% of black males are overweight or obese, compared with approximately 57% of white females and 67% of white males. In Mexican-Americans, approximately 72% of women and 75% of men are overweight or obese.

Evaluating weight

The National Heart, Lung, and Blood Institute (NHLBI) released the first federal guidelines on the identification, evaluation, and treatment of overweight and obesity in adults in 1998. According to these guidelines, assessment of overweight involves evaluation of three key measures: body mass index (BMI), waist circumference, and a patient's risk factors for diseases and conditions associated with obesity. The guidelines define overweight as having a BMI of 25 to 29.9 and obesity as a BMI of 30 or above.

Obesity is categorized into three classes:

• class I — BMI of 30 to 34.9
• class II — BMI of 35 to 39.9
• class III — BMI of 40 or more.

A complicated relationship

The relationship between body weight and good health is more complicated than simply comparing the number on the scale to a weight range table. Weight range tables aren't appropriate to use for all individuals because not all people who have a weight in the "healthy" range are necessarily at their healthy weight. For example, some people may have more fat and less muscle. In contrast, a weight above the healthy range may be fine if your patient has more muscle than fat. (See *Calculating BMI*, page 116.)

Weight distribution

Where your patients' body fat is may be a more important indicator of health problems than how much fat they have. People with a high distribution of fat around their waists (apple-shaped) as opposed to their hips and thighs (pear-shaped) are at greater risk for such diseases as type 2 diabetes, dyslipidemia, hypertension, and cardiovascular disease. (See *Pear- or apple-shaped?*)

Evaluating weight at the waist

To evaluate weight distribution, measure waist circumference. Locate the upper hip bone and the top of the iliac crest. Place a measuring tape in a horizontal plane around the abdomen at the level of the iliac crest. Before reading the tape measure, ensure that the tape is snug, but doesn't compress the skin, and is parallel to the floor. Measure at the end of expiration. If the measurement is greater than 35″ (88.9 cm) for women or 40″ (102 cm) for men with a normal BMI, your patient has a greater risk of health problems. If the BMI is 35 or higher, waist measurement is irrelevant because disease risk is already high based on the BMI alone.

Evaluating risk factors

Determining how many health risk factors your patient has will further help you assess his need for weight control. The more risk factors present, the more your patient will benefit from weight loss. Risk factors include:
• personal or family history of heart disease
• male older than age 45
• postmenopausal female
• cigarette smoking
• sedentary lifestyle
• hypertension
• high low-density lipoprotein (LDL) cholesterol or low high-density lipoprotein (HDL) cholesterol
• high triglycerides
• diabetes or impaired fasting glucose.

Treatment

Treatment of obesity can be long and difficult. No single treatment method or combination of methods is guaranteed to produce

Pear- or apple-shaped?

The illustrations below depict an apple-shaped person and a pear-shaped person. Studies indicate that where excess body fat is deposited may be a more important and reliable indicator of disease risk than degree of total body fat.

Pear-shaped

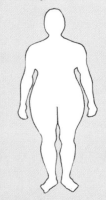

Apple-shaped

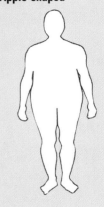

weight loss or maintain weight in all people. Treatment can be directed using guidelines from the NHLBI. (See *Treatment algorithm for obesity*, page 192.)

Before beginning any weight-loss therapy, it's important to determine a patient's motivation level. (See *Assessing motivation*.) Also, in 95% of cases in which weight loss occurs too rapidly, people regain the weight they lost. Explain to your patient that slow, steady weight loss will help with long-term weight management.

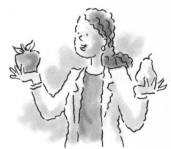

Benefits of weight loss

The benefits of weight loss include:
- reduced risk of diabetes and cardiovascular disease
- reduced risk of developing hypertension
- lower triglyceride levels
- higher HDL cholesterol levels
- lower LDL and total cholesterol levels
- lower blood glucose level in nondiabetic patients and some patients with type 2 diabetes.

Goals of weight loss

The general goals of weight loss and management are to:
- reduce body weight and maintain healthy body composition (percentage of fat mass versus lean mass)
- maintain a lower body weight over the long term
- prevent further weight gain.

10% reduction = health benefits

The initial goal of weight loss is to reduce body weight by 10% at a rate of 1 to 2 lb per week with a calorie deficit of 500 to 1,000 cal/day. Health benefits can be realized and obesity-related risk factors can be decreased with this moderate goal. After this goal is achieved, evaluation and goal setting can determine further weight loss. After 6 months of treatment, the rate of weight loss usually plateaus and the focus of treatment should turn to weight maintenance for the next 6 months. Then, after 6 months of weight maintenance, weight loss efforts can be resumed.

Success!

The clinician and patient must agree on weight-loss goals. Patient involvement is crucial to the treatment plan's success. In general, a successful weight loss plan yields weight regain of fewer than 6.6 lb in 2 years and a reduction in waist circumference of at least 1½″ (4 cm).

Assessing motivation

It's important to determine the patient's motivation level before beginning weight-loss therapy. A weight loss attempt will be more successful if the patient is motivated to make lifestyle changes. Factors to consider include:
- reasons for weight loss
- previous history of attempts at weight loss
- family and social support
- attitude towards exercise
- ability to exercise
- time availability
- understanding of the impact of obesity on disease risk
- financial considerations.

Treatment algorithm for obesity

This algorithm can help guide your treatment of an obese patient.

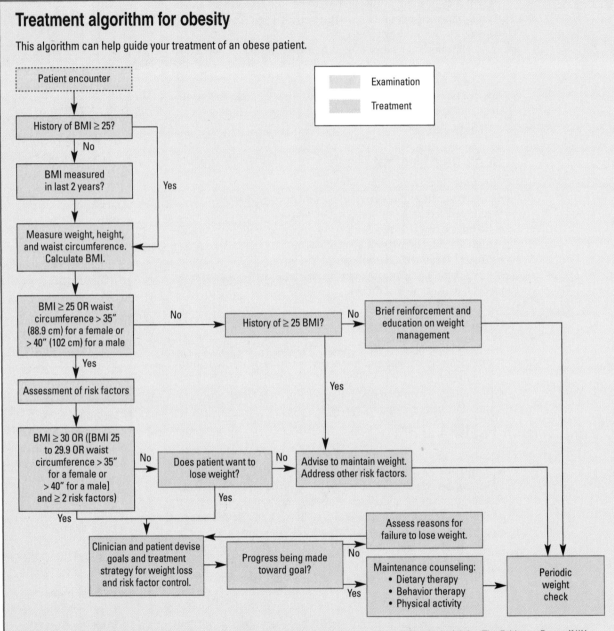

Source: *Clinical Guidelines on the Identification, Evaluation, and Treatment of Overweight and Obesity in Adults: The Evidence Report* (NIH Publication No. 98-4083). Rockville, Md.: U.S. Department of Health and Human Services, Public Health Service, National Institutes of Health, National Heart, Lung, and Blood Institute, 1998.

Components of weight loss

The three components of weight-loss therapy are:

 diet therapy

 increased physical activity

 behavioral therapy.

These methods should be used for at least 6 months before pharmacotherapy is attempted. Weight-loss surgery is an option for patients with extreme obesity.

Diet therapy

Diet, or nutrition, therapy includes instructing patients how to modify their diets to decrease caloric intake. A key element of the current recommendation is a moderated reduction in calories to achieve a slow, progressive weight loss of 1 to 2 lb per week. Calories should be reduced only to the level required to achieve the goal weight. (See *Serving up a weight-reducing diet*, page 194.)

How low to go?

An average sound diet for women is 1,200 cal/day; for larger women and men, it's about 1,400 to 1,600 cal/day. Eating plans that call for fewer than 1,200 cal/day may not provide adequate amounts of essential nutrients. In general, a decrease of 1,000 cal/day is needed to lose about 2 lb/week; a decrease of 500 calories is needed to lose 1 lb/week. In addition, reducing fat intake to less than 30% of total calories promotes greater weight loss and helps improve blood lipid levels.

Education is the key

Successful weight reduction is more likely to occur when the patient's food preferences are included in the menu and when dietary education is performed. (See *Controlling caloric intake.*)

When educating your patient, be sure to:
• cover the energy value of different foods as well as discuss food composition, such as fats, carbohydrates (including dietary fiber), and proteins
• encourage the reading of nutrition labels
• promote new habits of purchasing, especially a preference to low-calorie foods
• instruct on food preparation, especially the need to avoid adding high-calorie ingredients (such as fats and oils) during cooking
• warn against the overconsumption of high-calorie foods
• stress the importance of adequate water intake, reducing portion sizes, and limiting alcohol consumption.

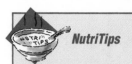

NutriTips

Controlling caloric intake

Include these tips when teaching your patient about caloric intake:
• Consume plenty of fresh fruits and vegetables; lean meats; whole-grain and high-fiber foods; skim milk; and low-fat dairy products.
• Eat sensible portions.
• Stick with steamed, broiled, or baked foods made without cheese or high-calorie sauces.
• Use oil and vinegar or lemon instead of prepared salad dressings.
• Request milk for coffee instead of cream.
• Use nonstick cooking spray and trim all visible fat before cooking.
• Replace high-fat ingredients with low-fat substitutes.
• Halve the amount of meat in stews and casseroles.
• Use herbs, spices, and cooking wine to enhance flavor.
• When food shopping, buy smart, read labels, and stick to your list.

Menu maven

Serving up a weight-reducing diet

This chart lists recommended nutrient intake to achieve a weight loss of 1 to 2 lb per week.

Nutrient	Recommended intake
Calories	Approximately 500 to 1,000 cal/day reduction from usual intake
Total fat	30% or less of total calories
Saturated fatty acids	8% to 10% of total calories
Monosaturated fatty acids	Up to 15% of total calories
Polyunsaturated fatty acids	Up to 10% of total calories
Cholesterol	Up to 300 mg/day
Protein	Approximately 15% of total calories
Carbohydrate	Up to 55% of total calories
Sodium chloride	No more than 100 mmol/day (approximately 2.4 g of sodium or approximately 6 g of sodium chloride)
Calcium	1,000 to 1,500 mg
Fiber	20 to 30 g

Diet doesn't mean don't eat. Patients should only reduce calories to the level necessary to achieve their goal weight.

Increased physical activity

Exercise plays a critical role in the loss and maintenance of body weight. Exercise is important for increasing energy expenditure, maintaining or increasing lean body mass, and promoting the loss of fat. These changes in body composition result in improved body dimensions and possibly in an increased metabolic rate.

Getting physical

Efforts to lose weight through physical activity alone generally produce an average weight loss of only 2% to 3%. Exercise affects the rate of weight loss based on frequency and duration of the activity. Sustained physical activity is helpful in maintaining weight loss and reducing cardiovascular and diabetes risks and may be helpful in inhibiting food intake. Even without weight loss, increasing physical activity lowers blood pressure, increases HDL-cholesterol levels, improves glucose tolerance, enhances the sense of well-being, reduces tension, and heightens alertness.

Slow is the way to go

For obese patients, exercise should be started slowly and increased in intensity gradually. Initial activities may simply include increasing activities of daily living, such as taking the stairs or walking at a slow pace. With time, depending on progress, the amount of weight lost, and functional capacity, the patient may engage in more strenuous activities. Moderate levels of physical activity for 30 to 45 minutes, 3 to 5 days per week should be encouraged. The long-term goal should be to accumulate at least 60 minutes of moderate-intensity exercise every day of the week.

Take a hike

Daily walking is an attractive form of physical activity, especially for obese patients. Tell your patient to start by walking 10 minutes, 3 days per week and to build to 30 to 45 minutes of more intense walking at least 5 to 7 days per week. With this regimen, an additional 100 to 200 cal/day can be expended. A moderate amount of physical activity that burns about 150 calories can be achieved in various ways. (See *Burning calories*, page 196.)

Reducing sedentary time, such as time spent watching television, is another way to increase activity. Patients should build physical activities into each day. For example, parking farther than usual from work or shopping and walking up stairs instead of taking elevators are easy ways to increase daily physical activity.

Behavior therapy

Behavior therapy is a useful adjunct to planned decreases in food intake and increases in physical activity. The goal of behavior therapy is to overcome barriers to compliance with eating and activity habits. Long-term weight reduction most likely won't succeed unless new habits are acquired. The primary assumptions of behavior therapy are listed here:
• Changing eating and physical activity habits makes it possible to change body weight.
• Eating and physical activity behaviors are learned and can be modified.
• Environment must be changed to change patterns.

Here's the plan

Various strategies must be used for behavior modification because no single method is superior:

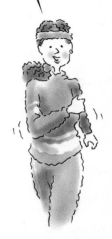

Don't move too fast! Exercise activities for obese patients should start off slow and gradually increase in intensity.

Burning calories

This chart shows the activity and duration needed to burn 150 calories for an average 154-lb (70-kg) adult.

Activity	Intensity	Duration (in minutes)
Volleyball, noncompetitive	Moderate	43
Walking, moderate pace (3 mph, 20 min/mile)	Moderate	37
Walking, brisk pace (4 mph, 15 min/mile)	Moderate	32
Table tennis	Moderate	32
Raking leaves	Moderate	32
Social dancing	Moderate	29
Lawn mowing (powered push mower)	Moderate	29
Jogging	Hard	18
Field hockey	Hard	16
Running	Very hard	13

• Self-monitoring of eating and physical activity — This strategy involves recording the amount, type of food, caloric value, and nutrient composition of food eaten and the frequency, intensity, and type of physical activity performed each day. Recording this information allows the patient to gain insight into his behavior.

• Stress management — Stress triggers dysfunctional eating habits. Using coping strategies, meditation, relaxation techniques, and exercise can help relieve stress.

• Stimulus control — This strategy involves identifying stimuli that encourage incidental eating and limiting those stimuli, for example, by keeping high-calorie foods out of the house, limiting times and places of eating, and avoiding situations in which overeating occurs.

• Problem solving — This strategy includes identifying weight-related problems and planning and implementing alternative behaviors.

• Contingency management — This strategy involves rewarding positive changes in behavior, such as increasing exercise or reducing consumption of a specific food.
• Cognitive restructuring — Cognitive restructuring involves changing self-defeating thoughts and feelings by replacing them with positive thoughts and setting of reasonable goals.
• Social support — A strong support system can help provide the emotional support needed to lose weight. Including friends and family in physical activity and diet or joining a support group can be beneficial.

Pharmacotherapy

Drug therapy should be considered as an adjunct to nutrition therapy, increased activity, and behavior therapy if, after 6 months, the patient hasn't lost the recommended 1 lb per week. Drugs produce a modest weight loss of 4.4 to 22 lb within the first 6 months and can help maintain weight loss. However, most studies show a rapid weight gain after the drugs are stopped. When drug therapy is effective and adverse effects are manageable, therapy can be continued for the long term; however, no one knows how long drug therapy can safely be maintained.

Because few long-term studies have been conducted on the safety and effectiveness of weight-loss medications, they should be used only by patients who are at an increased medical risk because of their weight. These patients include those with a BMI of 30 or more and those with one of the following disorders:
• hypertension
• dyslipidemia
• coronary artery disease
• type 2 diabetes
• sleep apnea.

Not for everyone

Not every patient responds to drug therapy. Tests show that initial responders tend to continue to respond, while nonresponders are less likely to respond even with increases in dosage. Drug therapy should be discontinued if adverse effects are unmanageable or therapy is ineffective. The decision to add a drug to an obesity treatment program should be made after consideration of all potential risks and benefits and only after all behavioral options have been exhausted. (See *Fat fighters*, page 198.)

Weight-loss surgery

Surgery is an option for some patients who are experiencing complications from severe and resistant obesity. Surgery should be considered if the risk of remaining obese is greater than the risk

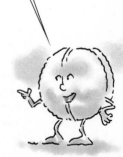

Drugs can help in the fight against fat, but make sure the adverse effects don't send your patient reeling.

Fat fighters

Two current medications used for weight loss are sibutramine and orlistat.

Sibutramine

Sibutramine (Meridia) is an appetite suppressant that works centrally by inhibiting the reuptake of norepinephrine, serotonin, and dopamine. The most common adverse effects are headache, insomnia, anorexia, constipation, and dry mouth. It may also increase blood pressure and heart rate.

Sibutramine should be used cautiously in patients who have a history of seizures or angle-closure glaucoma. It's contraindicated in patients taking monoamine oxidase inhibitors or other centrally acting appetite suppressants and in those with anorexia nervosa. It shouldn't be given to patients with severe renal or hepatic dysfunction, coronary artery disease, or a history of hypertension, heart failure, arrhythmias, or stroke.

Orlistat

Orlistat (Xenical) works peripherally to inhibit pancreatic lipase and, therefore, decreases fat absorption in the GI tract. It should be used in conjunction with a reduced-calorie diet with 30% of calories from fat. Adverse reactions include headache, flatus with discharge, fecal urgency, fatty or oily stool, and abdominal pain. Absorption of fat-soluble vitamins also is decreased.

of surgery. Long-term success of surgery depends on the patient's ability to change behavior and commit to life-long follow-up. About 70% of patients maintain a weight loss of 50% for 5 years. Two types of surgery are primarily used to promote weight loss: restrictive and malabsorptive/restrictive procedures.

Restrictive procedures

In gastric restriction, also known as *vertical banded gastroplasty* and *stomach stapling*, the size of the stomach is surgically decreased so that a patient feels full after eating a small amount of food. A vertical row of staples are inserted across the patient's stomach, decreasing the stomach's size to between 15 and 30 ml. A band decreases the opening from the upper pouch to about 1 cm, which delays gastric emptying. Over time, the pouch can stretch to hold more food. (See *Surgical weight loss procedures.*)

Inner-tube

In adjustable gastric banding, a silicone rubber band is placed around the upper portion of the stomach, creating a small pouch with a narrow opening into the larger portion of the stomach. The band can be inflated or deflated with saline solution through a tube attached to an access port under the skin, allowing the size of stomach opening to be adjusted. This procedure may be performed laparoscopically.

Surgical weight loss procedures

Two types of surgical procedures promote weight loss: restrictive and combination malabsorptive/restrictive procedures.

Restrictive procedures

Adjustable gastric banding

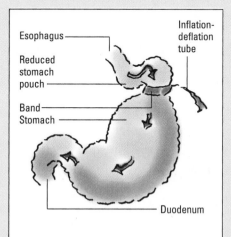

- Esophagus
- Reduced stomach pouch
- Band
- Stomach
- Inflation-deflation tube
- Duodenum

Vertical banded gastroplasty

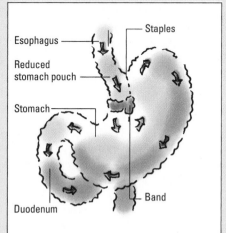

- Esophagus
- Reduced stomach pouch
- Stomach
- Duodenum
- Staples
- Band

Malabsorptive procedures

Gastric bypass

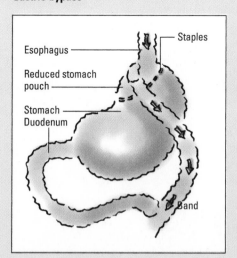

- Esophagus
- Reduced stomach pouch
- Stomach
- Duodenum
- Staples
- Band

Biliopancreatic diversion

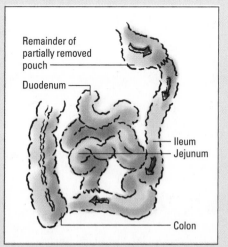

- Remainder of partially removed pouch
- Duodenum
- Ileum
- Jejunum
- Colon

Chew on these complications

Complications of gastric restriction may include bursting of the staples if too much food or liquid is consumed before the staple line heals and obstruction if food isn't chewed well. Nutritional complications include hypoalbuminemia and vitamin deficiencies as well as nausea and vomiting. A patient undergoing restrictive gastric procedures must understand the importance of eating small meals, eating slowly, chewing food thoroughly, progressing the diet gradually from liquid to pureed foods to soft foods, and using nutritional supplements.

Malabsorptive/restrictive procedures

Malabsorptive/restrictive procedures reduce stomach size as well as the number of calories and nutrients the body can absorb. Rapid dumping of food from the stomach into the small intestine limits calorie absorption, leading to weight loss. Nausea, diarrhea, and abdominal cramping may occur after this surgery, but these adverse effects improve over time. These procedures produce better weight-loss and maintenance results than gastric restriction.

Two for the road

Two types of malabsorptive/restrictive procedures are:
• gastric bypass — Also known as *Roux-en-Y gastric bypass*, this procedure combines gastric restriction with a bypass of the duodenum and the first portion of the jejunum. It's the most commonly performed surgical weight loss procedure and is recommended for long-term weight loss.
• biliopancreatic diversion — This is a more complicated surgery in which the lower part of the stomach is removed and the remaining pouch is connected to the terminal segment of the small intestine, thus bypassing the duodenum and jejunum. This surgery isn't commonly used because it can lead to nutritional deficiencies. Patients who have undergone biliopancreatic diversion must take fat-soluble vitamin (A, D, E, and K) supplements. In a modified version of the procedure, a larger portion of the stomach and pyloric valve are in place, allowing control of the movement of stomach contents into the duodenum. With this variation, the patient can eat more food than following other procedures.

A look at eating disorders

Eating disorders aren't a new problem; anorexia has its roots as far back as the 13th century, and bulimia dates as far back as 700 B.C. Binge eating disorder was first discussed in the literature in

1959. Eating disorders usually occur before or after the onset of puberty or after other major personal stressors, such as a parent's divorce, a broken relationship, or a death in the family. Dancers and gymnasts are prone to eating disorders and commonly control their eating to improve their performance.

Added risks

Between 90% and 95% of cases of anorexia and bulimia occur in females. These eating disorders are most likely to occur between ages 12 and 13 and between ages 19 and 20. Binge eating is slightly more common in women than in men, and most people with this eating disorder are overweight or obese. Women with eating disorders also have a higher incidence of drug and alcohol abuse. People with eating disorders are more affected by depression, irritability, suicidal tendencies, and passiveness, and they exhibit more health risk behaviors, such as tobacco, alcohol, and marijuana use; delinquency; unprotected sex; and suicide attempts.

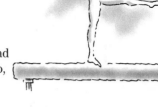

Dancers and gymnasts are prone to eating disorders.

Types of eating disorders

Three common eating disorders are anorexia nervosa, bulimia nervosa, and binge eating.

Anorexia nervosa

The main characteristic of anorexia nervosa is self-imposed fasting or dieting with severe weight loss or maintenance of a weight that's 15% below the recommended weight. Other characteristics of anorexia include compulsive exercise habits and laxative or diuretic use. In most cases, an anorexic patient is overly preoccupied with food and weight and perceives herself as fat. If left untreated, anorexia can lead to severe malnutrition, brain damage, sterility, damage to vital organs, heart failure, and death.

Bulimia nervosa

Bulimia nervosa is a disorder characterized by episodes of recurrent binge-purge cycles. During binges, the patient eats large amounts of food compulsively and quickly. Weight is controlled through vomiting, emetics, laxatives, diuretics, and diet pills.

The bulimic patient typically is of normal or above-normal body weight and has weight fluctuations. Because in most cases the undernutrition is less severe than that of a patient with anorexia, a bulimic patient may experience fewer medical complications. The most frequent cause of death for those with bulimia is gastric dilation and rupture.

Binge eating disorder

People with binge eating disorder eat very large amounts of food and feel that their eating is out of control. During a binge episode, the binge eating patient may eat faster than usual, eat until she feels overly full, and consume vast quantities of food even if she's not feeling hungry. The binge eating patient may also eat alone if she's embarrassed about the large quantity of food she consumes. Following a binge episode, the patient may feel repulsed, depressed, or guilty over her behavior. Unlike the bulimic patient, the patient with binge eating disorder doesn't engage in purging, fasting, or strenuous exercise after binging.

Assessment data

Assessing a patient for an eating disorder includes collecting historical data and performing a physical examination. (See also *Personal characteristics associated with eating disorders.*)

Historical data

During the health history, ask your patient about:
• current, usual, and ideal weight
• complaints of fatigue, tooth sensitivity, intolerance to cold, or dizziness
• abdominal complaints, such as constipation, indigestion, and nausea
• regularity or absence of menses
• history or current practice of self-induced vomiting
• use of laxatives, diet pills, or diuretics
• usual 24-hour food intake, including which foods are best or least tolerated
• use of vitamin, mineral, and other nutritional supplements as well as over-the-counter and prescription drugs
• significant medical history as well as history of drug or alcohol abuse
• psychosocial aspects, such as family or significant other support, emotional state, and body image
• physical activity patterns.

Focusing in on food

Assess cultural, ethnic, or religious influences on food intake as well as abnormal food eating practices, such as cutting food into tiny pieces, refusing high-calorie foods, disposing of food secretly, and bingeing and purging.

Physical findings

Anorexia and bulimia typically present with different signs and symptoms. Signs and symptoms of binge eating may not be as apparent.

Signs and symptoms of anorexia

Signs and symptoms of anorexia include:
- wasted appearance
- thinning hair or alopecia
- dry skin and brittle nails
- decreased heart rate or low blood pressure
- constipation
- cessation of menses
- reduced muscle mass and joint swelling.

Signs and symptoms of bulimia

Signs and symptoms of bulimia include:
- puffy cheeks due to enlarged salivary glands
- damaged tooth enamel due to excessive vomiting
- broken blood vessels in eyes
- scars on hands (from tooth injury during self-induced vomiting).

Signs and symptoms of binge eating

Signs and symptoms of binge eating include:
- normal weight or overweight with weight fluctuations
- fatigue
- hypertension
- joint pain.

Causes

Although eating disorders don't have an exact cause, many patients with eating disorders share common characteristics that may influence the development of the disease, including low self-esteem, feelings of helplessness, and fear of becoming fat.

Personal characteristics associated with eating disorders

Eating disorders are most common among young girls with low self-esteem. Other associated personal characteristics vary by disorder, as listed below.

Anorexia
- Perfectionism
- Concern with pleasing others
- Lack of maturity
- Family emphasis on high achievement
- History of bulimia

Bulimia
- Difficulty controlling impulses, stress, and anxiety
- Pattern of hiding binge and purge cycles from family
- History of anorexia

Binge eating disorder
- Tendency to eat quickly, eat until uncomfortably full, eat when not hungry, and eat alone
- History of depression
- Difficulty controlling impulses and stress
- Difficulty expressing feelings
- Family history of eating disorders

All in the family?

Girls who live in families that place a strong importance on physical attractiveness and weight control are at an increased risk for inappropriate eating behaviors. People who pursue professions that emphasize thinness, such as modeling or dancing, are also more likely to exhibit eating disorders.

Outcomes

Eating disorders can have serious health consequences. These consequences vary by the type of disorder.

Long-term effects of anorexia

Patients with anorexia typically have long-term health problems that result from the disorder. Malnutrition leads to irregular heart rhythms and heart failure as well as osteoporosis (due to a lack of calcium and reduced estrogen levels). A majority of people with anorexia also experience depression, anxiety, personality disorders, and substance abuse problems. About 1 in 10 women with anorexia dies of starvation, cardiac arrest, or other complications.

Long-term effects of bulimia

Due to repeated purging, patients with bulimia typically have health problems associated with electrolyte imbalances and loss of potassium, such as damage to the heart muscle and an increased risk of cardiac arrest. Excessive vomiting also causes esophageal inflammation. Patients with bulimia are also susceptible to drug addiction, obsessive-compulsive disorder, clinical depression, and anxiety.

Long-term effects of binge eating disorder

The weight gain associated with binge eating disorder can produce health problems including type 2 diabetes, hypertension, high blood cholesterol levels, gallbladder disease, heart disease, and certain types of cancer. Patients with binge eating may also have sleep disturbances, depression, alcohol abuse, and suicidal thoughts.

Treatment

There are no universally accepted treatment plans for anorexia, bulimia, or binge eating. An individualized multidisciplinary approach involving nutritionists, mental health professionals, and medical doctors (such as an endocrinologist) is most likely to be effective. Various types of therapy can be used, such as behavior modification, family and group therapy, and nutrition counseling. Antidepressants may also be helpful. Typically, eating disorders are treated on an outpatient basis; severe cases may require hospitalization.

Nutrition therapy for patients with anorexia

The goals of nutrition therapy for the patient with anorexia are to:
• reestablish normal eating behaviors
• restore nutritional status
• maintain reasonable weight.

Patient participation

Involving the patient in the planning of weight goals is imperative for patient cooperation and feelings of trust. (See *Tips for treating anorexia.*)

Keep in mind the following tips when preparing an eating plan for the anorexic patient:
• Be reasonable with calories, about 1,500 cal/day. (Larger amounts of calories may be tolerated poorly.) In some patients, you may need to start at a lower calorie level and increase by 200 cal/week.

> **Memory jogger**
>
> To remember the goals of nutrition therapy for the patient with anorexia, think of the 3 R's:
>
> **R**eestablishing normal eating behaviors
>
> **R**estoring nutritional status
>
> Maintaining **R**easonable weight.

Tips for treating anorexia

To help the patient with anorexia nervosa meet her nutritional goals, follow these tips:
• To create a better response to therapy, exclude high-risk binge foods (which vary with each patient) initially but reintroduce them into the eating plan later to prevent fear of that food.
• Provide small, frequent meals.
• Provide one-on-one supervision during meals.
• Whenever possible, give the patient control over food choices.
• Only use tube feedings or total parenteral nutrition if necessary to medically stabilize the patient. Because the patient with anorexia has control issues, using enteral nutrition unnecessarily may increase feelings of mistrust and body-image distortion and may make the patient feel a loss of control and identity.

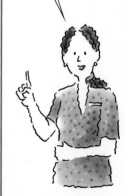

> Treatment of an eating disorder includes behavior modification, therapy, and nutrition counseling.

- Include small, frequent meals and snacks.
- Gradually increase calories, after the patient can tolerate a full meal.
- Limit gas-producing and high-fat foods.
- Include meals based on the patient's food preferences.
- Include nutritionally dense foods to meet caloric goals.
- Include high-fiber or low-sodium foods to control constipation and fluid retention.
- Include multivitamin and mineral supplements.
- Avoid caffeine.
- Use enteral support only if necessary.

Nutrition therapy for patients with bulimia

Goals for nutrition therapy for the patient with bulimia are to:
- identify food fears
- correct food misinformation
- reestablish normal eating patterns.

Promoting compliance

To promote patient compliance, nutrition therapy initially is structured and inflexible. Eating plans similar to those used for patients with diabetes can be used to specify meal portions, food groups, and the frequency of eating. Encourage the patient with bulimia to keep a food diary, recording intake before each meal, to help control the amount she eats. (See *Tips for treating bulimia.*)

Meal planning for the patient with bulimia should:
- be at least 1,500 cal/day, including snacks
- include fat, which helps delay gastric emptying and promotes satiety
- avoid large amounts of food eaten in a short amount of time
- introduce forbidden foods as appropriate.

Nutrition therapy for patients with binge eating disorder

Nutrition therapy for the patient with binge eating disorder focuses on changing unhealthy eating habits and achieving and maintaining a reasonable weight. To promote weight loss and healthy eating behaviors, nutritional interventions for the patient with binge eating disorder are similar to those for bulimia. Research is being conducted to evaluate the effectiveness of nutritional interventions. The binge eating patient who is mildly obese or not overweight doesn't need to diet since a stringent diet may aggravate binge eating.

Tips for treating bulimia

To help the patient with bulimia reach nutritional goals, encourage her to:
- sit down during each meal to increase awareness of eating and satiety
- eat meals slowly (at least 20 minutes) without distraction (such as television)
- use appropriate-sized utensils
- refrain from skipping meals or eating snacks.

When minor relapses occur, help the patient resume the structured eating plan immediately.

Teaching points

Promoting self-esteem in patients with eating disorders is important for positive treatment results. This can be done by fostering decision making, providing encouragement and support, offering choices, and using a positive approach throughout all areas. Help the patient eliminate her preoccupation with food and avoid preaching of rules.

Syllabus

Teach your patients with an eating disorder:
- the components of a healthy diet
- appropriate food intake patterns
- the dangers of dieting, bingeing, and purging
- how to recognize hunger and satiety
- how to identify food- and weight-related behaviors in themselves
- how the idealization of thinness in our society has resulted in distorted body images and unrealistic goals for beauty.

Prevention

Prevention is accomplished by early detection and treatment.

Get to them early

Because attitudes that influence the development of eating disorders develop as early as fourth grade, prevention needs to begin early. Parents and teachers can follow these steps to help prevent the formation of eating disorders:
- Help children develop a positive self-image and sense of worth.
- Avoid pressuring children to excel beyond their capabilities.
- Recognize stressors and provide encouragement and support.
- Teach how good nutrition and exercise can keep you healthy.
- Give children the correct amount of independence, responsibility, and accountability for their age-group.
- Discourage dieting. If a child needs to lose weight, do it with a medically supervised plan.
- Seek professional help if a child has the signs and symptoms of an eating disorder.

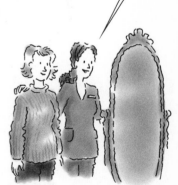

One of the most important things you can do for your patient is promote her self-esteem.

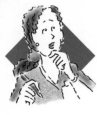

Quick quiz

1. Which of the following signs or symptoms doesn't indicate anorexia?

A. Decreased heart rate and blood pressure
B. Constipation and diarrhea
C. Puffy cheeks
D. Severe weight loss, under 15% ideal body weight

Answer: C. Puffy cheeks are a sign of bulimia.

2. The need for weight loss is determined by:

A. BMI, waist circumference, and risk factors.
B. risk factors, weight, and eating patterns.
C. waist circumference, weight, and motivation.
D. physical activity level, BMI, and risk factors.

Answer: A. The need for weight loss is determined by BMI, waist circumference, and risk factors.

3. The three major components of weight-loss therapy are:

A. medications, exercise, and diet therapy.
B. diet therapy, increased physical activity, and behavioral therapy.
C. diet therapy, medications, and surgery.
D. behavioral therapy, increased exercise, and surgery.

Answer: B. Diet therapy, increased physical activity, and behavioral therapy are the major components of weight-loss therapy.

4. Which of the following changes is a benefit of weight loss?

A. Lower HDL levels
B. Higher LDL levels
C. Increased blood pressure
D. Reduced risk of diabetes and cardiovascular disease

Answer: D. Benefits of weight loss include higher HDL levels, decreased blood pressure, and a reduced risk of diabetes and cardiovascular disease.

Scoring

☆☆☆ If you answered all four questions correctly, congratulations are in order! You've distinguished yourself when it comes to understanding eating disorders!

☆☆ If you answered three questions correctly, great! Your intake of knowledge is sure to help your brain stay properly nourished!

☆ If you answered fewer than three questions correctly, don't worry! The next chapter offers another chance to fuel up on nutritional info!

GI disorders

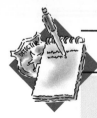

Just the facts

Nutritional therapy is a major component of care for patients with GI disorders. In this chapter, you'll learn:

♦ pathophysiology and treatment of common GI disorders

♦ effects of GI system malfunctions on nutritional status

♦ nutrition-based preventive and treatment measures for patients with common GI disorders.

A look at GI disorders

The digestive system, which is composed of the GI tract (or alimentary canal) and accessory glands and organs, acts as the body's food processing complex. It performs the critical task of supplying the essential nutrients that fuel other organs and body systems. A malfunction in the digestive system can have far-reaching metabolic effects, which can become life-threatening.

When the GI tract malfunctions, nutrition therapy is usually a major component of the treatment plan. That's because, in many cases, the effects of a disorder interfere with the body's ability to obtain nutrients or to use them appropriately. Therefore, nutrition therapy is used to control the disorder or to prevent or lessen the symptoms associated with it.

> I'm not trying to tell you that you can't order what you want. It's just that you know certain foods predispose you to disorders.

Assessment

As for any disorder, a focused assessment — including a health history, a physical examination, and diagnostic tests — is necessary to help confirm the presence of a GI disorder and to develop an appropriate care plan.

Health history

If you suspect your patient has a GI disorder, ask him about his major complaint. Be alert for such complaints as pain, heartburn, nausea, vomiting, and a change in bowel habits—these signs and symptoms are commonly associated with GI problems. If the patient reports one of these problems, be sure to question him about:

- its onset, duration, and severity
- measures used to treat or control it
- effectiveness of measures taken.

To determine if the patient's problem is new or recurring, ask him about past GI illnesses, such as ulcers, gallbladder or liver disease, and GI bleeding. Also inquire about a history of surgery or trauma, especially any involving the abdomen.

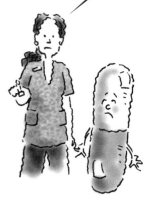

Be sure to ask your patient about recent drug use because many medications can cause adverse GI effects, such as nausea, vomiting, diarrhea, and constipation.

Current events

Follow up with questions about the patient's current health status. Be sure to inquire about medications—prescription and over-the-counter (including herbal preparations)—the patient is using or has used recently. Several medications, such as aspirin, sulfonamides, nonsteroidal anti-inflammatory drugs (NSAIDs), and some antihypertensive medications, can cause nausea, vomiting, diarrhea, constipation, and other GI signs and symptoms. Herbal preparations, such as ginkgo biloba and ginger, can cause stomach irritation. Also ask about the use of stool softeners, laxatives, or enemas because habitual use can lead to constipation or diarrhea.

Ask the patient if he's allergic to any medications or foods. Such allergies commonly cause GI problems. In addition, ask the patient about changes in appetite; difficulty chewing, eating, or swallowing; and changes in bowel habits. For example, has the patient noticed any changes in the color, amount, or appearance of his stool? Has he noticed any blood?

Unwanted souvenirs

Don't forget to question the patient about recent travel, especially travel to rural areas or foreign countries, because GI disorders may result from consumption of contaminated water or food.

A day in the life

Because GI function and nutrition are so closely intertwined, ask the patient to describe his typical day to provide clues about his routine activity level and eating habits. Ask him to recount what and how much he ate the previous day, how the food was cooked, and who cooked it. This information not only tells you about the patient's usual intake but also gives you clues about food preferences and eating patterns as well as the patient's memory and mental status.

Family matters

Ask the patient about his family's health. Some GI diseases and disorders show a familial tendency or are hereditary. Disorders with a familial link include:
• ulcerative colitis
• stomach ulcers
• Crohn's disease
• celiac disease.

Inquire about the patient's psychosocial status, including his occupation, home life, family and financial situation, stress level, and recent life changes. Studies show that stress threatens a person's emotional and physical well-being, increasing metabolism, catabolism, and the body's need for calories. Also ask about alcohol, caffeine, and tobacco use as well as food consumption, exercise habits, and oral hygiene.

As you proceed through the history, attempt to determine the patient's attitude and willingness to change if dietary modifications become necessary. In addition, be alert for information that might help you identify positive and negative effects that dietary interventions may have on the patient.

In conclusion...

Conclude the health history by conducting a review of body systems to gain further information for clues to the patient's problem.

Physical examination

Begin the physical examination by obtaining the patient's height and weight and comparing these findings to a standardized height and weight table. Note any recent changes in weight.

Assessing the accessories

Then assess the patient's mouth, abdomen, and rectum:
• Inspect the patient's mouth, noting any problems with the teeth, gums, or tongue and any unusual breath odor. Then inspect the pharynx for abnormalities, lesions, or exudate.
• Inspect the abdomen, noting symmetry, shape, contour, and skin appearance. Check for any bulges or masses. Observe for abdominal movements and pulsations. Peristaltic waves aren't usually visible; visible rippling waves may indicate a bowel obstruction. Also, measure the patient's abdominal girth.
• Auscultate the abdomen, noting the presence of bowel sounds—high-pitched, gurgling noises that occur intermittently from 5 to 34 times per minute. Hyperactive sounds (loud, high-pitched, tinkling sounds that occur frequently) may be caused by diarrhea, consti-

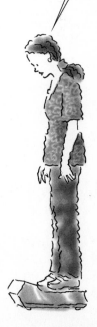

Begin your physical examination by obtaining the patient's height and weight.

pation, or laxative use. Conversely, hypoactive sounds are heard infrequently and indicate diminished peristalsis.

• Percuss the abdomen to detect the size and location of the abdominal organs and to detect air or fluid in the abdomen, stomach, or bowel. Remember that hollow organs, such as an empty stomach or bowel, should sound like a drum beating on percussion. This sound is called *tympany*. Dullness typically is heard when solid organs such as the liver are percussed. Also expect to hear dullness when the intestines are filled with feces.

• Palpate the abdomen to determine the size, shape, position, and tenderness of the major abdominal organs (including the liver) and to detect masses and fluid accumulation. Palpate all four quadrants, leaving painful and tender areas for last. After palpation, check for rebound tenderness.

• Use percussion to help estimate the size of the liver. Liver enlargement is commonly associated with such diseases as hepatitis.

• Inspect the perianal area, noting scars, fissures, discharge, or hemorrhoids.

• Palpate the rectum using a lubricated, gloved finger. The rectal walls should feel soft and smooth, without masses, fecal impaction, or tenderness. After palpating the rectum, test any stool adhering to the gloved finger for occult blood.

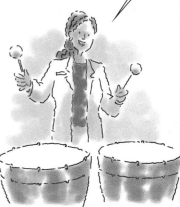

Listen to the music! The drum-beating sound of tympany is normal over a hollow organ.

Diagnostic tests

Numerous diagnostic tests may be performed for patients with GI disorders or in cases in which GI disorders are suspected. These tests may include:

• X-rays—flat plate of the abdomen, barium swallow, upper GI series, small bowel series, barium enema, and cholecystography

• ultrasound—abdominal ultrasound and ultrasound of the gallbladder

• endoscopy—upper GI endoscopy (esophagogastroduodenoscopy), sigmoidoscopy, and colonoscopy

• computed tomography scan of the abdomen

• magnetic resonance imaging of the abdomen

• GI motility studies

• stool testing—for example, for occult blood, fecal urobilinogen, ova and parasites, and nitrogen.

Getting specific

In addition, specific laboratory tests are used to help diagnose GI disorders. Some of these tests can provide information about the effect of the disorder on the patient's nutrition. Common laboratory tests may include:

- hemoglobin level
- hematocrit
- serum albumin
- serum transferrin
- liver function studies
- 24-hour urine for nitrogen balance.

Dysphagia

Dysphagia, or difficulty swallowing, is one of the most common problems associated with the esophagus. One possible cause is a mechanical obstruction, such as from a bolus of food, inflammation, edema, or surgery of the throat. Another possible cause is interference in esophageal motility caused by another disorder—for example, a neurologic disorder such as myasthenia gravis, amyotrophic lateral sclerosis, or stroke. Regardless of cause, dysphagia can severely impact the patient's nutritional intake and status as well as increase the risk of aspiration.

Pathophysiology

In preparation for swallowing, a person chews food after it's ingested. Gradually, this bolus of food is pushed toward the back of the mouth. Normally, when food reaches the back of the mouth, the receptors that surround the pharynx are stimulated and transmit impulses to the brain via the sensory portion of cranial nerves V (trigeminal) and IX (glossopharyngeal). The brain's swallowing center is activated and relays motor impulses to the esophagus via V, IX, X (vagus), and XII (hypoglossal). The bolus moves toward and into the esophagus. Peristaltic movements carry the bolus through the esophagus and to the stomach.

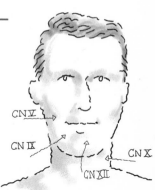

Appetite for obstruction

For the patient with dysphagia, this sequence of events becomes impaired. When a mechanical obstruction is present, although the impulses for swallowing are still at work, the obstruction physically blocks or narrows the passageway, making swallowing painful and difficult.

Obstructions can be intrinsic or extrinsic:

- *Intrinsic* obstructions originate in the esophagus itself and can result from tumors, strictures, and herniations.
- *Extrinsic* obstructions originate outside of the esophagus; for example, from a tumor or edema due to surgery. With this type of obstruction, the lumen becomes narrowed due to pressure exerted on the esophageal wall.

For the patient with a neural or muscular disorder, voluntary swallowing (from the time the food enters the mouth until it enters the esophagus) and peristalsis become impaired as the upper esophageal striated muscles malfunction. This type of dysphagia is called *functional dysphagia.*

What to look for

Patient complaints associated with dysphagia range from discomfort (feeling of something stuck in the throat) to severe acute pain on swallowing. Pain is most commonly due to distention and spasm at the site of the obstruction. If the obstruction is in the upper esophagus, pain typically occurs 2 to 4 seconds after swallowing. If the obstruction is in the lower esophagus, pain commonly occurs 10 to 15 seconds after swallowing. If a tumor is present, dysphagia begins with difficulty swallowing solids, eventually progressing to difficulty swallowing semisolid foods and liquids. If motor function is impaired, the patient reports difficulty swallowing liquids and solids.

Also be alert for these additional signs and symptoms:
- difficulty articulating words
- facial drooping
- drooling
- decreased gag reflex
- coughing or choking during or after meals
- gurgling voice
- pocketing of food in the mouth (such as in the cheeks).

> A patient with dysphagia may feel as if something is stuck in his throat.

Picking up the pieces

Note if a patient identifies specific foods that he prefers or avoids as a result of his discomfort. Some foods may be easier to swallow (for example, thickened semisolid foods), whereas such foods as meats may cause problems for the patient. The patient's nutritional status may suffer as a result of these self-imposed restrictions.

How it's treated

Treatment of dysphagia caused by obstruction focuses on removing or minimizing the cause of the obstruction, if possible, thereby allowing a more open and free passageway for food. For example, esophageal dilatation may be performed to stretch the narrowed area of the esophagus or surgery may be necessary to remove a tumor or strictures. Referral to a speech pathologist is important for a complete swallowing assessment and to provide therapeutic measures for dysphagia due to neurologic causes.

Nutrition therapy

Nutrition therapy is an important component of treatment for the patient with dysphagia because the difficulty encountered with swallowing commonly affects the types and amounts of food the patient consumes. Because the patient with dysphagia is at risk for aspiration, a speech therapist can recommend the types and consistency of foods that would be most appropriate and safe for the patient. (See *Dysphagia diets*, page 216.)

In addition to dietary recommendations, other interventions that can help ensure adequate intake include:
• providing mouth care immediately before meals to help improve taste
• ensuring adequate rest before meals to prevent fatigue from interfering with eating
• providing small frequent meals to prevent fatigue while maximizing intake
• placing the patient in semi-Fowler's to high Fowler's position and having him tilt his head forward to help ease swallowing
• minimizing or eliminating distractions so that the patient can focus his full attention on eating and swallowing
• using adaptive devices as necessary, such as mugs with spouts; avoiding the use of straws (can cause more liquid to flow into the mouth than the patient can handle, increasing the risk of aspiration)
• encouraging small bites and thorough chewing
• offering praise and encouragement during mealtimes
• providing foods that are cool or mildly warm to stimulate the swallowing reflex
• adding flavor as necessary to stimulate salivation, helping to moisten food
• helping the patient select nutritionally dense foods.

Keep in mind that enteral feedings may be necessary if the patient still can't meet his nutritional requirements with these modifications.

Gastroesophageal reflux disease

Popularly known as *heartburn*, gastroesophageal reflux disease (GERD) refers to backflow of gastric contents, duodenal contents, or both into the esophagus and past the lower esophageal sphincter (LES), without associated belching or vomiting. The reflux of gastric contents causes acute epigastric pain, usually after a meal.

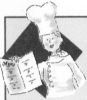

Menu maven

Dysphagia diets

Typically, a patient with dysphagia undergoes diagnostic testing to determine the underlying cause. In addition, a speech therapist is consulted to assist with a complete swallowing assessment and to provide recommendations for an appropriate diet.

Here are types of diets that may be recommended, based on assessment findings and multidisciplinary collaboration. Keep in mind that commercial thickeners are available for use by the patient at home.

Diet and description	Food examples
Thick liquids Blended or pureed liquids without lumps, grains, or solids (can run off spoon slowly)	Smooth, creamy soups; applesauce; puddings; liquids thickened to a puddinglike texture
Soft foods and thick liquids As above plus gelatin-like consistency or sticky foods without crumbs	Plain custards and yogurts, mashed potatoes, smooth cooked cereals (for example, cream of wheat), fruit nectars, eggnog, and liquids thickened to a puddinglike or nectar consistency
Semisolid foods, thick liquids, and carbonated beverages As above plus foods that are firm but not tough	Soft fruit, pasta, pureed entrees, soufflés, poached eggs, and liquids thickened to a nectar or honey consistency
Solid foods and thick liquids As above for thick liquids plus firm, chewy, crispy foods that aren't hard	Soft-cooked vegetables, soft fruit, diced meat, soft cookies, toast, and liquids thickened as necessary

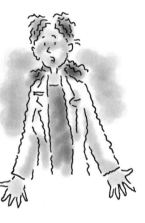

Causes of GERD include:
- weakened esophageal sphincter
- increased abdominal pressure such as with obesity or pregnancy
- hiatal hernia
- nasogastric intubation for longer than 4 days.

In addition, medications, such as morphine, diazepam, calcium channel blockers, meperidine, and anticholinergic agents; food; alcohol; and cigarettes may cause LES pressure to be decreased, resulting in GERD.

Pathophysiology

Normally, gastric contents don't back up into the esophagus because the LES creates enough pressure around the lower end of the esophagus to close it. Typically, the sphincter relaxes after each swallow to allow food to enter the stomach. In GERD, the sphincter doesn't remain closed — either because LES pressure is deficient or pressure within the stomach exceeds LES pressure. As a result, the normally contracted LES relaxes inappropriately and allows gastric acid or bile secretions to reflux into the lower esophagus, where the reflux irritates and inflames the esophageal mucosa. The high acidity of the stomach contents causes pain and irritation.

What to look for

Typically, the patient complains of burning epigastric pain that worsens with vigorous exercise, bending, or lying down. Pain also may radiate to the arms and chest. The patient may report that antacids or sitting upright relieve the pain. He may also describe a feeling of warm fluid traveling up the throat followed by a sour or bitter taste in the mouth due to hypersecretion of saliva.

Additional signs and symptoms may include:
• odynophagia (acute pain on swallowing), possibly followed by a dull substernal ache (suggestive of severe, long-term reflux dysphagia from esophageal spasm, stricture, or esophagitis)
• bright red or dark brown blood in vomitus
• chronic pain that mimics angina
• nocturnal salivation that awakens the patient with coughing, choking, and a mouthful of saliva (rare).

How it's treated

Effective treatment of GERD focuses on relieving the symptoms by reducing reflux through gravity, strengthening the LES with drug therapy, neutralizing gastric contents, and reducing intra-abdominal pressure. The patient should be instructed to sit up during and after meals and to sleep with the head of the bed elevated. Doing this helps to reduce intra-abdominal pressure and prevent reflux.

In addition, numerous medications may be ordered, including:
• antacids to neutralize the acidic content of the stomach and minimize irritation
• histamine-2 (H_2) receptor antagonists to inhibit gastric acid secretion

- proton pump inhibitors to reduce gastric acidity.

Surgery is typically reserved for the patient who doesn't respond to treatment or develops a serious complication, such as pulmonary aspiration, hemorrhage, or esophageal obstruction or perforation. Fundoplication, which may be performed laparoscopically, involves wrapping part of the fundus around the esophageal sphincter to strengthen the LES.

Nutrition therapy

Nutrition therapy is an important component of the treatment plan for patients with GERD. In mild cases, diet therapy may reduce the symptoms enough that no other treatment is required. Typically, diet therapy involves the use of small frequent meals, focusing on foods that increase LES pressure and avoiding foods that decrease LES pressure (see *Under pressure*). If the patient is obese, a weight-reduction diet is necessary.

The patient should refrain from eating before going to bed to reduce abdominal pressure and reflux. Substances that stimulate gastric acid secretion, such as coffee, caffeine, alcohol, and nicotine, should be avoided. If the patient avoids citrus products, such as orange juice, make sure he consumes other sources of vitamin C, such as strawberries, broccoli, and other green vegetables, to prevent deficiency.

Peptic ulcer disease

A peptic ulcer is a circumscribed lesion in the mucosal membrane of the upper GI tract. Peptic ulcers can develop in the lower esophagus, stomach, duodenum, or jejunum. (See *A close look at peptic ulcers.*)

Pathophysiology

There are two major forms of peptic ulcer, both of which are chronic conditions:

 duodenal

 gastric.

Upsetting the up-side

Duodenal ulcers affect the upper part of the small intestine. This type of ulcer accounts for about 80% of peptic ulcers, occurs mostly in men between ages 20 and 50, and follows a chronic

---

Under pressure

Various dietary substances can increase or decrease lower esophageal sphincter (LES) pressure. Keep them in mind when planning care for the patient with gastroesophageal reflux disease.

Increase LES pressure
- Protein
- Carbohydrate
- Nonfat milk

Decrease LES pressure
- Fat
- Whole milk
- Orange juice
- Tomatoes
- Chocolate
- Nicotine
- Alcohol

A close look at peptic ulcers

This illustration shows different degrees of peptic ulceration. Lesions that don't extend below the mucosal lining (epithelium) are called *erosions*. Lesions of acute and chronic ulcers can extend through the epithelium and may perforate the stomach wall. Chronic ulcers also have scar tissue at the base.

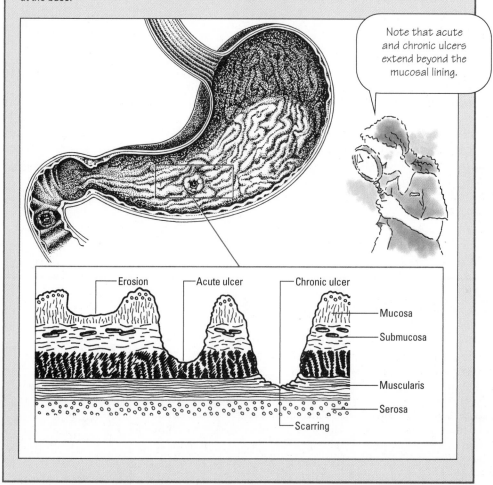

Note that acute and chronic ulcers extend beyond the mucosal lining.

course of remission and exacerbation. Between 5% and 10% of patients with duodenal ulcers develop complications that make surgery necessary. Duodenal ulcers are small (less than 1 cm in diameter), sharply demarcated, and usually deeper than gastric ulcers. These ulcers usually don't become malignant.

Mucosa corrosion

Gastric ulcers affect the stomach lining (mucosa). They're most common in men ages 50 to 60, especially those who are poor and undernourished. They commonly occur in chronic users of aspirin and alcohol. Gastric ulcers are more likely than duodenal ulcers to become malignant.

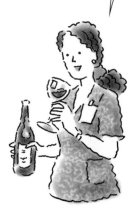

Everything in moderation! Chronic use of alcohol may cause gastric ulcers.

Peptic pep-squad

There are three major causes of peptic ulcers:

bacterial infection with *Helicobacter pylori* (causes 70% to 80% of peptic ulcers)

use of NSAIDs

hypersecretory states such as Zollinger-Ellison syndrome.

Researchers are still discovering the exact mechanisms of ulcer formation; however, predisposing factors include:
• type A blood (gastric ulcers)
• type O blood (duodenal ulcers)
• genetic factors
• exposure to irritants, such as alcohol and tobacco
• trauma
• stress and anxiety
• normal aging (see *Aging and ulcer formation*).

Resistance breaker

In a peptic ulcer caused by *H. pylori*, acid adds to the effects of the bacterial infection. *H. pylori* releases a toxin that destroys the stomach's mucous coating, reducing the epithelium's resistance to acid digestion that causes ulcer disease.

Getting complicated

A possible complication of severe ulceration is erosion of the mucosa. This can cause GI hemorrhage, which can progress to hypovolemic shock, perforation, and obstruction. Obstruction of the pylorus may cause the stomach to distend with food and fluid, block blood flow, and cause tissue damage.

Break out

The ulcer crater may extend beyond the duodenal wall into nearby structures, such as the pancreas or liver. This phenomenon, called *penetration*, is a fairly common complication of duodenal ulcers.

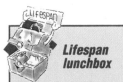

Lifespan lunchbox

Aging and ulcer formation

In the course of aging, the pyloric sphincter may wear down. As a result, bile can reflux into the stomach. This appears to be a common contributor to the development of gastric ulcers in the older adult.

What to look for

A patient with a gastric ulcer may report:
- recent loss of weight and appetite
- pain, heartburn, or indigestion
- feeling of abdominal fullness or distention
- pain triggered or aggravated by eating.

Painstaking problem

A patient with a duodenal ulcer may describe the pain as sharp, gnawing, burning, boring, aching, or hard to define. He may liken it to hunger, abdominal pressure, or fullness. Typically, pain occurs 90 minutes to 3 hours after eating. However, eating usually reduces the pain, so the patient may report a recent weight gain. The patient may also have pale skin from anemia caused by blood loss.

How it's treated

Treatment of peptic ulcer disease has changed dramatically over the past few decades. Dietary changes were once the focus. However, treatment now aims to eradicate the *H. pylori* infection. Drug therapy for this may include:
- antibiotics—tetracycline (Tetracyn), amoxicillin (Amoxil), metronidazole (Flagyl)
- H_2-receptor antagonist—famotidine (Pepcid)
- proton pump inhibitors—omeprazole (Prilosec)
- mucosal protectors—sucralfate (Carafate).

Smoke detector

Cigarette smoking encourages ulcer formation by inhibiting pancreatic secretion of bicarbonate. It also causes acceleration of gastric acid emptying into the duodenum, which promotes mucosal breakdown.

Nutrition therapy

Once a standard, a bland diet consumed in small frequent meals is no longer recommended for treatment of peptic ulcer disease; research shows that this type of diet is ineffective. Instead, encourage the patient to avoid or limit the intake of foods that cause GI discomfort. Some foods that commonly are irritating include:
- alcohol
- chili powder
- citric juices
- coffee

- cola
- hot peppers
- pepper
- tea.

In addition, tell the patient to avoid eating before bedtime to avoid dyspepsia during the night. Encourage vitamin C and protein intake to promote healing.

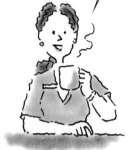

Such drinks as coffee, cola, and tea are commonly irritating and should be eliminated from the diet of a patient with peptic ulcer disease.

Dumping syndrome

Dumping syndrome occurs after certain types of gastric surgery in which part of the pyloric sphincter, or the entire pyloric sphincter, is removed or bypassed. Without proper sphincter function, food quickly passes from the stomach into the small intestine.

Pathophysiology

When the pyloric sphincter no longer functions, undigested food quickly passes into the small intestine. The presence of undigested food in the intestines raises the osmolarity (concentration of solutes) of the intestines. This increase in osmolarity causes fluid to shift from the bloodstream into the intestines, which dilutes the concentration of the intestines, leading to distention.

What to look for

The following symptoms may begin about 2 weeks after surgery and typically occur within 15 to 30 minutes after eating:
- pain
- cramping
- diarrhea
- physiologic changes brought about by the sudden fluid shift (orthostatic hypotension, tachycardia, dizziness, and diaphoresis).

Delayed reaction

A secondary reaction also occurs 2 to 3 hours later. Rapid absorption of carbohydrates causes a rapid rise in blood glucose levels. In response, the body produces excessive amounts of insulin, causing a rapid decrease in blood glucose levels. The rapid decrease in blood glucose level causes:
- dizziness
- nausea
- diaphoresis.

How it's treated

Because the patient is recovering from surgery, no food or fluids are allowed until peristalsis returns. Then treatment of dumping syndrome focuses primarily on nutrition therapy. In addition to nutrition therapy, an antispasmodic may be prescribed to delay gastric emptying.

Nutrition therapy

When peristalsis returns, the patient should eliminate simple sugars (sugar, cookies, gelatin, soft drinks) from his diet. (See *Serving up an antidumping diet.*) Encourage him to consume five or more small meals per day because the stomach's capacity has been reduced. Urge fat and protein intake because fat is considered isotonic and protein is broken down slowly. As a result, these won't increase the osmolarity of the intestinal contents. Instruct the patient to avoid fluids with meals and one hour before or after meals. Explain the importance of lying down for 30 to 60 minutes after meals to delay gastric emptying.

Serving up an antidumping diet

After gastric surgery, encourage the patient to adhere to dietary restrictions to successfully combat dumping syndrome. The patient can consume:
- beverages (coffee, tea, and artificially sweetened beverages)
- grains and starches (up to 5 servings of plain breads, crackers, rolls, unsweetened cereal, rice, pasta, corn, peas, and potatoes)
- meats
- unsweetened fruit and fruit juices (up to 3 servings)
- vegetables (unlimited cabbage, celery, cucumbers, lettuce, and radishes; up to 2½ servings of asparagus, beets, broccoli, carrots, cauliflower, eggplant, green pepper, mushrooms, onions, tomatoes, and zucchini).

   Encourage the patient to avoid:
- alcohol
- cereal (sweetened and those containing dried fruit)
- creamed vegetables
- desserts (cakes, cookies, gelatin, ice cream, and sherbet)
- fruit (dried and sweetened)
- milk and milk products (initially)
- sugar and high-sugar foods, such as honey, jam, jelly, and syrup.

Celiac disease

Celiac disease is a digestive disease that damages the small intestines and interferes with absorption of nutrients. People with celiac disease can't tolerate a protein called *gluten*, which is found in wheat, rye, barley, and oats.

A gluten for punishment

Because the body's own immune system causes the damage, celiac disease is considered an autoimmune disorder. However, it's also classified as a disease of malabsorption because nutrients aren't absorbed. Celiac disease is also known as *celiac sprue*, *nontropical sprue*, and *gluten-induced enteropathy*.

Celiac disease is genetic. Sometimes the disease is triggered or becomes active for the first time after surgery, pregnancy, childbirth, viral infection, or severe emotional stress.

Pathophysiology

In celiac disease, ingestion of gluten causes injury to the villi (tiny fingerlike protrusions that line the small intestine and are responsible for nutrient absorption) in the upper small intestine. This leads to decreased surface area and malabsorption of most nutrients. Inflammatory enteritis may also result, leading to osmotic and secretory diarrhea.

What to look for

The signs and symptoms of celiac disease include:
- recurring abdominal bloating and pain
- chronic diarrhea
- weight loss
- pale, foul-smelling stools
- unexplained anemia
- flatulence
- bone pain
- behavior changes
- fatigue
- tooth discoloration.

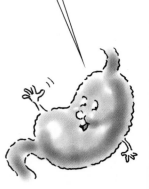

Gluten be gone! For patients with celiac disease, following a gluten-free diet restores my villi to working order!

How it's treated

Nutrition therapy is key to treatment of celiac disease.

Nutrition therapy

The only treatment of celiac disease is adherence to a gluten-free diet. For most people, following this diet stops symptoms, heals existing intestinal damage, and prevents further damage. Improvement occurs within days of starting the diet. The small intestine is usually healed, meaning the villi are intact and working, in 3 to 6 months. (It may take up to 2 years for older adults.)

Lifetime commitment

The gluten-free diet is a lifetime requirement. Eating any gluten, no matter how small the amount, can damage the intestine. This is true for anyone with celiac disease, including those who don't have noticeable symptoms. Depending on a person's age at diagnosis, such problems as delayed growth and tooth discoloration may not improve. (See *Celiac disease and child development.*)

A gluten-free diet requires avoiding foods that contain wheat (including spelt and triticale), rye, barley, and oats. This means restrictions on most grains, pasta, cereals, and many processed foods. (See *Serving up a gluten-free diet*, pages 226 and 227.)

Why so glum? Gluten-free isn't so grim!

Despite these restrictions, people with celiac disease can eat a well-balanced diet with various foods, including bread and pasta. For example, instead of wheat flour, people can use potato, rice, soy, or bean flour. They can buy gluten-free bread, pasta, and other products from special food companies. In addition, plain meat, fish, rice, fruits, and vegetables don't contain gluten, so people with celiac disease can eat as much of these foods as they like.

Are oats okay?

Research is currently under way to determine if patients with celiac disease can tolerate oats. Some people with the disease can eat oats without reactions. Until studies are complete, however, encourage your patient with celiac disease to follow his doctor's or dietitian's advice about eating oats.

Detection offers protection

The gluten-free diet is complicated. It requires a completely new approach to eating that affects a person's entire life. Advise a patient with celiac disease to be extremely careful about what he eats in all situations, including what he buys for lunch at work, eats at cocktail parties, and grabs from the refrigerator for a midnight snack. Eating out can also be a challenge. The person with celiac disease needs to scrutinize the menu for foods with gluten and question the waiter or chef about possible hidden sources of gluten, such as additives, preservatives, and stabilizers found in

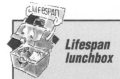

Lifespan lunchbox

Celiac disease and child development

Some evidence suggests that whether a person was breast-fed—and how long the person was breast-fed—plays an important role in the development of celiac disease. The longer a person was breast-fed, the later the occurrence is of symptoms of celiac disease and the more atypical the symptoms are. Other factors that influence celiac disease development include the age at which a person began eating foods containing gluten and how much gluten is eaten.

Menu maven

Serving up a gluten-free diet

Here are examples of foods that are allowed—and those that should be avoided—on a gluten-free diet. Note that this isn't a complete list. Encourage the patient and his family to discuss gluten-free food choices with the doctor and dietitian. Be sure to explain to your patient the importance of reading all food ingredient lists to make sure that the food doesn't include gluten.

Food groups	Daily servings*	Foods to eat	Foods to avoid
Grains	6 oz	Breads or bread products made from corn, rice, soy, arrowroot corn or potato starch, pea, potato or whole-bean flour, tapioca, cornmeal, buckwheat, millet, flax, sorghum and quinoa; hot cereals made from soy, hominy grits, brown and white rice; cold cereals such as puffed rice and corn; rice, rice noodles, and pasta made from allowed ingredients	Breads and baked products made with wheat, rye, triticale, barley, oats, wheat germ or bran, graham, gluten or durum flour, farina, bulgur, wheat-based semolina; cereals or pasta made from wheat, triticale, barley, and oats and cereals with added malt extract and malt flavorings; most crackers
Vegetables	2½ c	All plain, fresh, frozen or canned vegetables made with allowed ingredients	Creamed or breaded vegetables; canned baked beans; some french fries
Fruit	2 c	All fruits and fruit juices	Some commercial fruit pie fillings and dried fruit
Milk	3 c	All milk and milk products except those made with gluten additives; aged cheeses	Some milk drinks; flavored or frozen yogurt; malted milk
Meats and beans	5½ oz	All meat, poultry, fish, and shellfish; eggs, dry beans, peanut butter, soybeans; cold cuts, hot dogs, or sausage without fillers	Any prepared with wheat, rye, oats, barley, gluten stabilizers or fillers; self-basting turkey; some egg substitutes
Oils and sugar	Eat sparingly (6 tsp)	Butter, margarine, salad dressings, sauces, soups, and desserts made with allowed ingredients; sugar, honey, jelly, jam, plain chocolate, coconut; pure instant or ground coffee, carbonated drinks, wine made in the United States	Commercial salad dressing; prepared soups, condiments, sauces and seasonings prepared with above ingredients; hot cocoa mixes, nondairy creamers, flavored instant coffee, herbal teas, alcohol distilled from cereals such as gin, vodka, whiskey, and beer; licorice

(continued)

* For a 2,000-calorie diet

processed food. Medicines and mouthwash may also contain stabilizers. If ingredients aren't itemized, encourage the patient to check with the manufacturer. With practice, screening for gluten becomes second nature.

Serving up a gluten-free diet *(continued)*

What's on the menu
Here's a sample menu for a gluten-free diet.

Breakfast
- ½ c orange juice
- 1 oz puffed rice
- 2 slices gluten-free bread
- 1 egg (cooked any way)
- 1 c milk (preferably low-fat or fat-free)
- 1 tsp margarine
- 1 tsp jelly

Lunch
- Tuna salad
- 1 c salad greens with 1 tbs of fat-free dressing
- 1 c milk
- ½ c rice pudding

Snack
- 1 apple

Dinner
- Grilled chicken breast
- Baked potato with reduced fat sour cream
- 1 c steamed broccoli
- 1 c milk
- 1 pear

What if too much damage has occurred?

A small percentage of people with celiac disease don't improve on the gluten-free diet because the damage to the intestines is so severe that they can't heal even after eliminating gluten from the diet. These patients may need I.V. supplements because their intestines can't absorb enough nutrients.

Lactose intolerance

Lactose intolerance refers to an inability to digest significant amounts of lactose, the predominant sugar in milk. This deficiency results from a shortage of the enzyme lactase, which is usually produced by the cells that line the small intestine.

Pathophysiology

Lactase breaks down milk sugar into simpler forms that can be absorbed into the bloodstream. When there isn't enough lactase to digest the amount of lactose consumed, the results — although not usually dangerous — may be distressing. Although not all people deficient in lactase have symptoms, those who do are considered *lactose intolerant*.

Why the lack of lactase?

Some causes of lactose intolerance are well known. For instance, certain digestive diseases and injuries to the small intestine

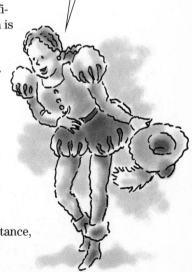

Alas! People who are lactose intolerant lack sufficient amounts of lactase and less lactase means more metabolic mishaps.

can reduce the amount of enzymes produced. In rare cases, children are born without the ability to produce lactase. For most people, lactase deficiency develops naturally over time. After about age 2, the body begins to produce less lactase. However, many people may not experience symptoms until they're much older. (See *Ethnicity and lactose intolerance.*)

What to look for

Common signs and symptoms of lactose intolerance include:
- bloating
- flatulence
- cramps
- diarrhea
- nausea.

These symptoms begin about 30 minutes to 2 hours after eating or drinking foods that contain lactose. The severity of symptoms varies depending on the amount of lactose each individual can tolerate.

How it's treated

Fortunately, lactose intolerance is relatively easy to treat. No treatment exists to improve the body's ability to produce lactase, but symptoms can be controlled through nutrition therapy.

Nutrition therapy

Young children with lactase deficiency shouldn't eat any foods containing lactose. Because individuals differ in the amounts of lactose they can handle as they grow older, most older children and adults need not avoid lactose completely. Dietary control of lactose intolerance depends on each person's learning — through trial and error — about how much he can handle.

Limiting lactase

For those who react to very small amounts of lactose or have trouble limiting their intake of foods that contain lactose, lactase enzymes are available over-the-counter. One example is a liquid form that can be used with milk. A few drops are added to a quart of milk and, after 24 hours in the refrigerator, the milk's lactose content is reduced by 70%. The process works faster if the milk is heated first. Doubling the amount of the liquid enzyme produces milk that's 90% lactose-free.

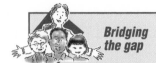

Bridging the gap

Ethnicity and lactose intolerance

Between 30 and 50 million Americans are lactose intolerant; however, certain ethnic and racial populations are more widely affected than others. As many as 75% of African Americans and Native Americans and 90% of Asian Americans are lactose intolerant. The condition is less common among persons of northern European descent.

A more recent development is a chewable lactase enzyme tablet that helps people digest solid foods that contain lactose. Three to six tablets should be taken just before a meal or snack.

Lactose-reduced milk and other products are available at many supermarkets. The milk contains all of the nutrients found in regular milk and remains fresh for about the same length of time or longer if it's super-pasteurized.

Balancing nutrition

Milk and other dairy products are a major source of nutrients in the American diet. The most important of these nutrients is calcium. Calcium is essential for the growth and repair of bones throughout life. In the middle and later years, a shortage of calcium may lead to thin, fragile bones that break easily (a condition called *osteoporosis*). A concern, then, for both children and adults with lactose intolerance is getting enough calcium in a diet that includes little or no milk.

Keeping calcium on the menu

When planning meals, making sure that each day's diet includes enough calcium is important, even if the diet doesn't contain dairy products. Many nondairy foods are high in calcium. Green vegetables, such as broccoli and kale, and fish with soft, edible bones, such as salmon and sardines, are excellent sources of calcium. (See *Sources of dietary calcium*, page 230.)

Recent research shows that yogurt with active cultures may be a good source of calcium for patients with lactose intolerance, even though it's fairly high in lactose. Evidence shows that the bacterial cultures used in making yogurt produce some of the lactase enzyme required for proper digestion.

Although milk and foods made from milk are the only natural sources, lactose is often added to prepared foods. People with a very low tolerance for lactose need to know about the many food products that may contain lactose, even in small amounts, including:

- bread and other baked goods
- processed breakfast cereals
- instant potatoes, soups, and breakfast drinks
- margarine
- lunch meats (other than kosher)
- salad dressings
- candies and other snacks
- mixes for pancakes, biscuits, and cookies.

Sources of dietary calcium

Here's a list of dietary sources of calcium that have little or no lactose. These items should become part of the diet of someone with lactose intolerance.

Food source	Calcium content
Broccoli (cooked), 1 c	94 to 177 mg
Chinese cabbage (cooked), 1 c	158 mg
Collard greens (cooked), 1 c	148 to 357 mg
Kale (cooked), 1 c	94 to 170 mg
Turnip greens (cooked), 1 c	194 to 249 mg
Oysters (raw), 1c	226 mg
Salmon with bones (canned), 3 oz	167 mg
Sardines, 3 oz	371 mg
Shrimp (canned), 3 oz	98 mg
Molasses, 2 tbsp	274 mg
Tofu (processed with calcium salts), 3 oz	225 mg

Hidden agenda

Some products labeled nondairy, such as powdered coffee creamer and whipped toppings, include ingredients that are derived from milk and therefore contain lactose. Encourage patients to learn to read food labels carefully, looking not only for milk and lactose among the contents but also for other ingredients that indicate that the item contains lactose, such as:
• whey
• curds
• milk by-products
• dry milk solids
• nonfat dry milk powder.

In addition, lactose is used as the base for more than 20% of prescription drugs and about 6% of over-the-counter medicines. Many types of birth control pills, for example, contain lactose, as do some tablets used to treat stomach acid and gas. However, these products typically affect only people with severe lactose intolerance.

Living with lactose intolerance

Even though lactose intolerance is widespread, it need not pose a serious threat to good health. People who have trouble digesting lactose can learn which dairy products and other foods they can eat without discomfort and which ones they should avoid. Many can enjoy milk, ice cream, and other such products if they take them in small amounts or eat other food at the same time. A carefully chosen diet is the key to reducing symptoms and protecting future health.

Diverticular disease

In diverticular disease, bulging pouches (diverticula) in the GI wall push the mucosal lining through the surrounding muscle. Although the most common site for diverticula is the sigmoid colon, they may develop anywhere, from the proximal end of the pharynx to the anus. Other common sites include the duodenum, near the pancreatic border or the ampulla of Vater, and the jejunum. Diverticular disease of the stomach is rare and is usually a precursor of peptic or neoplastic disease. Diverticular disease of the ileum (Meckel's diverticulum) is the most common congenital anomaly of the GI tract.

Who and where?

Diverticular disease is common in industrialized countries, suggesting that a low-fiber diet reduces stool bulk and leads to excessive colonic motility. This consequent increased intraluminal pressure causes herniation of the mucosa. (See *Diverticular disease around the globe*, page 232.)

Diverticular disease is most prevalent in men over age 40 and people who eat low-fiber diets. More than one-half of patients older than age 50 have colonic diverticula.

Type two

Diverticular disease has two forms:

diverticulosis, in which diverticula are present but don't cause symptoms

diverticulitis, in which diverticula are inflamed and may cause potentially fatal obstruction, infection, perforation, or hemorrhage.

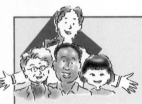

Bridging the gap

Diverticular disease around the globe

Diverticular disease is common in industrialized countries, such as the United States, England, and Australia, where people tend to eat diets low in fiber. It rarely occurs in Asia and Africa, where high-fiber vegetable diets are regularly consumed. Diverticular disease initially appeared in the United States in the early twentieth century, when processed foods became popular.

Pathophysiology

The etiology of diverticular disease hasn't been determined but it's thought to be caused by a disordered colonic motility pattern. Diverticula probably result from high intraluminal pressure on an area of weakness in the GI wall, where blood vessels enter. Diet may be a contributing factor, because insufficient fiber reduces fecal residue, narrows the bowel lumen, and leads to high intra-abdominal pressure during defecation.

In diverticulosis, the pouches formed by diverticula sometimes trap fecal material, which becomes hardened and irritates the surrounding cells. Inflammation develops, causing diverticulitis. In diverticulitis, retained undigested food and bacteria accumulate in the diverticular sac. This hard mass cuts off the blood supply to the thin walls of the sac, making them more susceptible to attack by colonic bacteria. Inflammation follows and may lead to perforation, abscess, peritonitis, obstruction, or hemorrhage. Occasionally, the inflamed colon segment may adhere to the bladder or other organs and cause a fistula.

What to look for

Typically the patient with diverticulosis is asymptomatic and will remain so unless diverticulitis develops.

With mild diverticulitis, signs and symptoms include:
- moderate left lower abdominal pain
- low-grade fever
- leukocytosis.

If diverticulitis is severe, signs and symptoms include:
- abdominal rigidity
- left lower quadrant pain
- high fever
- chills

- hypotension
- microscopic or massive hemorrhage.

How it's treated

If diverticulitis develops, administer antibiotics as prescribed to combat infection and minimize inflammation. Administer analgesics as prescribed to control pain and relax smooth muscle. Give antispasmodics to control muscle spasms. Encourage the patient to exercise to increase the rate of stool passage.

If diverticulitis is refractory to medical treatment, a colon resection with removal of the involved segment may be necessary. A temporary colostomy may be needed to drain abscesses and rest the colon if diverticulitis is accompanied by perforation, peritonitis, obstruction, or fistula. Blood transfusions may be necessary to treat blood loss from hemorrhage.

Nutrition therapy

For the patient with diverticulosis, encourage high fiber intake that includes 25 to 30 g of fiber per day. High-fiber diets produce soft, bulky stools that move easily through the colon, decreasing pressure within the colon.

During an acute phase of diverticulitis, a low-residue diet is recommended to reduce residue in the bowel. A liquid diet may be recommended in severe cases to rest the bowel.

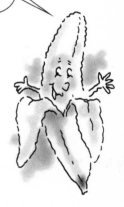

High-fiber fruits, which make good snacks for the patient with diverticulosis, include bananas, oranges, and peaches.

Irritable bowel syndrome

Irritable bowel syndrome (IBS) is characterized by chronic symptoms of abdominal pain, alternating constipation and diarrhea, and abdominal distention. This disorder is common, although about 20% of patients never seek medical attention. It occurs in women twice as often as men.

Mechanisms involved in IBS include visceral hypersensitivity and altered colonic motility. IBS is generally associated with psychological stress; however, it may result from such factors as diverticular disease, ingestion of irritants (coffee, raw vegetables, or fruits), laxative abuse, food poisoning, and colon cancer.

Pathophysiology

Typically, the patient with IBS has a normal-appearing GI tract. However, careful examination of the colon may reveal functional irritability—an abnormality in colonic smooth-muscle function marked by excessive peristalsis and spasms, even during remission.

Contractual obligations

To understand what happens in IBS, consider how smooth muscle controls bowel function. Normally, segmental muscle contractions mix intestinal contents while peristalsis propels the contents through the GI tract. Motor activity is most propulsive in the proximal (stomach) and distal (sigmoid) portions of the intestine. Activity in the rest of the intestines is slower, permitting nutrient and water absorption.

IBS appears to reflect motor disturbances of the entire colon in response to stimuli. Some muscles of the small bowel are particularly sensitive to motor abnormalities and distention; others are particularly sensitive to certain foods and drugs. The patient may be hypersensitive to the hormones gastrin and cholecystokinin. The pain of IBS seems to be caused by abnormally strong contractions of the intestinal smooth muscle as it reacts to distention, irritants, or stress.

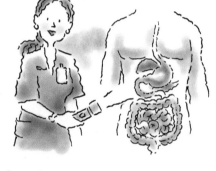

IBS pain is caused by abnormally strong contractions of the intestinal smooth muscle.

Developing a disturbing pattern

Some patients have spasmodic intestinal contractions that set up a partial obstruction by trapping gas and stools. This causes distention, bloating, gas pain, and constipation. Other patients have dramatically increased intestinal motility. Usually, eating or cholinergic stimulation triggers the small intestine's contents to rush into the large intestine, dumping watery stools and irritating mucosa. The result is diarrhea.

If further spasms trap liquid stools, the intestinal mucosa absorbs water from the stools, leaving them dry, hard, and difficult to pass. The result is a pattern of alternating diarrhea and constipation.

What to look for

The most commonly reported symptom is intermittent, cramping, lower abdominal pain that's relieved by defecation or passage of flatus. It usually occurs during the day and intensifies with stress or 1 to 2 hours after meals. The patient may experience alternating constipation and diarrhea, with one being the predominant problem. Mucus passage through the rectum may also occur. Abdominal distention and bloating are common.

How it's treated

Treatment of IBS aims to relieve symptoms and includes counseling to help the patient understand the relation between stress and his illness. Rest and heat applied to the abdomen are usually helpful.

In addition, some medications may be used:

• 5-HT$_3$ receptor antagonist (alosetron) is a selective antagonist used for short-term treatment of women with IBS who have severe diarrhea.

• 5-HT$_4$ receptor partial agonist (tegaserod) may be prescribed for short-term treatment of women with IBS whose primary symptom is constipation. It also relieves abdominal discomfort and bloating.

• Antidepressants have been effective, especially when diarrhea is a predominant symptom.

• Bulk-forming agents, such as psyllium (Metamucil), are effective when constipation is the predominant symptom. In the case of laxative overuse, bowel training is sometimes recommended.

• Antispasmodics, such as propantheline or diphenoxylate with atropine sulfate, are commonly prescribed.

• A mild barbiturate, such as phenobarbital, in judicious doses is sometimes helpful as well.

Nutrition therapy

Dietary restrictions haven't proven to be effective in treating IBS, but the patient is encouraged to be aware of foods that exacerbate symptoms. Advise the patient to chew food slowly and to eat small, frequent meals to reduce distention. Some people find a high-fiber diet effective; however, this type of diet isn't helpful for everyone. Consuming a low-fat diet has also proven beneficial for some patients.

Inflammatory bowel disease

Inflammatory bowel disease (IBD) is a chronic condition characterized by the formation of inflammatory and ulcerating lesions in the small intestine or colon. Patients commonly experience diarrhea, fever, and abdominal pain.

The two major types of IBD are:

• Crohn's disease
• ulcerative colitis.

Crohn's disease details

Crohn's disease is a type of IBD that may affect any part of the GI tract. Inflammation extends through all layers of the intestinal wall and may involve lymph nodes and supporting membranes in the area. Ulcers form as the inflammation extends into the peritoneum.

Crohn's disease is most prevalent in adults ages 20 to 40. It tends to run in families—up to 20% of patients have a positive family history.

When Crohn's disease affects only the small bowel, it's known as *regional enteritis.* When it involves the colon or affects only the colon it's known as *Crohn's disease of the colon.* Crohn's disease of the colon is sometimes called *granulomatous colitis;* however, not all patients develop granulomas (tumorlike masses of granulation tissue).

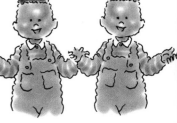

Although it isn't necessarily all in the family, Crohn's disease sometimes occurs in identical twins, and up to 20% of affected patients have relatives who also have the disease.

Ulcerative colitis particulars

Ulcerative colitis causes ulcerations of the mucosa in the colon. It commonly occurs as a chronic condition. As many as 1 in 1,000 people have ulcerative colitis. Peak occurrences are between ages 15 and 20 and between ages 55 and 60. It's more prevalent among women, people of Jewish ancestry, and whites. (See *Inflammatory bowel disease in Jewish people.*)

Pathophysiology of Crohn's disease

Although researchers are still studying Crohn's disease, possible causes include:
- lymphatic obstruction
- infection
- allergies
- genetic factors
- immune disorders, such as altered immunoglobulin A production and increased suppressor T-cell activity.

An inheritance you can't retire on

Genetic factors play an important role. Crohn's disease sometimes occurs in identical twins, and 10% to 20% of patients with the disease have one or more affected relatives. Researchers have identified a gene that predisposes people to the disease; however, no simple pattern of inheritance has been identified.

Groan! Crohn's

In Crohn's disease, inflammation spreads slowly and progressively. Here's what happens:

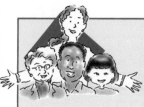

- Lymph nodes enlarge, and lymph flow in the submucosa is blocked.
- Lymphatic obstruction causes edema, mucosal ulceration, fissures, abscesses and, sometimes, granulomas. Mucosal ulcerations are called *skipping lesions* because they aren't continuous (as in ulcerative colitis).
- Oval, elevated patches of closely packed lymph follicles — called Peyer's patches — develop on the lining of the small intestine.
- Fibrosis occurs, thickening the bowel wall and causing stenosis, or narrowing of the lumen.
- Inflammation of the serous membrane (serositis) develops, inflamed bowel loops adhere to other diseased or normal loops, and diseased bowel segments become interspersed with healthy ones.
- Eventually, diseased parts of the bowel become thicker, narrower, and shorter.

Getting complicated

Severe diarrhea and corrosion of the perineal area by enzymes can cause an anal fistula, the most common complication. A perineal abscess may also develop during the active inflammatory state. Fistulas may develop to the bladder, vagina, or even skin in an old scar area.

Other complications include intestinal obstruction; nutrient deficiencies caused by malabsorption of bile salts and vitamin B_{12} and poor digestion; fluid imbalances; and inflammation of abdominal linings (peritonitis [rare]).

What to look for in patients with Crohn's disease

Initially, the patient experiences malaise and diarrhea, usually with pain in the right lower quadrant or generalized abdominal pain and fever. Chronic symptoms, which are more typical of the disease, are more persistent and less severe; they include diarrhea (four to six stools per day) with pain in the right lower quadrant, steatorrhea (excess fat in feces), and marked weight loss. The patient may complain of weakness and fatigue. The patient may also present with acute inflammatory signs and symptoms that mimic appendicitis, including steady, colicky pain in the right lower quadrant; cramping; tenderness; flatulence; nausea; fever; diarrhea; bleeding; (usually mild but may be massive); and bloody stools.

Pathophysiology of ulcerative colitis

The cause of ulcerative colitis is unknown; it may be related to an abnormal immune response in the GI tract, possibly associated with genetic factors. Lymphocytes (T cells) in people with ulcerative colitis may have cytotoxic effects on epithelial cells of the colon. Although no specific organism has been linked to ulcerative colitis, infection hasn't been ruled out. Stress doesn't cause the disorder, but it can increase the severity of an attack.

Surveying the damage

Ulcerative colitis damages the large intestine's mucosal and submucosal layers. Here's how it progresses:
• Usually, the disease originates in the rectum and lower colon. Then it spreads to the entire colon.
• The mucosa develops diffuse ulceration, with hemorrhage, congestion, edema, and exudative inflammation. Unlike Crohn's disease, ulcerations are continuous.
• Abscesses formed in the mucosa develop purulent drainage, become necrotic, and ulcerate.
• Sloughing occurs, causing bloody, mucus-filled stools.

Looking closer at the colon

As ulcerative colitis progresses, the colon undergoes these changes:
• Initially, the colon's mucosal surface becomes dark, red, and velvety.
• Abscesses form and coalesce into ulcers.
• Necrosis of the mucosa occurs.
• As abscesses heal, scarring and thickening may appear in the bowel's inner muscle layer.
• As granulation tissue replaces the muscle layer, the colon narrows, shortens, and loses its characteristic pouches (haustral folds).

Progression of ulcerative colitis may lead to intestinal obstruction, dehydration, and major fluid and electrolyte imbalances. Malabsorption is common, and chronic anemia may result from loss of blood in the stools.

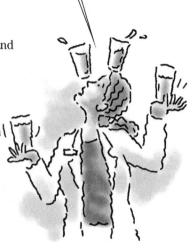

Progression of ulcerative colitis may lead to intestinal obstruction, dehydration, and major fluid and electrolyte imbalances.

What to look for in patients with ulcerative colitis

The hallmark of ulcerative colitis is recurrent bloody diarrhea—usually containing pus and mucus—alternating with symptom-free remissions. Accumulation of blood and mucus in the bowel causes cramping abdominal pain, rectal urgency, and diarrhea.

Other symptoms include:

- anorexia
- irritability
- nausea
- weakness
- weight loss
- vomiting.

How it's treated

For the patient with either type of IBD, the goals of treatment focus on reducing inflammation, relieving symptoms, and preventing malnutrition. Sulfasalazine is given to treat infection and decrease inflammation. Corticosteroids are prescribed to reduce inflammation and, subsequently, diarrhea, pain, and bleeding. Immunosuppressants and immunomodulators may be given if corticosteroids fail to control the disease. Antidiarrheal agents may be prescribed to relieve frequent diarrhea in patients whose IBD is otherwise under control. Opioid analgesics may be administered to control pain and diarrhea. I.V. therapy is administered to combat fluid losses.

Crohn's corrections

Patients with Crohn's disease may require surgery to repair bowel perforation and correct massive hemorrhage, fistulas, or acute intestinal obstruction. A colectomy with ileostomy may be necessary in patients with extensive disease of the large intestine and rectum.

Ulcerative colitis adjustments

If ulcerative colitis symptoms become unbearable or unresponsive to medications and supportive measures, the patient may require surgery to correct massive dilation of the colon. Proctocolectomy with ileostomy (to divert stool and to allow the rectal anastomosis to heal), ileoanal pull-through, or pouch ileostomy (Kock pouch or continent ileostomy) may be necessary if the patient doesn't respond to drugs and supportive measures.

Nutrition therapy

Malnutrition is a constant concern in patients with IBD. Anorexia, nausea, abdominal pain, and diarrhea discourage the patient from eating. Encourage the patient to eat and explain that eating aids healing and recovery.

A diet high in protein and calories is needed to promote weight gain and healing. Calorie consumption should be sufficient to reach and maintain an acceptable body weight. Protein intake should reach 1.5 to 2.5 g/kg/day. If the patient's fat digestion and absorption are impaired, he may need to restrict fat and lactose intake. Vitamin and mineral supplements may be necessary. Vitamin B_{12} injections may be administered to the patient with Crohn's disease. Omega-3 fatty acids (fish oils) may be ordered to help make the inflammatory response less severe.

Menu matters

Encourage the patient to consume small frequent meals, which are better tolerated than three larger meals. Also educate the patient to avoid these substances:
- alcoholic beverages
- caffeinated beverages
- iced beverages
- carbonated beverages
- simple sugars.

In some cases, patients also can't tolerate wheat and gluten, so these substances also need to be avoided.

How low can you go?

Those who have undergone surgical procedures are also at risk for nutritional deficiencies caused by malabsorption. (See *Colostomy and ileostomy concerns.*) Many are deficient in the fat-soluble vitamins A, E, and K. When portions of the ileum are resected, problems with vitamin B_{12} absorption may lead to deficiency. Patients also experience protein loss as protein-rich fluids are excreted with diarrhea.

Deficiencies must be corrected by providing nutrients in any way that the patient can tolerate them. Nutritional supplements may be necessary. Tube feedings may be necessary if the patient is experiencing an acute exacerbation. If complete bowel rest is required, parenteral nutrition (PN) may be prescribed.

Diarrhea

Diarrhea, the abnormally frequent passage of liquid stool, is a common disorder that results in excessive loss of fluid, elec-

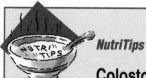

NutriTips

Colostomy and ileostomy concerns

Because fluid, potassium, and sodium are usually absorbed in the colon, patients with colostomies and ileostomies are at risk for nutritional deficiencies. The greater the portion of the colon removed, the greater the risk of deficiencies. (Therefore, ileostomies place the patient at higher risk than colostomies.) The patient with an ileostomy is also at risk for the malabsorption of bile, fat, and vitamin B_{12}.

Nutrition therapy

In the immediate postoperative period, the patient may be maintained on total parenteral nutrition. After healing takes place, nutrition therapy depends on tolerance as well as fluid and electrolyte status. A high fluid intake (64 to 80 oz/day) is recommended to replenish fluid losses. A high-calorie, high-protein diet is typically prescribed to promote healing and prevent weight loss. The patient with an ileostomy usually requires lifelong injections of vitamin B_{12}.

Patient teaching

A patient with an ileostomy or colostomy needs to be educated about the effects of certain foods so he can adequately control symptoms. Use the lists below to help your patient identify the effects of certain foods.

Gas-producing foods
- Apples
- Asparagus
- Beans
- Beer
- Bran
- Broccoli
- Cabbage
- Carbonated beverages
- Cauliflower
- Celery
- Coconut
- Cream sauces
- Cucumber
- Eggs
- Fish
- Fried food
- Garlic
- Honey
- Melon
- Milk
- Nuts
- Onions
- Prunes
- Radishes
- Wheat
- Yeast

Foods that increase the risk of stomal blockage
- Cabbage
- Celery
- Coconut
- Corn
- Cucumber
- Dried fruit
- Green peppers
- Lettuce
- Nuts
- Olives
- Peas
- Pickles
- Pineapple
- Popcorn
- Seeds

Stool-thickening foods
- Applesauce
- Bananas
- Breads
- Cheese
- Creamy peanut butter
- Pasta
- Starchy foods

Odor-producing foods
- Asparagus
- Eggs
- Fish
- Garlic
- Green pepper
- Mustard
- Onions
- Radish
- Spicy foods

Deodorizing foods
- Buttermilk
- Cranberry juice
- Parsley
- Yogurt

trolytes, and nutrients. Patients typically don't seek medical treatment; instead, they treat themselves with over-the-counter remedies. Diarrhea can be acute (present for less than 2 weeks) or chronic (present for more than 2 weeks).

Pathophysiology

Diarrhea can have numerous causes; however, the basic pathophysiology is the same regardless of the cause. Here's what happens:

A substance irritates the intestinal mucosa. In response, the mucosa secretes mucus to serve as a protective barrier.

Cells secrete water and electrolytes, washing the irritating substance toward the anus.

Neuromuscular stimulation causes increased peristalsis and quickly helps rid the body of the irritating substance.

Acute

Acute diarrhea is typically caused by pathogens or medications. When caused by pathogens, they're usually ingested through contaminated food or water. Acute infectious diarrhea has a rapid onset after exposure to the infectious organism. Abdominal pain and fever occur when the organisms overwhelm the intestinal tract's normal defenses.

Some bacteria release endotoxins that stimulate the intestinal cells to release sodium, chloride, and water, worsening fluid and electrolyte loss. Some endotoxins act directly on the innervation of the GI tract, increasing peristalsis and thereby worsening fluid and electrolyte loss.

Acute diarrhea can also be caused by medications. Some medications, such as antibiotics and NSAIDs, irritate the lining of the intestine. In response, the intestinal tract secretes mucus and fluid in an attempt to wash away the irritating substance. Some medications, such as antihypertensive agents, antiarrhythmics, bronchodilators, and antineoplastics, affect the nervous system, causing increased peristaltic action.

Diarrhea may also be caused by accidental ingestion of toxins, such as insecticides or mushrooms, or by host-transplant reactions.

Chronic

Chronic diarrhea may result from:
• ongoing infection by such organisms as *Giardia, Clostridium difficile, Entamoeba histolytica, Cryptosporidium,* and *Campylobacter*
• human immunodeficiency virus infection (although the specific cause is unknown)
• lactose intolerance
• adverse reaction to medications

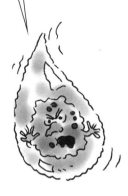

Pathogens like me can cause acute diarrhea if your patient ingests contaminated food or water.

- IBS
- IBD
- structural defects of the GI tract
- tumors.

Because chronic diarrhea typically occurs over a long time, nutritional deficiencies are common. The impaired absorption that occurs with diarrhea results in loss of electrolytes, minerals, vitamins, protein, and fats.

What to look for

The major manifestation associated with diarrhea is the frequent passage of watery stool. Abdominal pain and fever are seen with acute infectious diarrhea. In addition, dehydration and electrolyte imbalances are common.

How it's treated

Treatment of acute and chronic diarrhea differs.

Acute actions

Before initiating treatment of acute diarrhea, an accurate diagnosis must be made pinpointing the cause. Obtain a dietary history to determine where the patient has recently eaten. Question the patient about medical conditions that may reveal an organic cause. Also ask the patient about medications taken. A thorough physical examination and a stool culture are necessary to determine whether a pathogenic organism is present.

Antidiarrheal agents, such as diphenoxylate and atropine (Lomotil), can be given to slow peristalsis; however, these agents should be avoided in patients infected by pathogens. Slowing peristalsis in these patients allows pathogen overgrowth. Patients infected by pathogens require antibiotic therapy specific to the type of organism.

I.V. therapy is initiated if fluid and electrolyte imbalance is severe. If medication is the cause, the medication should be discontinued and an alternative medication prescribed. If an underlying disease process is the cause, measures should be taken to treat the disorder.

Chronic corner

For chronic diarrhea, treatment depends on the underlying cause. Stool cultures are obtained to check for and identify an infectious agent. If an infectious agent is identified, antibiotics are prescribed. If no infection is found, endoscopy

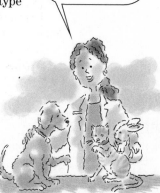

Unlike these guys, chronic diarrhea is never 'acute' problem.

may be performed to look for signs of inflammation or structural defects. A long-standing history of diarrhea may suggest irritable bowel syndrome.

Antidiarrheal medications, such as bismuth subsalicylate (Pepto-Bismol) or loperamide (Imodium), may be given to temporarily alleviate symptoms. Stronger antidiarrheals, such as opioid preparation, suppress peristalsis, allowing the absorption of water and electrolytes. These agents are especially effective in treating propulsive diarrhea.

Nutrition therapy

Nutrition therapy for acute diarrhea requires no intervention other than encouraging fluid intake to replace losses. I.V. fluid therapy may be necessary depending on the severity of acute diarrhea.

In patients with chronic diarrhea, withhold food intake for 24 to 48 hours. Administer I.V. fluid and electrolytes to treat fluid and electrolyte imbalances. After 48 hours, introduce a clear liquid diet. Provide a clear liquid diet for 1 to 2 days; then progress to a low-residue diet. Encourage the patient to consume the low-residue diet in small, frequent meals because they are better tolerated than three large meals. (See *Serving up a low-residue diet.*)

Encourage foods high in potassium, such as apricots, bananas, peaches, tomato juice, fish, potatoes, and meat, to replace losses. Patients with severe diarrhea who don't respond to medical treatment and nutrition therapy may require PN.

Constipation

Constipation, difficult or infrequent passage of stool, is a common complaint, especially among elderly patients. Constipation is exacerbated by poor nutrition, low fluid intake, and immobility. Individuals who complain of constipation experience prolonged periods of time between bowel movements and a sensation of incomplete evacuation after having one.

Despite what some people believe, it isn't necessary to have a bowel movement every day. Typically, people have at least three bowel movements per week.

Pathophysiology

Constipation occurs when decreased peristalsis results in prolonged transit time in the GI tract, allowing excessive fluid absorption. As a result, stool hardens, making it difficult to eliminate.

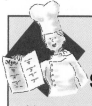

Menu maven

Serving up a low-residue diet

A low-residue diet restricts residue and fiber. It's effective against diarrhea because it slows transit time in the colon and reduces the frequency and volume of stool.

These foods may be included in a low-residue diet:
- meat, fish, or poultry (ground or well cooked)
- eggs
- milk (up to 2 c/day)
- fruit juices without pulp (excluding prune juice), canned fruits, and ripe bananas
- lettuce, vegetable juices without pulp, potatoes without skins, and most well-cooked vegetables without seeds
- breads (white, refined breads, rolls, biscuits, muffins, pancakes, crackers, and waffles)
- cereals (refined cereals, such as Cream of Wheat, Cream of Rice, and puffed rice)
- miscellaneous foods such as fruit ices, sherbet, ice cream (without nuts or coconut), gelatin, and marshmallows.

What's on the menu

Here's a sample menu containing low-residue foods.

Breakfast	*Lunch*	*Dinner*	*Snack*
• Apple juice	• Tomato juice	• Roasted chicken	• Melba toast
• Cream of rice	• Sandwich made with white	• Mashed potatoes	• ½ c milk
• Scrambled egg	bread, turkey, and mayon-	• Cooked carrots	
• White toast with butter and	naise	• French bread with butter	
jelly	• Canned peach halves	• Rice pudding	
• ½ c milk	• Gelatin	• ½ c milk	
• Coffee	• ½ c milk	• Cranberry juice	
	• Tea		

The longer stool remains in the colon, the more fluid is absorbed, making defecation more difficult and uncomfortable.

Predisposing factors include:
- sedentary lifestyle
- low-fiber diet
- dehydration
- depression
- aging
- systemic diseases (such as multiple sclerosis, Parkinson's disease, stroke, spinal cord injury, diabetes mellitus, thyroid disease, amyloidosis, systemic lupus erythematosus, and scleroderma)
- use of opioid analgesics (such as morphine)
- structural abnormalities (such as tumors, bowel obstruction, diverticulosis, and anal strictures).

What to look for

Signs and symptoms of constipation include:
- prolonged period of time between bowel movements
- abdominal cramping and bloating
- firm abdomen
- straining during defecation
- small, hard feces
- distant or muffled bowel sounds
- backache
- headache
- decreased activity level.

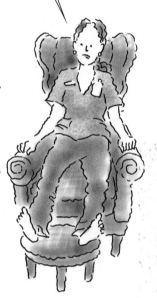

A sedentary lifestyle places patients at risk for constipation.

How it's treated

Before treating constipation, it's important to identify the underlying cause. Obtain an accurate health history. Question the patient about unexplained weight loss, rectal bleeding, or anemia. If present, diagnostic testing and follow-up treatment is warranted. Also ask the patient about medication usage.

Encouraging elimination

Lifestyle changes are successful in relieving constipation in most cases. Encourage regular aerobic exercise, which helps maintain neuromuscular function, control appetite, and enhance mood.

Explain the importance of establishing regular eating habits. Consuming food at the same times each day helps establish a regular pattern of intestinal stimulation and relaxation, which strengthens peristaltic contractions and decreases transit time through the colon. Moreover, when peristalsis becomes regular, a person can anticipate the urge to defecate and schedule around it.

Encourage the patient to increase fluid intake to at least eight 8-oz glasses per day. Drinks, such as hot coffee, tea, or lemon water help stimulate peristalsis. Inform the patient that prune juice has a laxative effect.

If diet and lifestyle changes are ineffective, fiber supplements such as Senna or Fibercon may be necessary. As a last resort, more potent medications, such as suppositories, osmotic laxatives, and stool softeners can be used temporarily. Stimulant laxatives should be avoided if possible. Rarely, an enema may be necessary.

Nutrition therapy

Typically a high-fiber diet is helpful in treating constipation because it increases stool bulk and speeds the passage of food

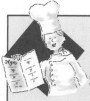

Menu maven

Serving up a high-fiber diet

A high-fiber diet substitutes high-fiber foods for those low in fiber. It alleviates constipation, lowers serum cholesterol levels, and improves glucose tolerance in diabetics. A high-fiber diet is also helpful in preventing and treating irritable bowel syndrome and diverticular disease. Encourage the patient to consume:

• breads and cereals—breads and cereals with an adequate fiber content provide 2 to 5 g of fiber per serving, and high-fiber cereals contain 7 to 11 g of fiber per serving.

• dry peas or beans

• fresh fruits and vegetables—fruits with the skin on should be eaten whenever possible. High-fiber fruits include apples, oranges, berries, nectarines, peaches, bananas, and pears. High-fiber vegetables include cabbage, greens, cauliflower, tomatoes, celery, and zucchini.

What's on the menu

Here's a sample menu containing high-fiber foods.

Breakfast	*Lunch*	*Dinner*	*Snack*
• Prune juice	• Bean soup	• Roast turkey	• Apple
• Milk	• Garden salad made with	• Brown rice	• Milk
• Multigrain toast with butter	lettuce, cheese, tomatoes,	• Zucchini	
• Apple	carrots, raw broccoli	• Fresh blueberries	
• Bran cereal	• Whole wheat roll	• Bran muffin with butter	
• Coffee	• Peach	• Milk	
	• Milk		

through the intestines. The American Dietetic Association recommends that adults consume 20 to 35 g of fiber daily. However, the average American adult typically consumes only one-half of the recommended amount. Adding the recommended amount of fiber to the diet isn't too difficult. (See *Serving up a high-fiber diet.*) For example, a slice of white bread has 1 g of fiber, whereas a slice of multigrain bread has 3 g. Substituting multigrain bread for white bread in a sandwich increases fiber intake by 4 g. Adding bran cereal, fruits, and vegetables to the diet can also greatly increase fiber intake.

Changing to a high-fiber diet may cause bloating, gas, or heartburn. Therefore, it's important for a patient to initiate a high-fiber diet slowly. Include these tips when teaching the patient to help ease his transition:

• Gradually add small amounts of fiber to the diet by making subtle changes in eating and cooking habits. Increase the size and number of portions slowly and cut back if symptoms appear.

- Read food nutrition labels and choose foods high in fiber. Switching to high-fiber breads and cereals can significantly increase fiber intake.
- Mix high-fiber foods with other foods; for example, try mixing cereals, adding fruit such as raisins or pears to salads, and using applesauce in recipes. Add bran or mashed beans to meat mixtures.
- Eat a meatless main dish with legumes at least once per week.
- Consume at least eight 8-oz glasses of fluid daily.

Viral hepatitis

Viral hepatitis is a common infection of the liver. In most patients, damaged liver cells eventually regenerate with little or no permanent damage. However, old age and serious underlying disorders make complications more likely.

Hepatitis may be caused by exposure to toxic substances such as carbon tetrachloride or medications that are toxic to the liver (excessive acetaminophen, for example).

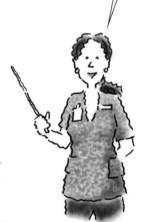

You read correctly, there's no hepatitis F. Non-hepatitis viral particles were mistakenly given this name. Now it's just a placeholder.

Pathophysiology

Viral hepatitis is marked by liver cell destruction, tissue death (necrosis), and self-destruction of cells (autolysis). It leads to jaundice, hepatomegaly, and anorexia. To date, six types of viral hepatitis have been identified: hepatitis A, B, C, D, E, and G. (See *Viral hepatitis from A to G*, pages 250 and 251.)

Different causes, same results

In general, the effects on the liver are usually similar among the different types of viral hepatitis. Varying degrees of liver cell injury and necrosis occur. However, the role hepatitis G plays in liver disease is unclear. This virus may cause a clinically similar systemic type of infection, affecting the liver.

What to look for

Early signs and symptoms of hepatitis infection include malaise, loss of appetite, nausea, diarrhea, and low-grade fever. As bilirubin excretion is impaired, urine becomes dark and jaundice develops. Tenderness over the right upper quadrant of the abdomen may also occur.

How it's treated

Interferon alpha, adefovir dipivoxil, and lamivudine have been approved for the treatment of patients with chronic hepatitis B. Interferon alpha and pegylated interferon in combination with ribavirin have been approved for the treatment of some patients with chronic hepatitis C. However, no specific drug therapy has been developed for the other forms of viral hepatitis. Treatment of viral hepatitis is mainly supportive:

- rest as needed
- I.V. hydration if vomiting is severe
- cholestyramine for severe pruritus.

Nutrition therapy

Providing nutrients to support recovery of hepatic tissue is the goal of nutritional therapy for hepatitis. A patient who's otherwise healthy should receive a well-balanced diet. A patient who was previously malnourished should be given a high-calorie, high-protein diet. Alcohol should be avoided to prevent further hepatic damage.

Calories

Between 25 and 30 cal/kg of body weight are recommended to meet energy needs and to avoid catabolism of protein. This intake also supports healing, such as correcting generalized dehabilitation and fever, and rejuvenates the body's strength and endurance.

Protein

Regeneration of tissue requires adequate protein intake. Protein is also responsible for manufacturing new hepatic tissues and cells. The recommended intake of protein is 75 to 100 g of protein daily. Because protein metabolism is sometimes impaired with liver disease, resulting in toxic concentrations of ammonia, this recommendation should be adjusted to individual tolerance. Usually hepatitis isn't so severe that it significantly impairs ammonia clearance. Protein should be restricted only if ammonia levels are elevated.

Carbohydrates

The diet should provide 300 to 400 g of carbohydrates daily. The glucose formed from carbohydrate metabolism helps to revitalize glycogen reserves in the liver. Glucose also prevents the breakdown of protein for energy and meets the increased energy demands brought about by the disease.

Viral hepatitis from A to G

This chart examines the features of each type of viral hepatitis.

Feature	Hepatitis A	Hepatitis B	Hepatitis C	Hepatitis D	Hepatitis E	Hepatitis G
Incubation	15 to 45 days	30 to 180 days	15 to 160 days	14 to 64 days	14 to 60 days	Unknown
Onset	Acute	Insidious	Insidious	Acute	Acute	Varies
Age-group most affected	Children, young adults	Any age	More common in adults	Any age	Age 20 to 40	More common in adults
Signs and symptoms	Symptomatic or asymptomatic; flulike symptoms, headache, malaise, fatigue, anorexia, fever, dark urine, jaundice of skin, tender liver	Symptomatic or asymptomatic, possible arthralgia, rash, jaundice	Similar to hepatitis B; less severe with less jaundice	Similar to hepatitis B	Similar to hepatitis A (very severe in pregnant women)	Similar to hepatitis C
Transmission	Fecal-oral, sexual (especially oral-anal contact), nonpercutaneous (sexual, maternal-neonatal), percutaneous (rare)	Blood-borne; parenteral route, sexual, maternal-neonatal (virus is shed in all body fluids)	Blood-borne; parenteral route	Parenteral route (sexual, maternal-neonatal, people infected with hepatitis D also infected with hepatitis B)	Primarily fecal-oral	Exposure to blood or body fluids; parenteral route
Severity	Mild	Often severe	Moderate	Possibly severe, leading to fulminant hepatitis	Highly virulent with common progression to fulminant hepatitis and hepatic failure, especially in pregnant patients	Unknown; questionable if leads to fulminant hepatitis

Viral hepatitis from A to G *(continued)*

Feature	Hepatitis A	Hepatitis B	Hepatitis C	Hepatitis D	Hepatitis E	Hepatitis G
Prognosis	Generally good	Worsens with age and debility	Moderate	Fair; worsens in chronic cases; can lead to chronic hepatitis D and chronic liver disease	Good unless pregnant	Unknown; results in chronic infection in 15% to 30% of adults
Progression to chronicity	None	Occasional	10% to 50% of cases	Occasional	None	Often a co-infection with hepatitis C; long-term significance associated with hepatitis C is unconfirmed

Fat

A moderate amount of fat in the diet encourages the patient to eat, which is necessary because of his poor appetite. This fat may come from vegetable oil or milk products. The amount of fat needed should range from 100 to 150 g daily.

Meal planning

Initially, treatment of hepatitis may require the administration of a liquid diet (as tolerated by the patient). As the patient's GI tolerance and appetite improve, advance to a solid diet. Be sure to obtain the patient's food preferences to optimize food intake.

In many cases, patients with hepatitis have poor appetites. Here are some tips for encouraging intake:
• Offer smaller meals more frequently.
• Find out dietary preferences and try to offer these foods in abundance.
• Use fats (in moderation) to make food appealing.
If the patient can't eat because of persistent vomiting, parenteral nutrition may be needed.

Cirrhosis

Cirrhosis, a chronic liver disease, is characterized by widespread destruction of hepatic cells. These cells are replaced by fibrous cells in a process called *fibrotic regeneration.* When a significant proportion of hepatic tissue is irreparably damaged, the liver can no longer perform its functions.

Cirrhosis may be caused by:

- excessive alcohol ingestion
- chronic hepatitis
- bile duct disease
- exposure to toxic chemicals, such as carbon tetrachloride
- late stage heart failure
- inherited metabolic disorders in which the body accumulates too much iron (hemochromatosis) or copper (Wilson's disease).

Cirrhosis is a common cause of death in the United States.

Pathophysiology

Cirrhosis is characterized by widespread destruction of hepatic cells; these cells are replaced by fibrous or fatty tissues. When this occurs, supporting structures are destroyed and strictures form, causing blockages of the hepatic blood flow.

There are different types of cirrhosis, each with its own etiology. The most common types are:

- postnecrotic cirrhosis—typically a result of a complication from viral hepatitis but also can be caused by exposure to a toxin (such as arsenic or phosphorus); more prevalent in women
- portal, nutritional, or alcohol-related cirrhosis—due to malnutrition and chronic alcoholism
- cardiac cirrhosis—due to prolonged venous congestion from right-sided heart failure
- biliary cirrhosis—caused by bile duct obstruction or inflammation of the bile duct
- idiopathic cirrhosis—unknown cause.

What to look for

In early stages of cirrhosis, signs and symptoms include loss of appetite, indigestion, nausea, vomiting, constipation, diarrhea, dull abdominal aching, fatigue, and jaundice. Later, signs and symptoms vary and reflect the resulting impairment of body functions and may include chronic dyspepsia, constipation, pruritus, weight loss, and bleeding tendencies. (See *Complications of cirrhosis.*)

Complications of cirrhosis

As cirrhosis progresses, impairment of other body systems and functions may occur.

Circulatory problems

Impedance of blood flow through the liver causes blood to back up into the veins that lead to the portal vein, causing portal hypertension. This has several serious consequences:

- esophageal varices form as blood backs up and causes the veins surrounding the esophagus to bulge into the esophageal lumen
- GI bleeding develops when esophageal varices burst and bleed into the esophagus and stomach
- ascites (abdominal edema) develops from portal hypertension as the higher pressures in the veins and low blood concentrations of protein (see below) allow diffusion of fluid from the blood into surrounding abdominal tissues; ascites causes early satiety and nausea and increases basal metabolic rate.

Metabolic problems

As the liver becomes unable to metabolize glucose, fats, and proteins, additional complications may include:

- impairment of protein metabolism, resulting in low concentrations of blood proteins (such as albumin)—These proteins are needed to maintain normal osmotic pressure in the circulatory system; without them, fluid diffuses from the blood into surrounding tissues, contributing to edema.
- impairment of bile production, resulting in loss of ability to digest fats—Bile is also an important excretory vehicle for bilirubin and, as bilirubin levels rise, jaundice ensues.

Coagulation problems

As cirrhosis progresses, the liver becomes unable to synthesize coagulating factors and store vitamin K, resulting in problems with blood clotting.

Vitamin deficiencies

Due to the liver's inability to create, utilize, and store certain vitamins (such as vitamins A, C, and K), evidence of deficiencies becomes apparent.

Anemia

Anemia results from the patient's poor dietary intake, impaired GI and liver function, and chronic gastritis. This, in turn, affects the patient's overall ability to carry out activities of daily living.

Mental impairment

Although the exact cause of mental deterioration isn't understood, it's believed to be linked to high ammonia levels. Ammonia is a natural by-product of protein metabolism, which occurs in the liver and intestine as normal bacteria break down long-chain amino acids. With cirrhosis, ammonia levels rise because the liver no longer converts ammonia into urea to be excreted in the urine.

Malnutrition

Due to inadequate intake, metabolism, and excretion, malnutrition is a prominent feature of cirrhosis. The situation is exacerbated in cases of chronic alcohol abuse, in which the GI tract may also be dysfunctional and unable to absorb certain nutrients.

How it's treated

Cirrhotic liver tissue can't be repaired, so the first goal of treatment of cirrhosis is to reduce further destruction by removing toxins (abstaining from alcohol, for example) or other causes. In addition, treatment aims to reduce blood pressure in the portal system and provide support for those functions the body can no longer perform.

Treatment commonly includes:
• antihypertensives and diuretics to treat portal hypertension and reduce edema
• oral antidiabetic agents to control blood glucose levels
• vitamin replacements
• coagulation factor replacement as needed
• electrolyte replacement (I.V. if necessary)
• blood transfusions if needed
• lactulose, an oral agent that draws ammonia into the intestine as an alternative method of excretion
• vasopressin, if necessary, to control esophageal varices
• antibiotics to decrease intestinal bacteria and reduce ammonia production, which causes encephalopathy
• paracentesis, infusions of salt-poor albumin, and salt and fluid restrictions to control ascites
• surgical procedures include treatment of varices by upper endoscopy with banding or sclerosis, splenectomy, esophagogastric resection, and splenorenal or portacaval anastomosis to relieve portal hypertension.

Nutrition therapy

Good nutritional intake is critical for the patient with cirrhosis. However, metabolism of nutrients is profoundly impaired in end-stage liver disease and difficult to achieve.

Calories

The patient with cirrhosis requires increased calories to meet the body's energy needs (120% to 175% of basal energy expenditure). The exact requirement depends on the presence of other factors, such as active infection and ascites. Caloric intake can be enhanced by using fats, such as butter on potatoes, bread, vegetables, and rice, and by using extra sugar in coffee. If steatorrhea develops (may result from lack of bile), fats may have to be restricted.

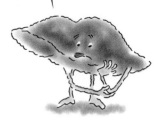

Oh dear! Damage to cirrhotic liver tissue can't be repaired so, initially, treatment is focused on preventing further destruction.

Protein

Protein intake can be a difficult aspect of nutritional therapy for the patient with cirrhosis because the body needs additional protein for healing and tissue building, but protein metabolism can lead to high levels of ammonia in the blood. Low protein intake (as low as 20 g/day) may be recommended if the patient has hepatic encephalopathy. Most patients can tolerate up to 1.5 g/kg/day. Monitor mental status and blood ammonia levels carefully.

Fluid

Fluids should be restricted to 1,000 to 1,500 ml/day initially to control edema. After edema subsides and blood protein levels rise, fluids may be increased to 2,000 ml/day or adjusted based on the patient's urine output (500 to 700 ml plus urine output/day).

Sodium

Sodium should also be restricted to control edema. Initially, sodium restriction may be as low as 2 g/day; it should gradually be increased as the patient's condition improves.

Vitamins and minerals

Nearly all vitamin stores are depleted in people with end-stage liver disease, so daily supplements are necessary. Calcium, magnesium, and zinc deficiencies are common.

Enteral and parenteral supplementation

At times, patients with cirrhosis can't meet their nutritional needs by oral ingestion, possibly as a result of mental impairment (encephalopathy), anorexia and vomiting, or GI bleeding. In these cases, enteral or parenteral nutrition may be necessary.

Formulas for patients with cirrhosis include those with branched-chain amino acids that, when metabolized, don't produce ammonia.

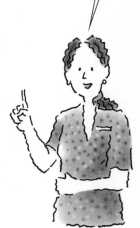

Initially, fluid and sodium should be restricted in the patient with cirrhosis to help control edema.

Gallbladder disease

Gallbladder disease typically refers to conditions involving the formation of stones (cholelithiasis) in the gallbladder. Stone formation can give rise to several related disorders. These include:
• cholecystitis (acute or chronic inflammation usually due to a stone becoming lodged in the cystic duct)
• choledocholithiasis (stones that pass out of the gallbladder and become lodged in the common bile duct)

• cholangitis (infection of the bile duct most commonly due to choledocholithiasis)
• gallstone ileus (obstruction of the small intestine by a gallstone).

Risky business

Certain risk factors predispose a person to stone formation. These include:
• high-calorie, high-cholesterol diet and associated obesity
• elevated estrogen levels from hormonal contraceptive use, postmenopausal hormone replacement therapy, or pregnancy
• use of clofibrate
• such diseases as diabetes mellitus, ileal disease, hemolytic disorders, hepatic disease, and pancreatitis.

Prognosis

Prognosis is usually good with treatment; however, if infection occurs, prognosis depends on the severity of the infection and the effectiveness of antibiotic treatment. (See *Gallbladder disease in middle age*.)

Lifespan lunchbox

Gallbladder disease in middle age

Generally, gallbladder disease occurs during middle age. In patients ages 20 to 50, occurrence is six times more common in women. After age 50, incidence in men and women equalizes and rises with each subsequent decade.

Pathophysiology

Gallbladder disease and its related disorders stem from a common cause: the formation of stones (calculi). Although the exact cause of stone formation is unknown, abnormal metabolism of cholesterol and bile salts clearly plays an important role.

Welcome to the stone age

Here's what's known about gallstone formation:
• The liver continuously makes bile, which the gallbladder concentrates and stores until it's needed for fat digestion.
• Changes in the composition of bile may cause gallstone formation. Changes in the gallbladder lining's absorptive ability may also play a part.
• Certain conditions, such as age, obesity, and estrogen imbalance, cause the liver to secrete bile that's abnormally high in cholesterol or that lacks the proper concentration of bile salts. When the gallbladder concentrates this bile, inflammation may occur. Excessive reabsorption of water and bile salts makes bile less soluble. Cholesterol, calcium, and bilirubin precipitate into gallstones.

Stone cold problems

When fat enters the duodenum, the intestinal mucosa secretes cholecystokinin, which stimulates gallbladder contraction and

Such factors as age and obesity can cause me to excrete bile that's high in cholesterol, which can result in gallstones.

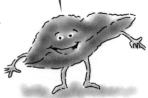

emptying. If stones are present, one can lodge in the cystic duct. The gallbladder then contracts but can't empty, causing it to become inflamed and distended. Bacteria growth, usually *Escherichia coli*, may contribute to the inflammation. Edema of the gallbladder obstructs bile flow, which irritates the gallbladder. Cells in the gallbladder wall may become oxygen starved and die as the distended organ presses on vessels and impairs blood flow. The dead cells slough off, causing the gallbladder to adhere to surrounding structures.

An alternative route

Alternatively, a stone can travel to the common bile duct and become lodged. When this happens, bile can't flow into the duodenum. Bilirubin is absorbed into the blood, causing jaundice. Biliary narrowing and swelling of the tissue around the stone can also cause irritation and inflammation of the common bile duct. This inflammation can travel the biliary tree into any of the bile ducts, causing scar tissue, fluid accumulation, cirrhosis, portal hypertension, and bleeding.

What to look for

Although the patient with gallbladder disease may be asymptomatic, acute cholelithiasis, acute cholecystitis, and choledocholithiasis produce these classic symptoms of a gallbladder attack:
• sudden onset of severe steady or aching pain in the midepigastric region or the right upper quadrant, possibly radiating to the back, the right shoulder or between the shoulders, or the front of the chest, that typically occurs after ingestion of a fatty meal or ingestion of a large meal after fasting for an extended time
• nausea and vomiting
• chills and low-grade fever
• jaundice (with common bile duct obstruction)
• dark-colored urine and clay-colored stools (with common bile duct obstruction and chronic cholecystitis).

Typically, the patient reports that milder GI symptoms preceded the acute attack. These symptoms may include indigestion, vague abdominal discomfort, belching, and flatulence after eating meals or snacks that are rich in fat.

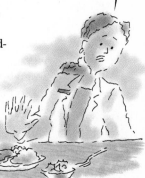

Hold the gravy! A gallbladder attack produces severe pain that typically occurs after eating a fatty meal.

How it's treated

During an acute attack, treatment focuses on administration of opioids for pain relief, antispasmodics and anticholinergic agents to relax smooth muscles and decrease ductal tone and spasm, and antiemetics to relieve nausea and vomiting. A nasogastric tube may be inserted and connected to low intermittent suction for abdominal decompression. I.V. fluids and antibiotics may be given to patients with severe acute chole-cystitis.

Lithotripsy (ultrasonic shock wave therapy) may be used to break up gallstones and to allow them to pass naturally. Oral urso-deoxycholic acid may be used to dissolve the stones.

Did someone say surgery?

Surgery, usually elective, remains the most common treatment of gallbladder disease. It's commonly recommended if the patient has symptoms frequent enough to interfere with his regular routine, if he has complications, or if he has had a previous attack of cholecystitis. Various surgical approaches may be used, including:
• cholecystectomy—removal of the inflamed gallbladder performed abdominally, laparoscopically, or percutaneously
• choledochostomy—creation of an opening into the common bile duct for drainage
• endoscopic retrograde cholangiopancreatography (ERCP)—for removal of gallstones.

Nutrition therapy

Nutrition therapy for patients with gallbladder disease focuses on minimizing stimulation of the gallbladder. Because fat is implicated in stimulating the gallbladder, a low-fat diet is typically suggested to reduce gallbladder stimulation and thus relieve pain. However, controversy exists about limiting fat in the diet. Several research studies demonstrate that the incidence of fat intolerance for patients with gallbladder disease is no greater than that for the general population. Therefore, dietary management is based on the individual's ability to tolerate specific foods.

If a patient is asymptomatic or has recovered from an initial attack of biliary colic, a low-fat diet usually is recommended. The amount of fat intake allowed varies, ranging from 20 to 60 g/day. (See *Serving up a low-fat diet.*)

Because of impaired bile secretion, deficiencies of fat-soluble vitamins may occur, necessitating vitamin replacement with water-soluble forms of vitamins A, D, E, and K. In addition, the patient is encouraged to eat small, frequent meals to prevent future attacks.

Coffee talk

Caffeinated and decaffeinated coffee have been shown to raise levels of cholecystokinin in the blood. Remember, cholecystokinin (released when fat enters the duodenum) stimulates the gallbladder to contract and empty; therefore, patients with gallbladder disease who are experiencing symptoms should avoid coffee.

Menu maven

Serving up a low-fat diet

When providing a low-fat diet for your patient, follow these suggestions for choosing foods:
- meat, poultry, fish, dry beans, eggs, and nut group—Use only lean cuts, skinless poultry, and egg whites or substitutes.
- milk, yogurt, and cheese group—Use fat-free milk products only.
- bread, cereal, rice, and pasta group—Use whole grains and enriched products.
- fruit and vegetable groups—All fruits and vegetables are allowed as long as they aren't prepared with fat.
- miscellaneous—Sherbet, gelatin, angel food cake, and graham crackers are allowed.

   The person on a low-fat diet should avoid:
- fatty or heavily marbled meats
- lunch meats
- egg yolks
- canned fish packed in oil
- fruits or vegetables prepared in butter or cream sauce
- whole, 2%, or 1% milk and milk products
- breads and bread products prepared with added fat, such as muffins, cakes, doughnuts, granola-type cereals, and buttered popcorn
- candy and most desserts
- creams and sauces.

What's on the menu
Here's a sample menu that's perfect for the low-fat diet:

Breakfast	*Lunch*	*Dinner*	*Snack*
• ½ c oatmeal (cooked)	• Tuna sandwich (3 oz of tuna salad prepared with 1 tbs of diet mayonnaise on 2 slices whole wheat bread)	• 3-oz grilled chicken breast	• 1 slice angel food cake
• Fat-free milk		• ½ c rice	• Fat-free milk
• Tea		• Peas and carrots	
• Whole wheat toast with 1 tsp margarine	• Tossed salad with fat-free dressing	• Tea	
	• 1 apple	• Fat-free milk	
	• Fat-free milk		

For acute cholecystitis
For the patient with acute cholecystitis, oral foods and fluids typically are withheld and I.V. fluid and electrolyte therapy is initiated. After 12 to 24 hours, the patient may be started on a clear liquid diet and may subsequently progress to a regular diet as tolerated.

After cholecystectomy

Controversy exists about the type of diet to follow after a cholecystectomy. Immediately after surgery, the patient should be given
nothing by mouth until bowel sounds return and then progress to
a regular diet as tolerated. In the postoperative period, some sur-
geons recommend a low-fat diet for 4 to 5 weeks whereas others
recommend a regular diet.

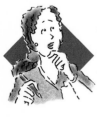

Quick quiz

1. Which intervention would be appropriate for a patient with
GERD?
  A.   Lying down immediately after eating
  B.   Eating chocolate
  C.   Drinking fat-free milk
  D.   Eating large, infrequent meals

Answer: C. A patient with GERD should consume foods that increase LES pressure, such as fat-free milk and nonfat milk.

2. Which factor is associated with the development of peptic ul-
cer disease?
  A.   *H. pylori* infection
  B.   Poor dietary habits
  C.   High-fat diet
  D.   Recent weight loss

Answer: A. *H. pylori* infection, NSAID use, and hypersecretory
conditions are the major causes of peptic ulcer disease.

3. A patient with dumping syndrome experiences light-headed-
ness, tachycardia, and diaphoresis 15 to 30 minutes after eating.
Which statement most likely explains these symptoms?
  A.   Hypoglycemia is occurring due to increased insulin se-
       cretion.
  B.   There's a sudden influx of stomach contents into the
       small intestine.
  C.   The patient has probably eaten too much too quickly.
  D.   The patient has eaten too many fatty foods.

Answer: B. Dumping syndrome is a complication of gastric
surgery that occurs when the pyloric sphincter is disturbed. Because the pyloric sphincter no longer functions, undigested food
is quickly dumped from the stomach into the small intestine. As
food digests in the jejunum, fluid shifts from the circulating blood

to the jejunum. The rapid decrease in circulating blood volume causes light-headedness, tachycardia, and diaphoresis.

4. Which of the following grains would be allowed on a diet specific for someone with celiac disease?
  A. Rye
  B. Wheat
  C. Corn
  D. Barley

Answer: C. Corn is the only grain listed here that doesn't contain gluten. A person with celiac disease needs to be on a gluten-free diet.

5. You're educating a patient with lactose intolerance about calcium-rich foods. Which of the following foods is a poor source of calcium?
  A. Sardines
  B. Yogurt
  C. Processed breakfast cereal
  D. Kale

Answer: C. Even though some breakfast cereals are calcium-fortified, most contain hidden lactose that would be unacceptable for the patient with lactose intolerance. Yogurt, despite being a dairy product, has been shown to be acceptable to patients with lactose intolerance because of its active cultures, which produce some of the lactase enzyme required for proper digestion.

6. A patient with chronic diarrhea is ordered to follow a low-residue diet. Which of the following foods would be an appropriate choice for this diet?
  A. Apples
  B. Rice pudding
  C. Zucchini
  D. Bran cereal

Answer: B. Rice pudding is a low-residue food.

7. A patient with cirrhosis would probably have which nutrient restricted to control ascites?
  A. Protein
  B. Calories
  C. Sodium
  D. Calcium

Answer: C. Sodium is restricted to reduce the edema associated with ascites.

Scoring

☆☆☆ If you answered all seven questions correctly, yippee! When it comes to understanding GI disorders, you're on the right tract.

☆☆ If you answered four to six questions correctly, keep up the good work! Your understanding of GI disorders is harmonious. It must be the tympany!

☆ If you answered fewer than four questions correctly, forge ahead. The malabsorption problems associated with this chapter won't hold you back from future intake.

Cardiovascular disorders

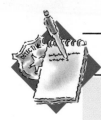

Just the facts

Nutrition can play a major role in the development of cardio-vascular disease. In this chapter, you'll learn:

♦ the role of nutrition in cardiovascular disease development

♦ modifiable and nonmodifiable risk factors for cardiovascular disease

♦ nutrition-based preventive and treatment measures for cardiovascular disease.

A look at cardiovascular disease

More than 61 million Americans have one or more forms of cardiovascular disease — the leading cause of death in the United States. Cardiovascular disease kills more people than cancer, chronic obstructive pulmonary disease, pneumonia, influenza, diabetes, and acquired immunodeficiency syndrome (AIDS) combined.

Assessment

To plan nutritional therapy for a patient with cardiovascular disease, first perform a nutrition-focused assessment that includes a health history, a physical examination, and diagnostic tests.

Health history

Obtain a history to assess the patient's cardiovascular status and evaluate cardiovascular risk factors. Gather information about the patient's:

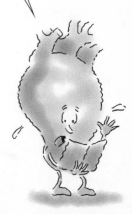

Yikes! Cardiovascular disease is the leading cause of death in the United States.

- dietary intake, especially of foods high in saturated fat and cholesterol
- use of low-fat or low-sodium products
- understanding of the nutrition facts panel on food labels
- knowledge of healthy eating habits
- willingness to change eating habits, if needed
- ability to buy and prepare healthy foods
- frequency of eating out
- physical activity and exercise
- religious and ethnic influences on food choices
- food allergies and intolerances
- use of alcohol, caffeine, tobacco, and recreational drugs
- use of nutritional supplements
- current and past medication use
- medical history
- personality traits, especially aggressiveness
- family history of heart disease and diabetes.

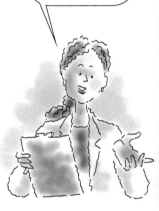

When taking your patient's health history for a nutritional assessment, be sure to gather information on his ability to buy and prepare healthy foods.

Assessing cardiovascular risk factors

The American College of Cardiology has identified four risk categories for cardiovascular disease, based on the effectiveness of treatments in reducing illness and death. Patients with categories I or II risk factors can lower their cardiovascular risks through such interventions as dietary changes, weight loss, blood pressure control, and smoking cessation.

Category I

Category I includes major risk factors for which interventions have been shown to lower cardiovascular risk. These risk factors include:
- cigarette smoking
- high total serum cholesterol level (200 mg/dl [SI, 5.18 mmol/L] or higher)
- high serum low-density lipoprotein (LDL) level (160 mg/dl [SI, 4.14 mmol/L] or higher)
- high dietary intake of saturated fats and cholesterol
- hypertension (140/90 mm Hg or higher).

Category II

Category II risk factors are those for which interventions are *likely* to lower cardiovascular risk. These risk factors include:
- diabetes mellitus
- low serum high-density lipoprotein (HDL) level (under 40 mg/dl [SI, 1.03 mmol/L])
- high serum triglyceride level (150 mg/dl [SI, 1.70 mmol/L] or higher)
- physical inactivity

- obesity
- postmenopausal status.

Category III

Category III risk factors are those for which interventions *may* lower cardiovascular risk. These risk factors include:
- psychological stress (hostility and social isolation are linked to a higher incidence of coronary artery disease [CAD])
- high blood homocysteine level (enzyme deficiency and inadequate intake of vitamins B_6, B_{12}, or folate are linked to a higher incidence of CAD)
- lipoprotein oxidation (vitamin E and other antioxidants may make LDL more resistant to oxidation, possibly helping to prevent CAD)
- excessive alcohol intake (moderate alcohol consumption may reduce cardiovascular risk by increasing HDL and flavanoids in the blood).

Category IV

Category IV risk factors are those that *can't* be modified or for which modification *isn't likely* to lower cardiovascular risk. These risk factors include:
- age — CAD risk increases with age (see *Age, gender, and cardiovascular risk*)
- gender — males have a higher risk
- race — Blacks and Mexican Americans have a higher risk (see *At greatest risk*)
- family history of early-onset heart disease.

Risk indicators
Diabetes, Framingham risk score, and metabolic syndrome are considered risk indicators for CAD.

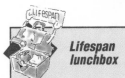

Lifespan lunchbox

Age, gender, and cardiovascular risk

Typically, coronary artery disease (CAD) appears in women 10 to 15 years later than it does in men, after age 65. When CAD occurs in younger women, it's generally due to the presence of multiple risk factors and metabolic syndrome. Although CAD is uncommon in both young men (age 20 to 35 years) and women (age 20 to 45 years), high cholesterol levels in this age-group may lead to the early onset of CAD in middle age. Early detection of and intervention for high low-density lipoprotein levels can slow or avert the appearance of CAD in the middle and later years.

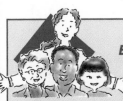

Bridging the gap

At greatest risk

Blacks, especially at younger ages, have a higher mortality rate and more out-of-hospital deaths due to coronary artery disease (CAD) than any other ethnic or racial group in the United States. This is partly due to the high number of CAD risk factors common in Blacks and genetic effects. High blood pressure, left ventricular hypertrophy, diabetes, cigarette smoking, obesity, and lack of physical activity are all common in this racial group.

CAD-diabetes link

Diabetes mellitus is considered a CAD risk equivalent because a patient with diabetes has the same risk of having a CAD event as someone who already has CAD.

Framing the risk with Framingham

If a person has two or more risk factors (other than high LDL levels) without CAD or a CAD risk equivalent, Framingham risk scoring is used to estimate the short-term (10-year) risk of heart disease. This scoring system considers the patient's age, total cholesterol level, smoking status, HDL level, and systolic blood pressure.

Metabolic mayhem

Metabolic syndrome, seen in about 25% of American adults, has emerged as an equal to cigarette smoking in contributing to early heart disease. Also called *syndrome X* or *insulin resistance syndrome*, metabolic syndrome encompasses a cluster of metabolic risk factors that significantly increase the risk of coronary events. The syndrome is diagnosed if the patient has three or more of the following factors:
• abdominal obesity (indicated by a waist circumference more than 40″ in men or 35″ in women)
• serum triglyceride level of 150 mg/dl (SI, 1.70 mmol/L) or higher
• HDL level below 40 mg/dl (SI, 1.03 mmol/L) in men or 50 mg/dl (SI, 1.29 mmol/L) in women
• blood pressure of 130/85 mm Hg or higher
• fasting serum glucose level of 100 mg/dl (SI, 5.6 mmol/L or higher).

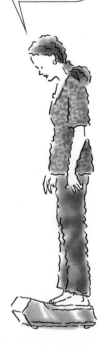

Focus the physical examination on nutrition-related aspects, such as weight and height.

A closer look at the risk factors

Central obesity, or fat contained within the abdominal cavity, is a strong predictor of metabolic syndrome. People with excess weight around their waists (apple-shaped bodies) are at increased risk for the syndrome--even more so than people who are equally overweight but with their weight distributed around the hips (pear-shaped bodies). The reason for this is that intraabdominal fat tends to be more resistant to insulin than does fat in the periphery of the body. Normally, insulin reduces the amount of free fatty acids in the liver. In people with insulin resistance, the excess free fatty acids that reach the liver cause apolipoprotein B levels to increase, low-density lipoprotein (LDL) levels to increase, high-density lipoprotein (HDL) levels to decrease, and triglyceride levels to increase, producing an abnormal endothelium and atherosclerosis, thereby increasing the risk of cardiovascular disease.

An elevated fasting blood glucose level greater than 100 mg/dl (SI, 5.6 mmol/L) is a hallmark for metabolic syndrome. People with diabetes commonly develop atherosclerotic heart disease at a young age, a condition that affects more diabetic women than men. Diabetes also increases the risk of macrovascular disease (ischemic heart disease, stroke, and peripheral vascular disease) and is a coronary heart disease risk equivalent.

In patients with insulin resistance, cells respond abnormally to insulin. For people who are genetically inclined to insulin resistance, abdominal obesity and sedentary lifestyle promote insulin resistance and metabolic syndrome. Insulin resistance leads to hyperinsulinemia, hyperglycemia, abnormal glucose and lipid metabolism, a damaged endothelium, and cardiovascular disease. The combination of insulin resistance, hyperinsulinemia, and abdominal obesity leads to hypertension and its harmful cardiovascular effects. Moreover, insulin resistance promotes salt sensitivity in people with high blood pressure.

Because metabolic syndrome is an independent risk factor in the development of cardiovascular disease as well as a strong predictor of type 2 diabetes, patients with this syndrome require intensive lifestyle modification. Changes that can prevent or reduce the effects of metabolic syndrome include weight loss, regular exercise, and dietary changes. (See *Ethnicities and metabolic syndrome.*)

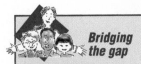

Bridging the gap

Ethnicities and metabolic syndrome

Metabolic syndrome is more common in Blacks and Mexicans. Among these ethnic groups, women are more susceptible than men to the disease. Other ethnic groups that are susceptible to metabolic syndrome include South Asians (from the Indian subcontinent), Southeast Asians (for example, people of Polynesian and Japanese descent), and Native Americans (such as Pima Indians).

Physical examination

Be sure to measure the patient's blood pressure and assess for signs and symptoms specific to cardiovascular disease. However, focus the physical examination on nutrition-related aspects, including:
• patient's height, current weight, usual weight, and weight history
• body mass index (BMI)
• waist circumference
• skinfold measurements
• body shape.

Body mass index

The BMI, which describes a person's weight relative to height, gives an acceptable estimate of body fat. (For instructions on calculating the BMI, see chapter 8, Assessing nutritional status.) According to 1998 federal guidelines, a BMI of less than 18.5 indicates underweight; 18.5 to 24.9, normal; 25 to 29.9, overweight; and 30 and above, obesity.

Waist circumference

Waist circumference reflects body fat distribution. A high distribution of abdominal fat is linked to greater cardiovascular risk than excess lower-body fat. A waist circumference over 40″ in men or 35″ in women indicates a higher risk of cardiovascular disease. (To determine the patient's waist circumference, see chapter 8, Assessing nutritional status.)

Waist circumference gives a more accurate picture of weight category in patients with large muscle mass, who might be classified as overweight in terms of BMI. For example, a female athlete has a BMI of 27 because of increased muscle mass (which adds to weight); as long as her waist circumference is under 35″, she wouldn't be considered overweight despite her high BMI.

Skin-fold measurements

Roughly one-half of total body fat is located directly under the skin. For this reason, measuring skin folds helps assess body fat percentage. Skin folds are measured with calipers that pinch the skin as it's pulled away from the underlying muscle. Skin fold may be measured at the triceps, biceps, thigh, calf, subscapular, or suprailiac areas.

Cardiovascular signs and symptoms

Assess your patient for physical indications of CAD, hypertension, and heart failure. Suspect CAD (or high risk of CAD) if the patient has an apple-shaped body or if you note xanthomas — fatty yellow nodules or tumors in the subcutaneous skin layer sometimes seen in patients with high blood cholesterol levels.

Inspect for edema and measure the patient's blood pressure. Presence of edema or high blood pressure may indicate hypertension. Edema, along with ascites and shortness of breath, also may accompany heart failure.

Diagnostic tests

To evaluate a patient for cardiovascular disease, the doctor may order various laboratory and diagnostic tests, including:
- total cholesterol, LDL, and HDL levels
- serum triglycerides
- C-reactive protein
- blood glucose
- electrocardiogram (ECG)
- stress test
- echocardiography

- cardiac catheterization.

For a patient with hypertension, the doctor may order tests to check for an underlying cause (such as kidney disease, diabetes, or adrenal dysfunction) and studies to detect cardiovascular damage and other complications, such as ECG and chest X-rays.

Diagnostic tests for a patient with suspected heart failure may include:

- ECG
- echocardiogram
- plasma b-type natriuretic peptide (BNP) assay
- chest X-ray
- pulmonary artery pressure monitoring.

Coronary artery disease

The most common form of cardiovascular disease, CAD impairs coronary blood flow, leading to a loss of oxygen and nutrients to myocardial tissue. This disease is nearly epidemic in the Western world. It's most prevalent in white, middle-aged men and in elderly patients. CAD is the leading cause of death in the United States in both men and women.

Pathophysiology

Atherosclerosis is the most common cause of CAD. In this condition, fatty fibrous plaques (possibly including calcium deposits) progressively narrow the lumen of the coronary arteries, reducing the flow of blood through them. This can lead to myocardial ischemia (decreased blood supply to the heart tissue) and infarction (a localized area of necrosis in the heart). (See *Acute coronary syndromes,* page 270.)

Atherosclerosis usually results from a high level of cholesterol and other fats in the blood. These fats build up within the arterial walls, causing narrowing of the lumen. The higher the patient's blood cholesterol level, the greater the chance that some cholesterol will be deposited along the arterial walls.

Attack of the plaques

In many people, atherosclerosis starts in childhood or adolescence and first appears as fatty streaks in the arteries. With age, these streaks worsen, becoming plaques, or atheromas, that protrude from the inside walls of the arteries and impede blood flow.

Because blood cholesterol is waxy and can't dissolve in water, it travels through the blood in lipoproteins. HDL—the "good" cho-

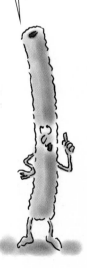

When plaques cause the lumen of the coronary artery to narrow, ischemia and infarction can occur.

Acute coronary syndromes

Acute coronary syndromes (ACS) is a general term that is used to describe a spectrum of disorders, including unstable angina and myocardial infarction (MI), that produce acute myocardial ischemia and, as a result, chest pain. Patients with ACS have some degree of coronary artery occlusion. The degree of blockage and the time that the affected vessel remains occluded are major determinants for the type of damage that occurs:

• If a patient has *unstable angina,* a thrombus partially occludes a coronary vessel. The partially occluded vessel may have distal microthrombi that cause necrosis in some myocytes. This condition may progress to *non-ST-segment elevation MI.*

• When a thrombus fully occludes the vessel for a prolonged time, this condition is known as a *ST-segment elevation MI.* In this type of MI, there's a greater concentration of thrombin and fibrin.

---

lesterol — gathers up excess cholesterol in the blood and carries it to the liver, which reprocesses or excretes it. HDL may also help remove some of the cholesterol deposited along the arterial walls. In contrast, LDL — the "bad" cholesterol — accumulates in body tissues.

Supply-side crisis

As atherosclerosis progresses, arterial narrowing is accompanied by vascular changes that impair the diseased vessel's ability to dilate. This causes a precarious balance between myocardial oxygen supply and demand, threatening the myocardium beyond the lesion. When oxygen demand exceeds what the diseased vessels can supply, localized myocardial ischemia results.

Transient ischemia leads to diminishing myocardial function; if left untreated, it can result in tissue injury or necrosis. Left ventricular function then becomes impaired. The strength of contractions in the affected myocardial region decreases as the fibers shorten inadequately with less force and velocity. As wall motion in the ischemic section becomes abnormal, less blood is ejected from the heart with each contraction.

Pressure and sympathy

Depression of left ventricular function may reduce stroke volume and thus lower cardiac output. Reduction in systolic emptying increases ventricular volumes. As a result, left-sided heart pressure

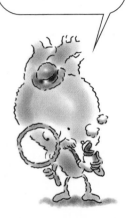

It's elementary, really — just a problem of supply and demand.

and pulmonary artery wedge pressure rise. Changes in wall compliance induced by ischemia magnify these pressure increases.

During ischemia, sympathetic nervous system response causes slight rises in blood pressure and heart rate before the onset of pain. With pain onset, further sympathetic activation occurs.

What to look for

Angina, the classic sign of CAD, may range from mild and intermittent to pronounced and steady. However, it isn't always present. Some people with CAD are symptom-free. The patient may describe angina as a burning, squeezing, or crushing pain or tightness in the substernal or precordial area that radiates to the left arm, neck, jaw, or shoulder blade.

Angina commonly follows physical exertion but may also follow emotional excitement, cold exposure, or a large meal. Sometimes, it develops during sleep and awakens the patient.

Stable or unstable?

If the pain is predictable and relieved by rest or nitrates, it's called *stable angina*. If it increases in frequency and duration and is more easily induced, it's called *unstable* or *unpredictable angina*. Left untreated, unstable angina may progress to myocardial infarction (MI).

Patients typically describe the symptoms of an MI as uncomfortable pressure, squeezing, burning, severe persistent pain or fullness in the center of the chest lasting several minutes (usually longer than 15 minutes). Pain may radiate to the left arm, shoulders, neck, or jaw or may occur in the back between the shoulder blades. The patient may clench his fist over his chest or rub his left arm when describing it. Pain may be accompanied by nausea, vomiting, fainting, sweating, and cool extremities.

Treatment

The primary goal of therapy for a patient with CAD is to lower serum LDL levels. Recent clinical trials confirm that lowering LDL reduces the short-term risk of heart disease by as much as 40% and brings even greater risk reduction over time.

Adult Treatment Panel III

In 2004, the Adult Treatment Panel III (ATP III), sponsored by the National Cholesterol Education Program of the National Institutes of Health (NIH), updated its guidelines on cholesterol management. ATP III recommends:

Classifying cholesterol levels

The Adult Treatment Panel III of the National Cholesterol Education Program (National Institutes of Health) has published guidelines for classifying levels of total, low-density-lipoprotein (LDL), and high-density-lipoprotein (HDL) cholesterol. Use the chart below when assessing your patient's lipoprotein profile.

Level	Profile
LDL cholesterol	
< 100 mg/dl (SI, < 2.59 mmol/L)	Optimal
100 to 129 mg/dl (SI, 2.59 to 3.34 mmol/L)	Near optimal/Above optimal
130 to 159 mg/dl (SI, 3.36 to 4.12 mmol/L)	Borderline high
160 to 189 mg/dl (SI, 4.14 to 4.90 mmol/L)	High
$\geq$ 190 mg/dl (SI, $\geq$ 4.92 mmol/L)	Very high
HDL cholesterol	
< 40 mg/dl (SI, < 1.03 mmol/L)	Low
$\geq$ 60 mg/dl (SI, $\geq$ 1.55 mmol/L)	High (desirable)
Total cholesterol	
< 200 mg/dl (SI, < 5.18 mmol/L)	Desirable
200 to 239 mg/dl (SI, 5.18 to 6.19 mmol/L)	Borderline high
$\geq$ 240 mg/dl (SI, $\geq$ 6.2 mmol/L)	High

Adapted from *High Blood Cholesterol.* National Institutes of Health, National Heart, Lung and Blood Institute: National Cholesterol Education Program, May 2001, no. 01-3670. *www.nhlbi.nih.gov/guidelines/cholesterol/atp3xsum.pdf.*

• more aggressive cholesterol-lowering treatment, which includes a therapeutic option to treat LDL to a lower end point in very-high-risk patients, and better identification of people at high risk for MI
• a complete lipoprotein profile as the first test for high cholesterol (see *Classifying cholesterol levels.*)
• increased focus on treating high triglyceride levels
• emphasis on the cutoff point at which a low HDL level becomes a major CAD risk factor
• new, more powerful lifestyle changes to improve cholesterol levels
• a sharper focus on metabolic syndrome.

Matching treatment to risk

The ATP III recommends that doctors tailor the intensity of LDL-lowering treatment to the patient's cardiovascular risk level. It divides patients with multiple risk factors into three categories based on their 10-year risk for CAD (see "Step 4" below).

ATP III guidelines focus on a stepped treatment plan, with nine steps progressing according to the patient's cholesterol profile and risk factors.

Step 1

Obtain a complete lipoprotein profile using blood samples drawn after a 9- to 12-hour fast.

Step 2

Identify clinical atherosclerotic disease that confers a high risk of CAD events or a CAD risk equivalent. These include clinical CAD, symptomatic carotid artery disease, abdominal aortic aneurysm, and peripheral arterial disease.

Step 3

Count the number of major risk factors a patient has, other than a high LDL level. Major risk factors include:
• cigarette smoking
• hypertension (blood pressure of 140/90 mm Hg or higher) or use of antihypertensive medication
• HDL level below 40 mg/dl (SI, 1.03 mmol/L) (HDL level greater than 60 mg/dl (SI, 1.55 mmol/L) removes a risk factor from the count)
• family history of premature CAD (CAD in a male first-degree relative under age 55 or in a female first-degree relative under age 65)
• age 45 or older (male) or 55 or older (female).

Step 4

Assess the patient's level of 10-year cardiovascular risk. (Presence of CAD or CAD risk equivalent automatically places the patient in the highest risk category.) Count the number of risk factors the patient has (excluding high LDL level and presence of CAD). If he has two or more risk factors, the Framingham scoring system is used to determine risk level and intensity of therapy.

The three risk categories are:
• above 20% (CAD and CAD risk equivalent)
• 10% to 20% (two or more risk factors)
• less than 10% (one or zero risk factors).

Memory jogger

To remember the major risk factors for CAD, think **ASHHH**:

Age (males 45 or older; females 55 or older)

Smoking

Hypertension

History of CAD in family

HDL level < 40 mg/dl.

Step 5

Determine the patient's LDL goal of therapy, need for therapeutic lifestyle changes (TLC), and LDL level at which drug therapy should be considered:

• *Risk above 20%*—LDL goal is less than 100 mg/dl (SI, 2.59 mmol/L). Begin TLC if LDL is 100 mg/dl or higher. Begin drug therapy if LDL is 130 mg/dl (SI, 3.36 mmol/L) or higher. The ATP III 2004 update adds an LDL goal of less than 70 mg/dl (SI, 1.81 mmol/L) for very-high-risk patients (such as patients with recent MIs or those who have cardiovascular disease and diabetes, poorly controlled risk factors, or metabolic syndrome). The update also recommends consideration of drug therapy and the therapeutic lifestyle changes if LDL level is 100 mg/dl or higher in high-risk patients. Drug therapy is optional in patients with LDL levels less than 100 mg/dl. The update also advises that the goal of drug therapy is to reduce the LDL level by 30%.

• *Risk of 10% to 20%*—LDL goal is less than 130 mg/dl (SI, 3.36 mmol/L). Begin TLC if LDL is 100 mg/dl or higher. Begin drug therapy if LDL is 130 mg/dl or higher. The ATP III 2004 update adds the option of setting an LDL goal at less than 100 mg/dl (SI, 2.59 mmol/L) and starting drug therapy if LDL level is 100 to 129 mg/dl (SI, 3.34 mmol/L). The goal is to reduce the LDL level by 30%.

• *Risk below 10%*—LDL goal is less than 160 mg/dl (SI, 4.14 mmol/L). Begin TLC therapy if LDL is 160 mg/dl or higher. Begin drug therapy if LDL is 190 mg/dl (SI, 4.92 mmol/L) or higher. Consider drug therapy optional if LDL level is 160 to 189 mg/dl (SI, 4.90 mmol/L).

Step 6

If the patient's LDL is above the goal for his risk level, initiate TLC, including the TLC diet, weight management, and increased physical activity. The TLC diet recommends eating only enough calories to maintain a desirable weight and avoid weight gain. Other highlights include:

• restricting saturated fats to less than 7% of daily calories
• keeping cholesterol intake under 200 mg/day
• as an option, increasing soluble fiber intake (from the recommended 5 to 10 g/day to 10 to 25 g/day) and intake of plant stanols or sterols (2 g/day) to enhance LDL lowering. (See *Nutrient composition of TLC diet.*)

Step 7

Consider starting drug therapy if the patient's LDL exceeds the levels specified in step 5. To maximize cholesterol lowering, TLC should always be maintained when drug therapy is prescribed.

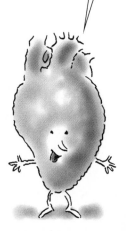

To lower your patient's cholesterol, try a little TLC!

Nutrient composition of TLC diet

Nutrient	Recommended intake
Saturated fat*	Less than 7% of total calories
Polyunsaturated fat	Up to 10% of total calories
Monounsaturated fat	Up to 20% of total calories
Total fat	25 to 35% of total calories
Carbohydrate**	50 to 60% of total calories
Fiber	20 to 30 g/day
Protein	Approximately 15% of total calories
Cholesterol	Less than 200 mg/day
Total calories (energy)***	Balance energy intake and expenditure to maintain desirable body weight/prevent weight gain

* Trans fatty acids are another LDL-raising fat that should be kept at a low intake.
** Carbohydrates should be derived predominantly from foods rich in complex carbohydrates, including grains, especially whole grains, fruits, and vegetables.
*** Daily energy expenditure should include at least moderate physical activity (contributing approximately 200 kcal per day).

Source: U.S. Department of Health and Human Services, National Institutes of Health, National Heart, Lung, and Blood Institute (*www.nhlbi.nih.gov/guidelines/cholesterol/atp3xsum.pdf*). "Third Report of the National Cholesterol Education Program (NCEP) Expert Panel on Detection, Evaluation, and Treatment of High Blood Cholesterol in Adults (Adult Treatment Panel III)." NIH Publication No. 01-3670, May 2001.

Drug therapy may include:
• statin drugs (such as lovastatin, pravastatin, and simvastatin), which have been shown to be effective in persons with or without CAD (in clinical trials, lowering of LDL levels with statins decreased the rate of MI and deaths from CAD by roughly 30%); these drugs may be used in combination with other lipid-lowering drugs
• bile acid sequestrants (such as cholestyramine and colestipol), which also lower LDL levels and may be used alone or in combination with statins

• nicotinic acid (niacin), which lowers LDL and triglyceride levels and raises HDL levels (however, when taken in doses large enough to lower cholesterol, it can cause adverse effects, so it should be used only under a doctor's supervision)
• fibric acids (such as gemfibrozil and fenofibrate), which are used mainly to treat high triglyceride levels and low HDL levels
• cholesterol absorption inhibitors (ezetimibe) reduce total cholesterol and LDL levels and may slightly increase HDL levels
• combination cholesterol absorption inhibitor and statin (ezetimibe/simvastatin) reduces LDL and triglyceride levels and increases HDL levels.

Step 8

Assess the patient for the indicators of metabolic syndrome. A patient who meets diagnostic criteria should receive treatment for metabolic syndrome after 3 months of TLC. Therapies center on addressing obesity, increasing physical activity, lowering blood pressure and serum triglyceride levels, raising HDL levels, and using aspirin to reduce prothrombotic states in patients with CAD.

Step 9

A patient with elevated triglyceride levels (150 mg/dl or higher) should take steps to manage weight, increase physical activity and, if needed, start an LDL-lowering drug, nicotinic acid, or fibric acid.

Nutrition therapy

A heart-healthy diet is essential to controlling and managing CAD. This diet can slow the progression of atherosclerosis. When combined with other heart-healthy strategies, it may even stop or reverse narrowing of arteries. What's more, a heart-healthy diet can help reduce total cholesterol and LDL levels, lower blood pressure and blood glucose levels, and aid weight management. (See *Sample menu for the TLC diet.*)

Focus on fat

To help your patient reduce high cholesterol levels, recommend a diet that's low in fat. Advise him to restrict total fat intake (saturated, trans-, monounsaturated, and polyunsaturated fats) to 25% to 35% of total daily calories and to restrict saturated and trans-fat intake to less than 7%. Instruct him to keep dietary cholesterol intake under 200 mg daily.

Remind the patient that lowering dietary fat intake promotes weight loss. If the patient is overweight, losing excess weight can help lower blood cholesterol as well as high blood pressure — another risk factor for atherosclerosis and heart disease. If the patient eats out a lot, maintaining a heart-healthy diet can pose a

Menu maven

Sample menu for TLC diet

The therapeutic lifestyle change (TLC) diet aims to reduce low-density-lipoprotein levels by promoting intake of foods low in saturated fat and cholesterol. Here's a sample menu of traditional American cuisine for a male age 25 to 49. Less than 7% of daily calories should come from saturated fat, and cholesterol intake is limited to no more than 200 mg of dietary cholesterol per day.

Breakfast
Oatmeal (1 cup)
 Fat-free milk (1 cup)
 Raisins (¼ cup)
English muffin (1 medium)
 Soft margarine (2 tsp)
 Jelly (1 Tbsp)
Honeydew melon (1 cup)
Orange juice, calcium fortified
 (1 cup)
Coffee (1 cup) with fat-free
 milk (2 tbsp)

Lunch
Roast beef sandwich
 Whole-wheat bun
 (1 medium)
 Roast beef, lean (2 oz)
 Swiss cheese, low fat
 (1 oz slice)
 Romaine lettuce (2 leaves)
 Tomato (2 medium slices)
 Mustard (2 tsp)
Pasta salad
 Pasta noodles (¾ cup)
 Mixed vegetables (¼ cup)
Olive oil (2 tsp)
Apple (1 medium)
Iced tea, unsweetened
 (1 cup)

Dinner
Orange roughy (3 oz) cooked
 with olive oil (2 tsp)
 Parmesan cheese (1tbsp)
Rice* (1½ cup)
Corn kernels (½ cup)
 Soft margarine (1 tsp)
Broccoli (½ cup)
 Soft margarine (1 tsp)
Roll (1 small)
 Soft margarine (1 tsp)
Strawberries (1 cup) topped
 with low-fat frozen yogurt
 (½ cup)
Fat-free milk (1 cup)

Snack
Popcorn (2 cups) cooked with
 canola oil (1 tbsp)
Peaches, canned in water
 (1 cup)
Water (1 cup)

Nutrient analysis

Calories	2,523	Total fat, % calories	28
		Saturated fat, % calories	6
Cholesterol (mg)	139	Monounsaturated fat, % calories	14
		Polyunsaturated fat, % calories	6
Fiber (g)	32	Trans fat (g)	5
Soluble (g)	10	Omega 3 fat (g)	0.4
Sodium (mg)	1,800	Protein, % calories	17
Carbohydrates, % calories	57	*Higher fat alternative	
		Total fat, % calories	34

*For a higher fat alternative, substitute ⅓ cup unsalted peanuts, chopped (to sprinkle on the frozen yogurt) for 1 cup of the rice.

Source: U.S. Department of Health and Human Services, National Institutes of Health, National Heart, Lung, and Blood Institute (*www.nhlbi.nih.gov/guidelines/cholesterol/atp3full.pdf*). "Third Report of the National Cholesterol Education Program (NCEP) Expert Panel on Detection, Evaluation, and Treatment of High Blood Cholesterol in Adults (Adult Treatment Panel III)." NIH Publication No. 01-3670, May 2001.

NutriTips

Tips for eating out

If your patient eats out a lot, pass on these hints to help him eat healthier when dining out:
• Choose restaurants that offer low-fat, low-cholesterol menu choices. As a paying customer, don't be afraid to make special requests.
• Don't let the restaurant dictate your portion size, and don't feel compelled to eat everything because you're paying for it. Ask for a small serving, share a dish with a friend, or take some home for another meal.
• Limit such extras as gravy, butter, rich sauces, and salad dressings. Ask that these items be served on the side so you can control the amount.
• Avoid fried foods in favor of foods that are baked, broiled, grilled, or stir-fried.
• Choose extra vegetables and salad whenever possible.

• If you must have dessert, split it so you only eat half the portion.
• At a buffet, choose mostly low-fat foods. If you just can't resist a few higher-fat items, keep portions small.
• When attending a potluck dinner, bring low-fat options. That way, you'll have a few healthy items to add to those that may not be as low in fat.
• At parties, don't fixate on food. Instead, focus on the people and activities.
• Encourage others to help you reduce your fat intake. If you're invited to a friend's home for dinner, ask the friend to include low-fat dishes.
• If you eat too many high-fat foods, don't feel guilty and go on a binge. Just eat lightly the next day to get back on track.

---

challenge. Provide appropriate suggestions. (See *Tips for eating out.*)

Cut the cholesterol

Point out to the patient that cholesterol comes in two different types—blood (serum) cholesterol and dietary cholesterol. Dietary cholesterol is found in foods of animal origin, including egg yolks, organ meats, and full-fat dairy products. Blood cholesterol is a waxy substance that occurs naturally in the body.

Many patients think that just avoiding foods high in cholesterol will lower their serum cholesterol level. However, the body continues to make cholesterol no matter what kind of diet a person eats. Controlling *total* fat intake—and saturated fat in particular—has a more direct impact on blood cholesterol levels.

Dish out the dietary do's, not the don'ts

To help the patient succeed with a heart-healthy diet, focus on what he *can* eat rather than what he can't. Stress that a well-balanced diet—one that relies on fruits, vegetables, whole grains, legumes, lean meat, low-fat dairy products, and a minimum amount of added fat—is the key. Emphasize that the goal is to *lower* fat intake—not eliminate fats entirely. Fats play an impor-

> If it sounds too good to be true, it probably is. Make sure your patient understands that fat-free usually doesn't mean calorie-free.

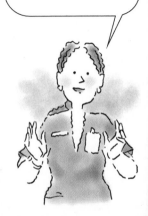

tant role in the body, providing storage of calories for energy, insulation, and a means for transporting fat-soluble vitamins.

Fat-free fallacies

Tell the patient that limiting calories is important, too — especially if he must lose excess weight. Point out that fat-free foods aren't calorie-free. Many fat-free and low-fat foods and beverages have added sugars to make them taste better. These sugars increase calories — that's why a fat-free or low-fat food may still be high in calories. In fact, some fat-free foods contain nearly the same number of calories as their high-fat counterparts.

Serving savvy

When teaching your patient about a heart-healthy diet, recommend the following measures:
• Eat at least two servings of fruits or vegetables at each meal. Choose fruits as between-meal snacks. They're the healthiest "fast food." (In cultures where people consume a lot of fruits, vegetables, and grains and relatively little meat, CAD rates are far lower than in cultures that consume a lot of meat and high-fat, high-sugar foods.)
• Eat more whole grains, such as whole grain breads, brown rice, barley, oatmeal, and soluble fiber.
• Pay attention to total fat intake. Choose low-fat dairy products and lean meats. Watch out for high-fat desserts and snacks.
• Reduce intake of saturated fat and fats that act like saturated fat, such as hydrogenated fat and trans-fat. (See *Fat facts: The good, the bad, and the ugly*, page 280.)
• Use more monounsaturated fats (canola oil and olive oil).
• Taste food before adding salt. A yen for salt is a learned taste — it can be unlearned, too. Getting used to less salty foods takes about 6 weeks.
• Mind portion size. Just about any food can be consumed in moderation.
• Make balanced meals. The meat portion should take up no more than one-third of the plate. Two servings of vegetables and one serving of starch should accompany the main course. Adding a green, leafy salad with additional raw vegetables tossed in, topped with a light or fat-free salad dressing, earns an "A."

Vitamins for healthy vessels

Numerous studies from around the world suggest that getting enough folic acid and vitamins B_6 and B_{12} can help maintain a healthy heart and blood vessels. Folic acid and vitamins B_6 and B_{12} work in combination to reduce the blood level of homocysteine, a natural product of protein breakdown in the blood. Scien-

Fat facts: The good, the bad, and the ugly

Fats (fatty acids) come in many varieties—some good, some bad, and some really bad. To help your patient plan a heart-healthy diet, make sure you understand the various types.

Good

Monounsaturated fats
Monounsaturated fats are found mainly in canola oil, olive oil, peanut oil, and avocados. These fats are liquid at room temperature.

Polyunsaturated fats
Polyunsaturated fats are found in soybean, sesame, sunflower, and safflower seeds and their oils. They're also the main fats found in seafood. These fats are liquid or soft at room temperature. Specific polyunsaturated fatty acids, such as linoleic acid and alpha-linoleic acid, are called *essential fatty acids* because they're necessary for cell structure and making hormones. Essential fatty acids must be obtained from foods.

Bad

Saturated fats
Saturated fats are found chiefly in animal sources, such as meat, poultry, whole or reduced-fat milk, and butter. Some vegetable oils, such as coconut, palm kernel oil, and palm oil, are saturated. Saturated fats are usually solid at room temperature.

Dietary cholesterol
Dietary cholesterol is found in foods of animal origin, such as meat, pork, poultry, fish, eggs, and full-fat dairy products.

Ugly

Trans fatty acids
Trans fatty acids (trans-fats, for short) form when vegetable oils are processed into margarine or shortening. Sources of trans-fats in the diet include snack foods and baked goods made with partially hydrogenated vegetable oil or vegetable shortening. Trans fatty acids also occur naturally in some animal products, such as dairy products.

---

tific evidence shows that lower blood homocysteine levels are associated with reduced risk of heart disease.

The leading sources of folic acid are ready-to-eat cereals, enriched breads, fruits, vegetables, citrus juice, and dry beans. In 1998, the Food and Drug Administration (FDA) required that folic acid be added to enrich grain-based staples such as bread, pasta, and rice. At the same time, the FDA authorized ready-to-eat-cereals to be fully fortified up to 100% of the daily value of folic acid (400 mcg)—the only food permitted to contain this high level.

Vitamin B_6 is widely distributed in foods. Significant sources include meats, whole wheat products, vegetables, and nuts. Vitamin B_{12} is found in animal products only—particularly meat, milk, eggs, fish, and cheese.

Fiber-ific facts

Only plant foods, such as fruits, vegetables, and grains, contain fiber. The part of the plant fiber that's consumed, called *dietary fiber*, is an important part of a heart-healthy diet.

Dietary fiber comes in two main types—insoluble and soluble. Soluble fiber forms a gel when mixed with liquid, whereas insoluble fiber passes through the GI tract largely intact. Both types of fiber are important in the diet and help maintain regular bowel movements.

Soluble fiber has additional cardiovascular health benefits. It has been proven to reduce blood cholesterol levels, which may help reduce the risk of heart disease.

Set your sights on psyllium

Soluble fiber is found in oats, peas, beans, certain fruits, and a grain called *psyllium*, found in some cereal products, dietary supplements, and bulk fiber laxatives. Instruct the patient to read food, supplement, and drug labels carefully to check for psyllium. (See *How much fiber?*)

Judging a food by its label

Food labels have two important parts: the Nutrition Facts panel and the ingredients list. Instruct the patient to read the Nutrition Facts panel to check the amount of saturated fat, transfat, total fat, cholesterol, and calories in one serving of the product and then compare similar products to find the one with the lowest amounts. If he has high blood pressure, he should do the same for sodium.

Tell the patient that the ingredients are listed in descending order by weight. For instance, if sugar is listed first on a cereal product, the cereal has more sugar than any other ingredient. To choose foods low in saturated fat or total fat, advise the patient to limit food products that list any fat or oil first—or that list many fat and oil ingredients. If he's watching his sodium intake, tell him to do the same for sodium or salt.

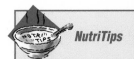

NutriTips

How much fiber?

Health experts recommend that Americans eat 25 to 38 g of fiber each day, including soluble and insoluble fiber. The average American eats only 12 to 17 g/day; about one-fourth is soluble fiber. This means the average American eats only 3 to 4 g/day of soluble fiber—less than half of the recommended 5 to 10 g/day. Daily intake of 3 g of soluble fiber from oats or 7 g from psyllium has been shown to lower blood cholesterol levels.

Hypertension

Hypertension (high blood pressure) is a consistent blood pressure of 140/90 mm Hg or higher. The major types of hypertension are essential (also called *primary* or *idiopathic*) and secondary.

The cause of essential hypertension, the most common type, involves several interacting homeostatic mechanisms. Hypertension is classified as secondary if it's related to a systemic disease that raises peripheral vascular resistance or cardiac output. Malignant hypertension is a severe fulminant form of the disorder that may arise from either primary or secondary hypertension.

> Tell your patient to read the fine print! If sugar is listed first, there's more sugar than any other ingredient!

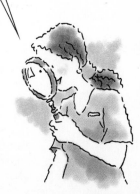

No news isn't good news

Hypertension is often called a *silent killer* because it causes few, if any, symptoms. A person may have it for years without knowing it. Of the roughly 65 million Americans who have hypertension, about one-third don't know it. Uncontrolled hypertension can damage the kidneys and lead to stroke, MI, and heart failure.

In 2003, the National Institutes of Health created a new category, called prehypertension, which includes blood pressure readings of 120 to 139/80 to 89 mm Hg, levels previously considered normal or high-normal. Normal blood pressure is defined as less than 120/80 mm Hg. Research indicates that people with prehypertension are twice as likely to develop cardiovascular disease than people with blood pressure values less than 120/80 mm Hg. For each increase of 20/10 mm Hg, the risk of developing cardiovascular disease doubles. The risk of death from heart disease and stroke rises with increasing blood pressure readings, starting as low as 115/75 mm Hg. It's estimated that 60 million people in the United States previously thought to have normal blood pressure readings are now considered prehypertensive. (See *Classifying blood pressure readings.*)

Pathophysiology

Hypertension may result from increases in cardiac output, total peripheral resistance, or both. Cardiac output rises from conditions that increase the heart rate or stroke volume. Peripheral resistance rises from factors that increase blood viscosity or reduce vessel lumen size. (See *Isolated systolic hypertension in elderly patients.*)

Essentially preventable

Essential hypertension usually starts insidiously as a benign disease and progresses slowly to a malignant state. If untreated, even mild cases can cause major complications and death. Carefully managed treatment, which may include lifestyle changes and drug therapy, improves prognosis.

In theory...

Various theories help explain the development of hypertension. For example, it's thought to arise from:
• changes in the arteriolar bed that cause increased resistance
• abnormally increased tone in the sensory nervous system that arises in the vasomotor centers, increasing peripheral vascular resistance
• greater blood volume resulting from renal or hormonal dysfunction

Classifying blood pressure readings

In 2003, the National Institutes of Health issued *The Seventh Report of the Joint National Committee on Prevention, Detection, Evaluation, and Treatment of High Blood Pressure (The JNC 7 Report)*. Modifications since the *The JNC 6* report include a new category of hypertension, prehypertension, and the combination of stage 2 and stage 3 hypertension. Categories now include normal, prehypertension, and stages 1 and 2 hypertension.

The revised categories are based on the average of two or more readings taken on separate visits after an initial screening. They apply to adults ages 18 and older. (If the systolic and diastolic pressures fall into different categories, use the higher of the two pressures to classify the reading. For example, a reading of 160/92 mm Hg should be classified as stage 2.)

Normal blood pressure with respect to cardiovascular risk is characterized by a systolic reading below 120 mm Hg and a diastolic reading below 80 mm Hg. Patients with prehypertension are at increased risk for developing hypertension and should follow health-promoting lifestyle modifications to prevent cardiovascular disease.

In addition to classifying stages of hypertension based on average blood pressure readings, clinicians should also take note of target organ disease and additional risk factors, such as diabetes, left ventricular hypertrophy, and chronic renal disease. These additional factors are important in assessing the patient's true cardiovascular health.

Category	Systolic		Diastolic
Normal	< 120 mm Hg	AND	< 80 mm Hg
Prehypertension	120 to 139 mm Hg	OR	80 to 89 mm Hg
Hypertension Stage 1	140 to 159 mm Hg	OR	90 to 99 mm Hg
Stage 2	≥ 160 mm Hg	OR	≥ 100 mm Hg

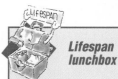

Lifespan lunchbox

Isolated systolic hypertension in elderly patients

In elderly people, systolic blood pressure may be elevated, even when diastolic blood pressure is not. This condition, known as *isolated systolic hypertension* (ISH), was once believed to be a normal part of aging and commonly went untreated. However, atherosclerosis causes a loss of elasticity in large arteries, which can cause ISH. Results of the Systolic Hypertension in the Elderly Program found that treating ISH with antihypertensive drugs lowered the incidence of stroke, coronary artery disease, and left-sided heart failure.

- increase in arteriolar thickening caused by genetic factors, leading to increased peripheral vascular resistance
- abnormal renin release, resulting in the formation of angiotensin II, which constricts the arterioles and increases blood volume.

Not-so-secondary considerations

Secondary hypertension may result from pre-existing diseases or use of certain drugs:
- renal vascular or parenchymal disease
- pheochromocytoma
- primary hyperaldosteronism
- Cushing's syndrome

- diabetes mellitus
- dysfunction of the thyroid, pituitary, or parathyroid gland
- aortic coarctation
- preeclampsia—a significant blood pressure rise during the last 3 months of pregnancy
- neurologic disorders
- use of certain cold remedies, decongestants, over-the-counter pain relievers, and prescription drugs (including hormonal contraceptives)
- cocaine and amphetamine use.

The pathophysiology of secondary hypertension varies with the underlying disorder. For example, in chronic renal disease, insult to the kidney from renal artery stenosis or chronic glomerulonephritis interferes with sodium excretion, the renin-angiotensin-aldosterone system, or renal perfusion. As a result, blood pressure rises.

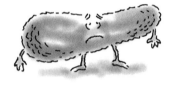

Oh my! Diabetes mellitus is a risk factor for CAD and secondary hypertension.

Out of my hands

Four major risk factors for hypertension can't be controlled. They include:

 increasing age

 race (hypertension is more common in Blacks than Whites)

 gender (in young adulthood and early middle age, more men have high blood pressure; rates are equal from ages 55 to 64; at age 65 and older, women have higher rates)

family history of hypertension.

In the driver's seat

Hypertension risk factors that a person can control or manage include:

- obesity
- inactivity
- tobacco use (chemicals in tobacco damage the lining of the arterial wall, causing the arteries to accumulate plaques; nicotine constricts blood vessels and forces the heart to work harder)
- sodium sensitivity (increased sensitivity to sodium causes increased sodium retention, leading to fluid retention and higher blood pressure)
- low potassium levels (potassium helps balance the amount of sodium in cells)
- excessive alcohol intake
- stress (high stress levels can lead to a temporary but steep blood pressure rise).

Chronic illnesses—including hypercholesterolemia, diabetes mellitus, sleep apnea, and heart failure—also can increase the risk of hypertension.

What to look for

Patients with hypertension may complain of a dull ache in the back of the head when they awaken in the morning. Some patients also experience dizziness and nosebleeds. However, these symptoms typically don't occur until hypertension is severe. In fact, most people with hypertension—even those with the highest blood pressure readings—have no signs or symptoms until vascular changes in the heart, brain, or kidneys occur. As severely elevated blood pressure damages the inner lining of small blood vessels, fibrin accumulates in the vessels and local edema occurs. Some patients also experience intravascular clotting. Signs and symptoms depend on the location of the damaged vessels:
- brain—stroke, transient ischemic attacks
- retina—blindness
- heart—MI
- kidneys—proteinuria, edema and, eventually, renal failure.

Because hypertension increases the heart's workload, the patient may also experience left ventricular hypertrophy and, later, left-sided heart failure, pulmonary edema, and right-sided heart failure.

Treatment

Treatment of secondary hypertension focuses on correcting the underlying cause and controlling hypertensive effects. For essential hypertension, the NIH recommends the following approach:
- Help the patient make necessary lifestyle changes, such as weight loss, sodium restriction, moderation of alcohol intake, regular physical exercise, smoking cessation, and adoption of the **D**ietary **A**pproaches to **S**top **H**ypertension (DASH) eating plan.
- Thiazide-type diuretics, alone or in combination with other classes of antihypertensive drugs, are recommended for most patients with uncomplicated hypertension. If a patient has compelling indications, other antihypertensive drugs may be used first, such as angiotensin-converting enzyme (ACE) inhibitors, beta-adrenergic blockers, calcium channel blockers, and angiotensin receptor blockers. A combination of two or more drugs may be necessary to achieve blood pressure control.

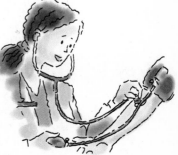

This patient hasn't lost weight or reduced his sodium intake, yet his blood pressure is lower. DASH does it again!

Other drugs that can be used include angiotensin II antagonists, alpha₁-receptor blockers, alpha-beta blockers, and vasodilators. (See *Antihypertensive therapy in Blacks.*)

• If the patient fails to achieve the desired blood pressure or make significant progress, the doctor may increase the drug dosage, substitute a drug in the same class, or add a drug from a different class.

Nutrition therapy

Nutrition therapy for hypertension focuses on reducing sodium intake, losing any excess weight, moderating alcohol intake, and increasing physical activity.

Make a splash with DASH

The recommended regimen is based on a clinical study by the National Heart, Lung, and Blood Institute that investigated the blood pressure effects of whole dietary patterns called *DASH*. The study found that high blood pressure can be lowered — without weight loss or reduced sodium intake — through an eating plan that's low in total fat, saturated fat, and cholesterol and rich in fruits, vegetables, and low-fat dairy products.

The DASH eating plan centers meals around plant foods instead of meat. Also, it's high in fiber and allows about two to three times the amounts of potassium, magnesium, and calcium that most Americans consume. It includes an additional food group — nuts, seeds, and dried peas and beans — from which four to five servings per week are recommended. (See *Slashing blood pressure with DASH.*)

Another DASH of success

More recently, another landmark study, DASH-Sodium, showed that combining the DASH eating plan with sodium reduction can lower blood pressure even more. The DASH-Sodium plan is twice as effective for Blacks because they're at greater risk for hypertension than Whites. (See *Tips to reduce sodium intake*, page 288, and *Get smart about salt terms*, page 289.)

Heart failure

Heart failure refers to the inability of the myocardium to pump effectively enough to meet the body's metabolic needs. Typically, loss in pumping action reflects an underlying heart problem such as CAD. Pump failure usually occurs in a damaged left ventricle but may also affect the right ventricle. Usually, left-sided heart failure develops first.

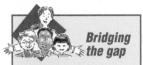

Bridging the gap

Antihypertensive therapy in Blacks

Black patients with hypertension commonly have a reduced response to single-drug therapy using beta-adrenergic blockers, angiotensin-converting enzyme (ACE) inhibitors, and angiotensin receptor blockers as compared with diuretics and calcium channel blockers. The use of combination drugs that include a diuretic removes this difference in response. Moreover, Blacks with hypertension are two to four times more likely than patients in other racial groups to develop angioedema when taking ACE inhibitors.

Slashing blood pressure with DASH

The Dietary Approaches to Stop Hypertension (DASH) eating plan, which is used to treat hypertension, is based on a daily 2,000 calorie diet. Use the chart below to help your patient plan menus or buy food to follow the DASH diet. Keep in mind that the number of daily servings in a food group may vary from those listed, depending on the patient's caloric needs.

Food group	Daily servings (except as noted)	Serving sizes	Examples	Significance to DASH plan
Grains and grain products	7 to 8	• 1 slice bread • 1 oz (28 g) dry cereal* • ½ cup cooked rice, pasta, or cereal	Whole wheat bread, English muffin, pita bread, bagel, cereals, grits, oatmeal, crackers, unsalted pretzels and popcorn	Major sources of energy and fiber
Vegetables	4 to 5	• 1 cup raw leafy vegetable • ½ cup cooked vegetable • 6 oz (177 ml) vegetable juice	Tomatoes, potatoes, carrots, green peas, squash, broccoli, collards, kale, spinach, green beans, lima beans, sweet potatoes	Rich sources of potassium, magnesium, and fiber
Fruits	4 to 5	• 6 oz (177 ml) fruit juice • 1 medium fruit • ¼ cup dried fruit • ½ cup fresh, frozen, or canned fruit	Apricots, bananas, dates, grapes, oranges, orange juice, melons, peaches, pineapples, prunes, strawberries, raisins, tangerines	Important sources of potassium, magnesium, and fiber
Low-fat or fat-free dairy foods	2 to 3	• 8 oz (237 ml) milk • 1 cup yogurt • 1½ oz (43 g) cheese	Fat-free or low-fat (1%) milk, fat-free or low-fat buttermilk, fat-free or low-fat regular or frozen yogurt, low-fat or fat-free cheese	Major sources of calcium and protein
Meats, poultry, and fish	2 or less	• 3 oz (85 g) cooked meat, poultry, or fish	Poultry (remove skin), fish, and lean meat	Major sources of protein and magnesium
Nuts, seeds, and dry beans	4 to 5 per week	• ⅓ cup or 1½ oz (43 g) nuts • 2 tbsp or ½ oz (14 g) seeds • ½ cup cooked dry beans	Almonds, mixed nuts, peanuts, walnuts, sunflower seeds, kidney beans, lentils, peas	Rich sources of protein, magnesium, potassium, and fiber
Sweets	5 per week	• 1 tbsp sugar • 1 tbsp jelly or jam • ½ oz (14 g) jelly beans • 8 oz (237 ml) lemonade	Sugar, jelly, jam, fruit-flavored gelatin, jelly beans, hard candy, fruit punch, sorbet, maple syrup, flavored ices	Sweets should be low in fat
Fats and oils**	2 to 3	• 1 tsp soft margarine • 1 tbsp low-fat mayonnaise • 2 tbsp light salad dressing • 1 tsp vegetable oil	Soft margarine, low-fat mayonnaise, light salad dressing, vegetable oil (such as olive, corn, canola, or safflower)	Allows 27% of calories as fat, including fats in or added to foods

* Equals ½ to 1¼ cup, depending on cereal type. Check product's nutrition label.
** Fat content changes serving counts for fats and oils. For example, 1 tbsp of regular fat-free dressing equals 0 servings; salad dressing equals 1 serving; 1 tbsp of low-fat dressing equals ½ serving.

Adapted from *Facts about the DASH Eating Plan.* Bethesda, MD: U.S. Department of Health and Human Services, National Institutes of Health, National Heart, Lung and Blood Institute, Revised May 2003, no.03-4082.

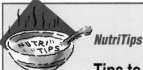

NutriTips

Tips to reduce sodium intake

Only a small amount of sodium occurs naturally in foods. Most sodium is added to foods during processing. To help your patient cut down on sodium intake, provide the following suggestions.

Read those labels
• Read food labels for sodium content.
• Use food products with reduced sodium or no added salt.
• Be aware that soy sauce, broth, and foods that are pickled or cured have high sodium contents.

Now you're cookin'
• Instead of cooking with salt, use herbs, spices, cooking wines, lemon, lime, or vinegar to enhance food flavors.
• Cook pasta and rice without salt.
• Rinse canned foods, such as tuna, to remove some sodium.
• Avoid adding salt to foods, especially at the table.
• Avoid condiments such as soy and teriyaki sauces and monosodium glutamate (MSG)—or use lower-sodium versions.

You are what you eat
• Eat fresh poultry, fish, and lean meat rather than canned, smoked, or processed versions (which typically contain a lot of sodium).
• Whenever possible, eat fresh foods rather than canned or convenience foods.
• Limit intake of cured foods (such as bacon and ham), foods packed in brine (pickles, olives, and sauerkraut) and condiments (mustard, ketchup, horseradish, and Worcestershire sauce).
• When dining out, ask how food is prepared. Ask that your food be prepared without added salt or MSG.

Heart failure is classified in the following ways:
• acute or chronic
• left-sided or right-sided
• diastolic or systolic.

Systolic or diastolic?

Systolic failure occurs when the heart's ability to contract decreases. The heart can't pump with enough force to pump a sufficient amount of blood into circulation. Diastolic failure occurs when the heart has a problem relaxing. The heart can't properly fill with blood because the muscle has become stiff.

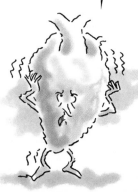

I'm a diastolic failure – I can't relax!

Get smart about salt terms

Food manufacturers use various terms to indicate that a product has a low sodium content. The chart below lists interpretations of these terms.

What the label says	What it means
Sodium-free or salt-free	5 mg or less of sodium per serving
Very low sodium	35 mg or less of sodium per serving
Low sodium	140 mg or less of sodium per serving
Reduced or less sodium	At least 25% less sodium than the regular version (some items, such as canned soup or soy sauce, may still contain significant amounts of sodium)
Light in sodium	At least 50% less sodium than the regular version
Unsalted or no salt added	No salt added during processing, which doesn't guarantee that the product is sodium-free

Adapted from *DASH Eating Plan*. National Institutes of Health, National Heart, Lung and Blood Institute. *www.nhlbi.nih.gov/health/public/heart/hbp/dash/index.htm*.

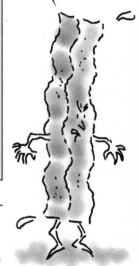

I don't want to sound bitter but your patients should keep the salt off me!

Pathophysiology

Heart failure may result from a primary abnormality of the heart muscle, such as MI, that impairs ventricular function and prevents the heart from pumping enough blood. It can also result from problems unrelated to MI, including:
• mechanical disturbances in ventricular filling during diastole, which occur because blood volume is too low for the ventricle to pump
• systolic hemodynamic disturbances (such as excessive cardiac workload caused by volume or pressure overload) that limit the heart's pumping ability.

Failure factors

Certain conditions can predispose a patient to heart failure, especially if he has underlying heart disease. These conditions include:
• arrhythmias that reduce ventricular filling time, disrupt filling synchrony, or reduce cardiac output
• pregnancy and thyrotoxicosis, which increase cardiac output

• pulmonary embolism, which raises pulmonary arterial pressures, causing right ventricular failure
• infections, which increase metabolic demands and further burden the heart
• anemia, which leads to increased cardiac output to meet tissue oxygen needs
• heart valve problems
• heart infections
• genetic abnormalities
• increased salt or water intake, emotional stress, or failure to comply with a prescribed treatment regimen for underlying heart disease.

Core complications

Eventually, fluid may enter the lungs, causing pulmonary edema, a life-threatening condition. Decreased perfusion to the brain, kidneys, and other major organs may cause them to fail. MI also may result because the oxygen demands of the overworked heart can't be met.

Worth the risk?

Heart failure is closely associated with major risk factors for CAD: smoking, high cholesterol levels, hypertension, diabetes mellitus, and obesity. A single risk factor may be sufficient to cause heart failure, but a combination of factors dramatically increases the risk. Advanced age adds to the potential impact of any heart failure risk.

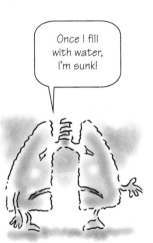

What to look for

Early signs and symptoms of heart failure include:
• fatigue
• exertional, paroxysmal, and nocturnal dyspnea
• neck vein engorgement
• hepatomegaly.
    Later signs and symptoms include:
• tachypnea
• palpitations
• dependent edema
• unexplained, steady weight gain
• nausea
• chest tightness
• slowed mental response
• anorexia
• hypotension
• diaphoresis

- narrow pulse pressure
- pallor
- oliguria
- gallop rhythm and inspiratory crackles on auscultation
- dullness over the lung bases
- hemoptysis
- cyanosis
- marked hepatomegaly
- pitting ankle edema
- sacral edema in bedridden patients.

Treatment

The goal of therapy is to improve pump function by reversing the compensatory mechanisms producing the signs and symptoms. Heart failure may be controlled quickly through treatment consisting of:
- ACE inhibitors to decrease peripheral vascular resistance
- carvedilol, a nonselective beta-adrenergic blocker with alpha-receptor blockade, to reduce mortality and improve quality of life
- inotropic agents, such as dobutamine and milrinone, to improve the heart's ability to pump
- nesiritide, a recombinant form of endogenous human B-type natriuretic peptide, to reduce sodium through its diuretic action.
- diuresis to reduce total blood volume and circulatory congestion
- digoxin to strengthen myocardial contractility and improve cardiac output
- vasodilators to raise cardiac output by reducing impedance to ventricular outflow
- antiembolism stockings to prevent venostasis and thromboembolism.

When symptoms fail to respond to medical therapy, implanted devices such as the left ventricular assist device can provide temporary assistance until the patient's condition stabilizes or surgery is performed. Biventricular pacing has been successful in reducing symptoms and improving the quality of life in patients with advanced heart failure. Left ventricular remodeling surgery may be performed, resulting in a smaller organ that's able to pump blood more efficiently. Heart transplantation may be another option for some people. (See *Ethnicity and drug response*.)

Lifestyle changes and drug therapy can improve the patient's quality of life and survival. For instance, the patient can minimize the effects of heart failure by controlling cardiovascular risk factors, stopping smoking and losing weight if necessary, abstaining

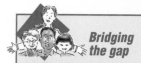

Bridging the gap

Ethnicity and drug response

A patient's ethnicity may affect how his body responds to the drugs used to treat heart failure. For example, almost half of all Asian patients develop a cough while taking an angiotensin-converting enzyme (ACE) inhibitor. Although the majority of antihypertensive drugs work well in Black patients, some of these drugs are more dependable and produce effects with lower dosages in this population. When using monotherapy, Black patients have a better response to diuretics than to beta-adrenergic blockers and ACE inhibitors. Moreover, labetalol (an alpha-beta blocker) produces a better response than propranolol in Blacks.

from alcohol, and reducing dietary sodium and fat intake. (See *Treatment of heart failure in Black patients.*)

Nutrition therapy

Nutrition therapy for a patient with heart failure centers on restricting sodium, easing edema (fluid retention), and minimizing the cardiac workload. To reduce edema, sodium intake typically is restricted to 2,000 mg/day initially. If this doesn't significantly reduce edema, the patient may need to cut back to as little as 1,000 mg/day. (To visualize this, keep in mind 1 tsp of table salt contains about 2,400 mg of sodium.) Adherence to a diet that's restricted to less than 1,000 mg/day is extremely difficult without the use of low-sodium foods, especially bread, and limiting milk to no more than 2 cups per day. The sodium allowance may be eased progressively as edema subsides. However, not all patients require strict sodium restriction; a no-added-salt diet (3 to 4 g/day of sodium) may be sufficient. (See *Sample menu for a sodium-restricted diet.*)

Most patients who restrict sodium adequately don't require fluid restriction. But if edema persists despite a low-sodium diet, the doctor may restrict fluids to 2 qt/day (2 L/day) or less.

Pour on the potassium

If your patient is taking a thiazide (potassium-wasting) diuretic or a cardiac glycoside, make sure the diet provides adequate potassium to replace losses. Foods high in potassium include:
- bananas
- citrus fruits and their juices
- melons
- raisins
- apricots
- avocados
- potatoes
- tomatoes and tomato products
- dried peas and beans
- green leafy vegetables
- spinach
- carrots
- corn
- whole grains
- fresh meat
- milk
- yogurt
- ice cream.

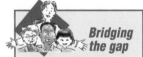
Bridging the gap

Treatment of heart failure in Black patients

In June 2005, the Food and Drug Administration approved the drug BiDil for the treatment of heart failure in Black patients. Although other patients with severe heart failure showed no improvement with this drug, Black patients had a 43% decline in mortality and a 39% drop in hospitalization for heart failure when compared with the results of a placebo. BiDil is a combination of two drugs, hydralazine and isosorbide dinitrate.

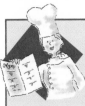

Menu maven

Sample menu for a sodium-restricted diet

If your patient must restrict his sodium intake, provide a sample menu such as the one below. Be sure to emphasize that he shouldn't add any sodium to these items.

Breakfast
- Orange juice
- Rice cereal with banana
- Whole wheat toast with margarine and jelly
- Coffee with 2 tsp sugar and 1% milk

Lunch
- Apple or cranberry juice (1 glass)
- Roast turkey sandwich with lettuce and tomato
- Carrot and raisin salad (no salt added)
- Low-fat frozen yogurt (vanilla)

Dinner
- Pork tenderloin
- Baked sweet potato
- Fresh steamed green beans
- Dinner roll with margarine
- Gelatin dessert
- Decaffeinated coffee with 2 tsp sugar and 1% milk

Snack
- Unsalted pretzels
- Apple juice

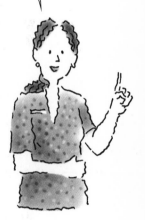

Drug therapy can be used in conjunction with other treatments to control heart failure quickly. For longer-term effects, though, tell your patient to consider quitting smoking and cutting down on salt intake.

Some patients may be advised to use potassium-containing salt substitutes, sold under such brand names as Morton Salt Substitute, Morton Lite Salt Mixture, No Salt, and Adolph's Salt Substitute.

Spice, not salt

Advise the patient to use no-salt spices and seasonings instead of table salt. Tell him to avoid food products whose labels state "convenient," "instant," or "prepared." The high sodium content of most of these products makes them nearly impossible to work into a low-sodium diet.

Caution the patient that various nonfood products also contain sodium—including certain medications, toothpastes, mouthwash, and drinking water. (See *Sodium content of nonprescription drugs*, page 294.)

Other ways to ease the workload

If your patient is overweight, recommend a low-calorie diet to help reduce cardiac workload. Provide five to six small meals per day, with no more than 3 qt/day (3 L/day) of fluid (or as specified by the doctor) to increase intake without overstressing the heart. Recommend nonirritating and non-gas-forming foods to minimize gastric distention and pressure on the heart.

Sodium content of nonprescription drugs

The chart below lists the sodium content of some commonly used nonprescription (over-the-counter) drugs.

Medication	Dosage	Sodium content (mg)
Alka-Seltzer	2 tablets	1,040
Di-Gel	2 tablets	21
Maalox	1 tbsp	8
Mylanta II	1 tbsp	24
Phillips Milk of Magnesia	2 tbsp	3
Rolaids	2 tablets	106
Tums	2 tablets	6
Vicks Cough syrup	5 ml	54
Vicks Formula 44 D	5 ml	68

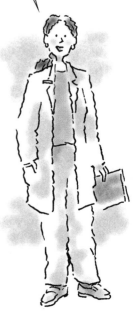

Fluid restriction is a key component to nutrition therapy for heart failure.

Advise the patient to restrict caffeine intake to avoid stimulating the heart. Tell him to avoid alcohol.

Stop those fluids

Edema that resists treatment may call for fluid restriction to half the amount of calories required. In other words, a patient on a 2,400-cal/day diet would be allowed to have 1¼ qt (1,200 ml) of fluid per day. An obese patient requires a calorie-controlled diet.

Advise the patient to plan fluid consumption throughout the day. Recommend that he fill a clear pitcher each morning with the amount of fluid he's permitted to have daily. Each time he consumes fluid, he should pour the same amount of water out of the pitcher so he can keep track of his remaining fluid allowance.

No roughage in the house

To lessen heartburn, abdominal distention, and flatulence, encourage the patient to eat slowly and avoid gulping food. To reduce the amount of chewing required, encourage the patient to eat a soft diet — one consisting of plain, soft foods that are low in roughage.

Less is more

Patients with heart failure commonly complain of feeling congested and, as a result, find it difficult to muster an appetite. If your patient has a poor appetite, instruct him to try smaller, more frequent meals — but tell him he should never force himself to eat. Consider recommending a high-calorie oral supplement (350 cal/8 oz [237 ml]) to increase the nutrient density of his diet. Remember, though, that a patient who can eat solid foods shouldn't use oral supplements.

Perplexing cachexia

If the patient has poor nutritional intake and has been using medication long-term, he may develop cardiac cachexia—a type of malnutrition that causes anorexia and fat and muscle wasting with edema. Patients with cardiac cachexia need a diet high in calories, protein, and nutrients but still need to restrict sodium. A calorie- and nutrient-dense diet maximizes intake.

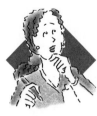

Quick quiz

1. Janet, age 60, is a white female with no family history of heart disease. Her LDL level is 163 mg/dl, HDL level 35 mg/dl, and blood pressure 148/96 mm Hg. How many risk factors for CAD does Janet have?
   A. 1
   B. 2
   C. 3
   D. 4

Answer: D. Risk factors for CAD include a high LDL level (160 mg/dl or higher), a low HDL level (under 40 mg/dl), hypertension, and postmenopausal status.

2. The DASH diet is the most effective plan for lowering which of the following values?
   A. Blood pressure
   B. LDL
   C. Total serum cholesterol
   D. HDL

Answer: A. The DASH diet has been proven effective in lowering blood pressure.

3. The TLC diet recommends that calories from saturated fat should be what percentage of total intake?
   A. Less than 7%
   B. Less than 10%
   C. 12%
   D. 20%

Answer: A: The TLC diet recommends that less than 7% of calories come from saturated fat.

Scoring

☆☆☆ If you answered all three questions correctly, hopping hearts! You perform well under pressure!

☆☆ If you answered two questions correctly, keep it up! DASH to the fridge and grab a snack; then move on to the next chapter.

☆ If you answered fewer than two questions correctly, don't get disheartened. Take a break and then review the chapter!

Renal disorders

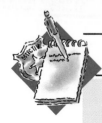

Just the facts

The renal system is responsible for the excretion of body wastes. In this chapter, you'll learn:

♦ the structure and functions of the renal system

♦ pathophysiology, signs and symptoms, and treatments for common renal disorders

♦ nutrition therapy for common renal disorders and kidney transplant.

A look at the renal system

The renal system, teamed with the urinary system, serves as the body's water treatment plant. These systems work together to collect the body's waste products and expel them as urine.

Filtration system

The kidneys, located on each side of the abdomen near the lower back, contain an amazingly efficient filtration system that filters about 45 gallons of fluid per day. (See *Kidney function declines with age*, page 298.) The byproduct of this filtration is urine, which contains water and waste products. After it's produced by the kidneys, urine passes through the urinary system and is expelled from the body.

Other structures of the system, extending downward from the kidneys, include:

• ureters—muscular tubes that contract rhythmically (peristalsis) to transport urine from each kidney to the bladder

• urinary bladder—a sac with muscular walls that collects and holds urine that's expelled from the ureters every few seconds

• urethra—a narrow passageway, surrounded by the prostate gland in men, from the bladder to the outside of the body through which urine is excreted.

> We kidneys are good at taking out the trash!

Renal role

The kidneys perform vital functions, including:
- maintaining fluid and acid-base balance
- regulating electrolyte concentration
- detoxifying the blood and eliminating wastes
- regulating blood pressure
- aiding red blood cell (RBC) production (erythropoiesis)
- regulating vitamin D and calcium formation.

Assessment

To plan nutritional therapy for a patient with renal disease, first perform a nutrition-focused assessment. This assessment should include a health history, a physical examination, and diagnostic tests.

Health history

Obtain a history to assess the patient's renal status. Focus the health history on the patient's eating habits, weight, blood pressure, past illnesses, and preexisting conditions. Gather information about the patient's:
- dietary intake, especially of high-sodium foods
- use of low-protein or low-sodium products
- understanding of the Nutrition Facts panel on food labels
- knowledge of healthy eating habits
- willingness to change eating habits, if needed
- ability to buy and prepare healthy foods
- frequency of eating out
- physical activity and exercise
- religious and ethnic influences on food choices
- food allergies and intolerances
- use of alcohol, caffeine, tobacco, and recreational drugs
- use of nutritional supplements
- use of herbal supplements
- current and past medication use
- medical history
- family history of renal disease and hypertension.

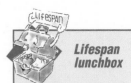

Lifespan lunchbox

Kidney function declines with age

After age 40, renal function may diminish. If a person lives to age 90, renal function may have decreased by as much as 50%. This change is reflected by a decline in the glomerular filtration rate caused by age-related changes in renal vasculature that disturb glomerular hemodynamics. Renal blood flow decreases by 53% from reduced cardiac output and age-related atherosclerotic changes. Tubular reabsorption and renal concentrating ability also decline because the size and number of functioning nephrons decrease.

Additionally, as a person ages, the bladder muscles weaken, which can result in incomplete bladder emptying and chronic urine retention, predisposing the bladder to infection.

Physical examination

Focus the physical examination on nutrition-related aspects, such as the patient's weight and height, vital signs, skin condition, and mental status.

Weighing in on renal health

Weighing the patient can provide information about fluid status and is important for patients with renal disorders or renal failure, especially those receiving dialysis. Ask the patient about recent weight changes.

They ain't called *vital* for nothin'

Evaluate your patient's vital signs, which can provide clues about renal dysfunction. For example, a patient's vital signs might reveal hypertension, which can cause renal dysfunction if it's uncontrolled. Be sure to check blood pressure in each arm.

Get the skinny on the skin

Examine your patient's skin. Inspect for edema especially. Presence of edema could indicate fluid retention and renal dysfunction.

Stable status?

Observing the patient's behavior can give you clues about his mental status. Does he have trouble concentrating, have memory loss, or seem disoriented? Renal dysfunction can cause those symptoms. Progressive, chronic renal failure can cause lethargy, confusion, disorientation, stupor, convulsions, and coma.

Diagnostic tests

To evaluate a patient for renal disease, the doctor may order various laboratory and diagnostic tests, including:
- blood urea nitrogen (BUN) level
- creatinine level
- albumin level
- electrolyte levels
- hemoglobin level
- hematocrit
- parathyroid hormone level
- phosphorus and calcium levels
- renal scan
- urinalysis.

Renal calculi

Renal calculi, or kidney stones, may form anywhere in the urinary tract but usually develop in the renal pelvis or calices. Calculi form when substances that normally dissolve in the urine precipitate. They vary in size, shape, and number.

About 1 in 1,000 Americans requires hospitalization at some time for renal calculi. They're more common in men than women and rare in Blacks and children.

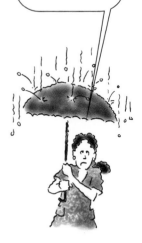

Hail stones and kidney stones are both forms of precipitation.

Pathophysiology

Renal calculi are particularly prevalent in specific geographic areas such as the southeastern United States. Although their exact cause is unknown, there are several predisposing factors:
- *Dehydration* — Decreased water and urine excretion concentrates calculus-forming substances.
- *Infection* — Infected, scarred tissue, such as that formed from a urinary tract infection, provides a site for calculus development. Calculi may become infected if bacteria are the nucleus in calculi formation. Calculi that result from *Proteus* infections may lead to the destruction of kidney tissue.
- *Changes in urine pH* — Consistently acidic or alkaline urine provides a favorable medium for calculus formation.
- *Obstruction* — Urinary stasis allows calculus constituents to collect and adhere, forming calculi. Obstruction also encourages infection, which compounds the obstruction.
- *Immobilization* — Immobility from spinal cord injury or other disorders allows calcium to be released into the circulation and, eventually, to be filtered by the kidneys.
- *Diet* — Increased intake of calcium or oxalate-rich foods encourages calculi formation.
- *Metabolic factors* — Hyperparathyroidism, renal tubular acidosis, elevated uric acid (usually with gout), defective oxalate metabolism, a genetic defect in cystine metabolism, and excessive intake of vitamin D or dietary calcium may predispose a person to renal calculi.

Disturbing a delicate balance

Renal calculi usually arise because the delicate excretory balance breaks down. Here's how it happens:

 Urine becomes concentrated with insoluble materials.

Crystals form from these materials and then consolidate, forming calculi. These calculi contain an organic mucoprotein framework and crystalloids, such as calcium, oxalate, phosphate, urate, uric acid, struvite, cystine, and xanthine.

Mucoprotein is reabsorbed by the tubules, establishing a site for calculi formation.

Calculi remain in the renal pelvis and damage or destroy kidney tissue, or they enter the ureter.

Large calculi in the kidneys may cause tissue damage (pressure necrosis).

In certain locations, calculi obstruct urine, which collects in the renal pelvis (hydronephrosis). These calculi also tend to recur. Intractable pain and serious bleeding can result.

Initially, hydrostatic pressure increases in the collection system near the obstruction, forcing nearby renal structures to dilate as well. The farther the obstruction is from the kidney, the less serious the dilation because the pressure is diffused over a larger surface area.

With a complete obstruction, pressure in the renal pelvis and tubules increases, the glomerular filtration rate (GFR) falls, and a disruption occurs in the junctional complexes between tubular cells. If left untreated, tubular atrophy and destruction of the medulla leave connective tissue in place of glomeruli, causing irreversible damage.

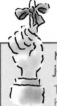

> **Memory jogger**
>
> To remember how renal calculi formation happens, think **U**nusual **C**hanges **M**ean **T**hat **L**iquid **U**nder **P**ressure **G**athers:
>
> **U**rine concentrates.
>
> **C**rystals form.
>
> **M**ucoprotein is reabsorbed.
>
> **T**issue is damaged.
>
> **L**arge calculi may form.
>
> **U**rine collects.
>
> **P**ressure builds.
>
> **G**FR falls.

> Ninety percent of renal calculi may pass naturally with vigorous hydration. So, bottoms up!

What to look for

The key symptom of renal calculi is severe pain, which usually occurs when large calculi obstruct the opening of the ureter and increase the frequency and force of peristaltic contractions. Pain may travel from the lower back to the sides and then to the pubic region and external genitalia. Pain intensity fluctuates and may be excruciating at its peak.

The patient with calculi in the renal pelvis and calices may complain of more constant, dull pain. He also may report back pain from an obstruction within a kidney and severe abdominal pain from calculi traveling down a ureter. Severe pain is typically accompanied by nausea, vomiting and, possibly, fever and chills.

It isn't just painful

Other signs and symptoms include:
• hematuria (when stones abrade a ureter)

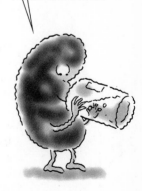

- abdominal distention
- oliguria (from an obstruction in urine flow).

Treatment

Ninety percent of renal calculi are smaller than 5 mm in diameter and may pass naturally with vigorous hydration (more than 3 qt/day [3 L/day]). Other treatments may include drug therapy for infection or other effects of illness and measures to prevent recurrence of calculi. If calculi are too large for natural passage, they may be removed by surgery or other means.

Drug duty

Drug therapy may include:
- antimicrobial agents for infection (varying with the cultured organism)
- analgesics, such as morphine, for pain
- diuretics to prevent urinary stasis and further calculi formation
- thiazides to decrease calcium excretion in the urine
- methenamine mandelate to suppress calculi formation when infection is present.

Canning the calculi

Calculi lodged in the ureter may be removed by inserting a cystoscope through the urethra and then manipulating the calculi with catheters or retrieval instruments. A flank or lower abdominal approach may be needed to extract calculi from other areas, such as the kidney calyx or renal pelvis. Percutaneous ultrasonic lithotripsy and extracorporeal shock wave lithotripsy shatter the calculi into fragments for removal by suction or natural passage.

Prevention techniques

Measures to prevent recurrence of renal calculi include:
- oxalate-binding cholestyramine for absorptive hypercalciuria
- parathyroidectomy for hyperparathyroidism
- allopurinol for uric acid calculi.

Nutrition therapy

Increasing fluid intake, thereby diluting urine, is the most effective nutritional therapy for treating and preventing renal calculi. High urine output helps flush calculi from the urinary system and also decreases the risk of recurrence. Fluid intake should be increased to 2½ to 3 qt/day (2.5 to 3 L/day). At least 8 oz (237 ml) of water should be consumed before bedtime because urine becomes more concentrated at night. (See *Cranberry juice controversy*.)

Cranberry juice controversy

Cranberry juice may be effective in preventing urinary tract infections, which can lead to calculi formation. An ingredient in the juice prevents bacteria such as *Escherichia coli* from adhering to the lining of the urinary tract, promoting their excretion. Unfortunately, not all bacteria are sensitive to the juice. Also, the juice's protective feature only lasts as long as the juice is consumed regularly.

Hold the oxalate

Patients with calculi typically need to restrict their intake of oxalate. Foods high in oxalate include:

- beets
- blueberries
- brewed tea
- cocoa
- draft beer
- instant coffee
- nuts
- nut butters
- purple grapes
- rhubarb
- spinach
- strawberries
- tofu
- wheat bran.

In addition, vitamin B_6 supplements have been shown to reduce oxalate production by 50%. Therefore, supplementation may be helpful.

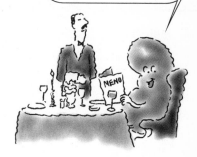

Garçon, give me the special but hold the beets, nuts, and spinach and put the tofu on the side. While you're at it, can you throw in a little extra B_6?

Other limits

Animal protein intake should be limited to 8 oz/day (227 g/day), and sodium should be limited to 2 g/day.

Acute renal failure

Acute renal failure is the sudden interruption of renal function. It can be caused by obstruction, poor circulation, or kidney disease. It's potentially reversible; however, if left untreated, permanent damage can lead to chronic renal failure.

Pathophysiology

Acute renal failure may be classified as prerenal, intrarenal, or postrenal. Each type has its own causes:

- *Prerenal failure* results from conditions that diminish blood flow to the kidneys. Examples include hypovolemia, hypotension, vasoconstriction, or inadequate cardiac output. One condition, prerenal azotemia (excess nitrogenous waste products in the blood), accounts for 40% to 80% of all cases of acute renal failure. Azotemia occurs as a response to renal hypoperfusion. Usually, it can be rapidly reversed by restoring renal blood flow and glomerular filtration.

• *Intrarenal failure*, also called *intrinsic* or *parenchymal renal failure*, results from damage to the filtering structures of the kidneys, usually from acute tubular necrosis (a disorder that causes cell death) or from nephrotoxic substances such as certain antibiotics.

• *Postrenal failure* results from bilateral obstruction of urine outflow, as in prostatic hyperplasia or bladder outlet obstruction.

> In acute renal failure, early intervention improves the chance of recovery.

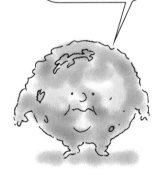

Phasing out

With treatment, each type of acute renal failure passes through three distinct phases:

    oliguric (decreased urine output)

    diuretic (increased urine output)

    recovery.

Going down

The oliguric phase is marked by decreased urine output (less than 400 ml/24 hours). Prerenal oliguria results from decreased blood flow to the kidney. Before damage occurs, the kidney responds to decreased blood flow by conserving sodium and water. Once damage occurs, the kidney's ability to conserve sodium is impaired. Untreated prerenal oliguria may lead to acute tubular necrosis.

During this phase, BUN and creatinine levels rise and the ratio of BUN to creatinine falls from 20:1 (normal) to 10:1. Hypervolemia also occurs, causing edema, weight gain, and elevated blood pressure.

Going up

The diuretic phase is marked by urine output that can range from normal levels to as high as 5 L/day. High urine volume has two causes:

    inability of the kidney to conserve sodium and water

    osmotic diuresis produced by high BUN levels.

During this phase, BUN and creatinine levels slowly rise, and hypovolemia and weight loss result. This phase lasts from several days to 1 week. These conditions can lead to deficits of potassium, sodium, and water that can be deadly if left untreated. If the cause of the diuresis is corrected, azotemia gradually disappears and the patient improves greatly—leading to the recovery phase.

> During the oliguric phase of acute renal failure, hypervolemia occurs. Boy am I full!

Riding the road to recovery

The recovery phase is reached when BUN and creatinine have returned to normal and urine output is between 1 and 2 L/day.

Getting complicated

Primary damage to the renal tubules or blood vessels results in kidney failure (intrarenal failure). The causes of intrarenal failure are classified as nephrotoxic, inflammatory, or ischemic.

When the damage is caused by nephrotoxicity or inflammation, the delicate layer under the epithelium (basement membrane) becomes irreparably damaged, commonly proceeding to chronic renal failure. Severe or prolonged lack of blood flow (ischemia) may lead to renal damage (ischemic parenchymal injury) and excess nitrogen in the blood (intrinsic renal azotemia).

What to look for

The signs and symptoms of prerenal failure depend on the cause. If the underlying problem is a change in blood pressure and volume, the patient may have:
- oliguria
- tachycardia
- hypotension
- dry mucous membranes
- flat neck veins
- lethargy progressing to coma
- decreased cardiac output and cool, clammy skin in a patient with heart failure.

As renal failure progresses, the patient may show signs and symptoms of uremia, including:
- confusion
- GI complaints
- fluid in the lungs
- infection.

About 5% of all hospitalized patients develop acute renal failure. The condition is usually reversible with treatment but, if it isn't treated, it may progress to end-stage renal disease, excess urea in the blood (prerenal azotemia or uremia), and death.

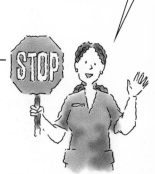

Stop uremia in its tracks to avoid hemodialysis, renal replacement therapy, and peritoneal dialysis.

Treatment

Supportive measures for acute renal failure include:
- establishment and maintenance of fluid and electrolyte balance
- diuretic therapy during the oliguric phase
- renal-dose dopamine to increase renal perfusion
- monitoring for signs of uremia
- antibiotics to prevent or treat infection.

If the above measures fail to control uremia, the patient may require hemodialysis, continuous renal replacement therapy, or peritoneal dialysis.

Halting hyperkalemia

Meticulous electrolyte monitoring is needed to detect excess potassium in the blood (hyperkalemia). Symptoms include malaise, anorexia, numbness and tingling, muscle weakness, and electrocardiogram changes. If these symptoms occur, hypertonic glucose, insulin, and sodium bicarbonate are given I.V., and sodium polystyrene sulfonate (Kayexalate) is given by mouth or rectum.

Nutrition therapy

Adequate calories are required in patients with acute renal failure to prevent weight loss and body protein catabolism. Caloric needs for most adults with acute renal failure are 30 to 50 kcal/kg/day.

Patients with acute renal failure may require enteral or parenteral feedings if they're unable to consume enough calories orally. Special enteral and parenteral formulas are available for patients with renal failure. These formulas are low in potassium and phosphorus and high in calories.

Patients who have acute renal failure accompanied by diabetes mellitus frequently must have their insulin or antidiabetic drug dosages adjusted to meet the nutritional demands of renal failure.

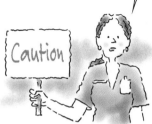

Be sure to adjust insulin or antidiabetic drug dosages for diabetic patients who also have acute renal failure!

Protein controversy

Some health care providers believe that protein should be restricted in acute renal failure because restricting protein may help preserve kidney function. Others believe that high-protein intake is important to correct the negative nitrogen balance. Those who aren't receiving dialysis are typically restricted to 0.8 g/kg/day. As the patient's renal function returns to normal or dialysis begins, the protein allowance is increased to 1.1 to 2.5 g/kg/day.

Fluid in phases

Fluid intake for patients in the oliguric and diuretic phases of acute renal failure should be 400 to 500 ml greater than their 24-hour urine output. For example, if the patient's urine output is 2,500 ml, then the patient should consume at least 2,900 ml of fluid.

Hold the potassium

Hyperkalemia may occur during the oliguric phase of acute renal failure. This electrolyte imbalance results when potassium is retained and tissue catabolism occurs, causing potassium to leave the cells and enter the serum. During this phase, the patient should restrict the intake of potassium to 2 g or less per day. During the diuretic phase, potassium is excreted and supplementation may be necessary.

The salt story

During the oliguric phase of acute renal failure, sodium may be restricted to 500 to 1,000 mg/day. Sodium intake is adjusted according to the patient's urine output, serum sodium level, and need for dialysis. Sodium is excreted during the diuretic phase and supplementation may be required.

Chronic renal failure

Chronic renal failure, a usually progressive and irreversible deterioration, is the end result of gradual tissue destruction and loss of kidney function. Occasionally, chronic renal failure results from rapidly progressing disease of sudden onset that destroys the nephrons and causes irreversible kidney damage.

Pathophysiology

Chronic renal failure typically progresses through four stages:

Reduced renal reserve — GFR is 35% to 50% of the normal rate.

Renal insufficiency — GFR is 20% to 35% of the normal rate.

Renal failure — GFR is 20% to 25% of the normal rate.

End-stage renal disease — GFR is less than 20% of the normal rate.

It may result from:
• chronic glomerular disease, such as glomerulonephritis, which affects the capillaries in the glomeruli
• chronic infections, such as chronic pyelonephritis and tuberculosis
• congenital anomalies such as polycystic kidney disease
• vascular diseases, such as hypertension and nephrosclerosis, which causes hardening of the kidneys
• obstructions such as renal calculi
• collagen diseases such as lupus erythematosus

- nephrotoxic agents such as long-term aminoglycoside therapy
- endocrine diseases such as diabetic neuropathy.

Nephrons lose the battle

Nephron damage is progressive. Once damaged, nephrons can no longer function. Healthy nephrons compensate for destroyed nephrons by enlarging and increasing their clearance capacity. The kidneys maintain relatively normal function until about 75% of the nephrons are nonfunctional.

Eventually, the healthy glomeruli are so overburdened they become sclerotic and stiff, leading to their destruction. If this condition continues unchecked, toxins accumulate and produce potentially fatal changes in all major organ systems.

Everlasting effects

Even if the patient can tolerate life-sustaining maintenance dialysis or a kidney transplant, he may still have anemia, nervous system effects (peripheral neuropathy), cardiopulmonary and GI complications, sexual dysfunction, and skeletal defects.

What to look for

Few symptoms develop until more than 75% of glomerular filtration is lost. Then the remaining normal tissue deteriorates progressively. Symptoms worsen as kidney function decreases. Profound changes affect all body systems. Major findings include:

- hypervolemia (abnormal increase in plasma volume)
- hyperkalemia
- hypocalcemia
- hyperphosphatemia
- azotemia
- metabolic acidosis
- anemia
- peripheral neuropathy.

The progression of chronic renal failure can sometimes be slowed, but it's ultimately irreversible, culminating in end-stage renal disease. Although it's fatal without treatment, dialysis or kidney transplant can sustain life.

Treatment

Treatment for chronic renal failure consists of hemodialysis, peritoneal dialysis, or renal transplantation and drug therapy. Drugs used to treat chronic renal failure include:

- loop diuretics such as furosemide (if some renal function remains) to maintain fluid balance
- cardiac glycosides to increase the heart's contractility and mobilize fluids that cause edema
- antihypertensives to control blood pressure and edema
- antiemetics to relieve nausea and vomiting
- histamine-2-receptor antagonists such as famotidine to reduce gastric irritation
- stool softeners such as docusate to prevent constipation
- iron and folate supplements or RBC transfusions to treat anemia
- synthetic erythropoietins to stimulate bone marrow to produce RBCs
- antipruritics such as trimeprazine to relieve itching
- phosphate binders to lower serum phosphorus levels
- calcimimetic drugs to treat secondary hyperparathyroidism in patients on dialysis.

Emergency measures

Potassium levels in the blood must be monitored closely to detect hyperkalemia. Emergency treatment includes dialysis therapy, oral or rectal administration of cation exchange resins such as sodium polystyrene sulfonate, and I.V. administration of calcium gluconate, sodium bicarbonate, 50% hypertonic glucose, and regular insulin.

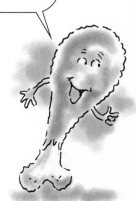

Half of the protein consumed by the patient with chronic renal failure should be high-biological-value protein, which can be found in such foods as beef, egg whites, fish, milk, pork, and poultry.

Nutrition therapy

The National Kidney Foundation has published clinical practice guidelines for nutrition in chronic renal failure. The foundation outlines requirements for those patients who don't require dialysis (pre-end-stage renal disease) and those who do (end-stage renal disease).

Nutrition for those with pre-end-stage renal disease depends on diagnostic test results. Daily protein requirements range from 0.8 to 1 g/kg. Half of the protein consumed should consist of high-biological-value protein. These high-biologic proteins contain all the essential amino acids that can be made by the body. Foods that contain such protein include beef, egg whites, fish, milk, pork, and poultry. Foods containing low-biological-value protein include legumes, nuts, and nut butters. Patients who require dialysis are instructed to consume 1.2 to 1.5 g/kg of protein daily.

Counting on calories

Adequate calorie intake is necessary to prevent weight loss and protein catabolism. Failure to consume adequate calories can cause BUN levels to rise because body protein is broken down for energy. Those who don't require dialysis should consume 35 cal/kg/day. Patients receiving peritoneal dialysis should decrease their calorie intake by 680 cal/day to compensate for the calories absorbed from the dialysate.

Sweet tooths, celebrate!

In many cases, patients with chronic renal failure must consume simple carbohydrates in order to provide enough calories without adding extra protein to the diet. Sources of protein-free calories include fruit drinks and punches, chewy fruit snacks, sorbet, lemonade, honey, corn syrup, and butter or margarine. (See *Slowed growth.*)

How much water and salt?

Sodium and fluid restrictions are determined by the patient's blood pressure, electrolyte levels, urine output, and weight. Most patients can successfully consume 2 to 4 g of sodium daily. (See *Spicing up foods.*)

In patients who have normal blood pressure, no edema, and normal serum sodium levels, fluid intake should be 500 ml greater than the patient's 24-hour urine output. For example, if the patient's urine output is 600 ml over the past 24 hours, then the patient can safely consume 1,100 ml of fluid. If the patient is receiving dialysis, the goal is to limit weight gain to 2 lb (0.9 kg) between treatments. (See *Dining out,* page 312.)

Potassium parity

Typically, patients with renal insufficiency and those receiving peritoneal dialysis don't need to restrict their potassium intake. Patients who have hyperkalemia and undergo hemodialysis should restrict their potassium intake to 2 to 3 g/day. (See *Avoiding potassium-rich foods,* page 313.)

Bone protection

Vitamin D deficiency is common in patients with chronic renal failure because the kidneys are unable to convert vitamin D to its active form. Calcium, magnesium, and phosphorus metabolism are altered, leading to hyperphosphatemia, bone demineralization, bone pain, and possible soft tissue calcification. These complications may be prevented by limiting the intake of phosphorus and providing vitamin D supplements and phosphorus binders. (See

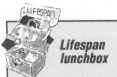

Lifespan lunchbox

Slowed growth

Children with chronic renal failure typically experience growth retardation. This failure to grow may be permanent if not corrected before puberty. Aggressive calcium and vitamin D supplementation may be used to boost calcium uptake by the bones and subsequent bone growth. Phosphate binders and human growth hormone may also be prescribed.

Whew! patients with renal insufficiency don't usually need to restrict their potassium intake.

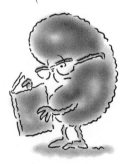

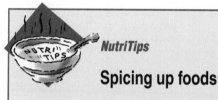

NutriTips

Spicing up foods

Because patients with renal failure must limit sodium intake, food commonly tastes bland. Inform the patient that the following seasonings can be used to spice up foods in place of salt:

- allspice
- anise
- basil
- bay leaf
- caraway seed
- chives
- cilantro
- cinnamon
- cloves
- cumin
- curry
- ginger
- horseradish root
- nutmeg
- onion powder
- oregano
- paprika
- pepper
- poppy seed
- rosemary
- saffron
- sage
- savory
- sesame seeds
- tarragon
- thyme
- turmeric
- vinegar.

Avoiding phosphorus-rich foods, page 314, and *Commonly prescribed phosphorous binders*, page 315.)

Vital vitamins

Patients with chronic renal failure usually have deficiencies of the water-soluble vitamins. Inadequate intake caused by anorexia and dietary restrictions, altered metabolism caused by uremia and medications, or increased losses of vitamins caused by dialysis are responsible.

Both dialyzed patients and those who don't require dialysis should receive supplementation according to Recommended Dietary Allowances (RDAs). Patients should receive vitamin B_6 and folic acid in amounts greater than the RDA to promote RBC production. Vitamin C intake should be limited to 100 mg to prevent the occurrence of kidney stones.

They may be trace, but they're important

Deficiencies in trace minerals such as zinc may occur in those patients undergoing dialysis. Supplementation is suggested if a zinc deficiency is identified. Iron supplements may be necessary to

Boy, could I go for a tall glass of B_6 right about now.

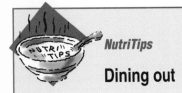

NutriTips

Dining out

Patients with chronic renal failure can still enjoy dining out. However, they need to plan ahead and make wise menu choices. Here are a few tips to help make dining out easier.

Menu choices
• Instruct the patient to choose meats without sauces or gravies.
• Explain that baked or grilled fish, broiled steaks, chicken, hamburgers, prime rib, roast beef, and turkey are all good choices.
• Cold cuts, such as pastrami and salami, and hot dogs should be avoided.
• Tell the patient that a small house salad is acceptable; however, it shouldn't contain tomatoes and should be served with oil and vinegar dressing. A serving of cooked vegetables without sauce is an acceptable alternative.
• When choosing bread products, the patient should choose French, Italian, white, rye, or sour-dough bread. English muffins and bagels are also acceptable.
• The choice of starches is somewhat limited. Instruct the patient to choose plain rice, plain noodles, or mashed potatoes.

Restaurant choices
• Eating at a Mexican restaurant is acceptable; however, avocados, beans, sour cream, and fresh tomatoes should be avoided. Fajitas, tacos, beef or chicken enchiladas, and meat-filled burritos are wise choices.
• Eating at an Italian restaurant is somewhat difficult. Tomato sauces and cream sauces should be avoided. Plain pasta can be ordered with butter or olive oil and meat.
• Chinese food is acceptable; however, it should be made without monosodium glutamate. Extra soy sauce should be avoided. The patient should be instructed to avoid courses containing nuts.

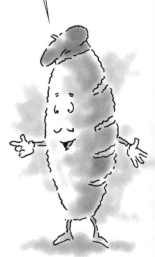

C'est magnifique! A patient with chronic renal failure can safely eat several kinds of bread — including me!

treat anemia. However, they shouldn't be taken with calcium supplements.

Nutrition therapy for transplant recipients

Transplant recipients are typically malnourished. In the immediate postoperative period, the patient should be encouraged to consume a diet high in protein and calories to promote healing. After healing is complete, the goal of nutrition therapy is to help reduce adverse effects and complications related to immunosuppressant therapy.

If temporary or permanent rejection occurs, resulting in uremia, the patient must resume dietary restrictions for chronic renal failure.

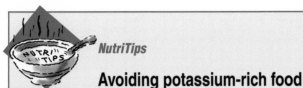

NutriTips

Avoiding potassium-rich food

When preparing the patient with chronic renal failure for discharge, make sure he understands the importance of avoiding foods rich in potassium. The list below contains some examples of potassium-rich foods.

Fruits
- Avocados
- Bananas
- Cantaloupe
- Grapefruit juice
- Honeydew melon
- Oranges
- Orange juice
- Fresh peaches
- Dried fruit

Beans
- Baked beans
- Black beans
- Black-eyed peas
- Butter beans
- Chickpeas
- Crowder peas
- Great Northern beans
- Kidney beans
- Lentils
- Lima beans
- Navy beans
- Pinto beans
- Split peas

Vegetables
- Broccoli
- Greens
- Spinach
- Tomatoes
- Tomato soup
- Tomato juice

Potatoes
- Baked white potato
- Baked sweet potato
- Potato chips
- French fries
- Instant potato mixes
- Home fries
- Yams

Miscellaneous foods
- Molasses
- Nuts
- Salt substitutes

Consumed with calories

Calories should be consumed in amounts necessary to maintain moderate body weight. Certain drugs cause anorexia, nausea, vomiting, and diarrhea, which cause weight loss. Corticosteroids, on the other hand, contribute to obesity. Fat intake should be limited to 30% of the total calories.

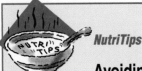

NutriTips

Avoiding phosphorus-rich foods

Advise patients with chronic renal failure to avoid foods high in phosphorus. Examples of high-phosphorus foods are listed here.

Bread group
- Bran

Vegetable group
- Artichoke (boiled)

Milk group
- Milk (1%, 2%, skim, and whole)
- Yogurt
- Cheese
- Ice cream

Meat and beans group
- Kidney beans
- Split peas
- Lentils
- Beef
- Salmon
- Chicken
- Pork
- Nuts
- Peanut butter

Miscellaneous
- Cocoa, beer, and cola beverages

How much protein?

Patients typically require 1 to 1.2 g/kg of protein daily. Protein intake should be adjusted as needed. Higher amounts may be necessary to surpass the catabolic effects of corticosteroid therapy. Lower amounts may be necessary if symptoms of uremia return.

Old salt

Sodium intake should be limited to 3 to 4 g/day to help prevent fluid retention and hypertension. Patients should be cautious of salt substitutes because many replace sodium with potassium.

Adjusting potassium

Potassium intake should be adjusted according to serum potassium levels and diuretic therapy.

Got milk?

Patients should be encouraged to consume 800 to 1,500 mg of calcium per day to prevent bone demineralization. The patient with hyperphosphatemia may need to limit intake of milk and other dairy products.

Commonly prescribed phosphorus binders

Phosphorus binders, alone or in combination, may be prescribed to reduce high phosphorus levels in a patient with chronic renal failure. Some common phosphorus binders include:
- calcium carbonate
- calcium acetate
- sevelamer hydrochloride
- lanthanum carbonate.

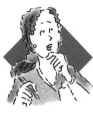

Quick quiz

1. Which of the following foods is high in oxalate and should be avoided in patients with renal calculi?
- A.   Green beans
- B.   Beets
- C.   Peaches
- D.   Apples

Answer: B. Beets should be avoided in patients with renal calculi because they contain high levels of oxalate.

2. A patient develops renal failure that's complicated by hyperkalemia. Which high-potassium food should the patient avoid?
- A.   Rhubarb
- B.   Strawberries
- C.   Honeydew melon
- D.   Grapes

Answer: C. Honeydew melon is very high in potassium and should be avoided in patients with hyperkalemia.

3. Teaching about sodium restriction has been effective for the kidney transplant patient when he states that he should restrict his sodium intake to what amount?
- A.   2 to 3 g/day
- B.   3 to 4 g/day
- C.   4 to 5 g/day
- D.   5 to 6 g/day

Answer: B. Renal transplant recipients should restrict sodium intake to 3 to 4 g/day to control hypertension and weight gain.

Scoring

☆☆☆ If you answered all three questions correctly, what a whiz! You really know your renal!

☆☆ If you answered two questions correctly, great! You're skilled at transplanting knowledge!

☆ If you answered fewer than two questions correctly, don't worry. Unlike chronic renal failure, these results are reversible. Review the chapter and try again!

Neurologic disorders

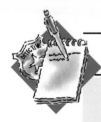

Just the facts

Because the neurologic system coordinates the functions of all other body systems, nutrition can be a major component of neurologic care. In this chapter, you'll learn:

♦ the structure and function of the neurologic system

♦ pathophysiology, signs and symptoms, and treatments for common neurologic disorders

♦ nutrition therapy for common neurologic disorders.

A look at the neurologic system

The neurologic, or nervous, system is the body's communication network. It coordinates and organizes the functions of all other body systems. This intricate network has two main divisions:

The central nervous system (CNS), made up of the brain and spinal cord, is the body's control center.

The peripheral nervous system, containing cranial and spinal nerves, provides communication between the CNS and remote body parts.

Neuron your own

The neuron, or nerve cell, is the nervous system's fundamental unit. This highly specialized conductor cell receives and transmits electrochemical nerve impulses. Delicate, threadlike nerve fibers called *axons* and *dendrites* extend from the central cell body and transmit signals. Axons carry impulses away from the cell body; dendrites carry impulses to the cell body. Most neurons have multiple dendrites but only one axon.

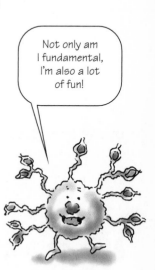

Not only am I fundamental, I'm also a lot of fun!

Living computer network

This intricate network of interlocking receptors and transmitters, along with the brain and spinal cord, forms a living computer that controls and regulates every mental and physical function. From birth to death, the nervous system efficiently organizes the body's affairs, controlling the smallest actions, thoughts, and feelings.

Central intelligence

The CNS consists of the brain and spinal cord. The fragile brain and spinal cord are protected by the bony skull and vertebrae, cerebrospinal fluid (CSF), and three membranes—the dura mater, the arachnoidea mater, and the pia mater.

Leading role

The *cerebrum*, the largest part of the brain, houses the nerve center that controls sensory and motor activities and intelligence. The outer layer of the cerebrum, the cerebral cortex, consists of neuron cell bodies (gray matter). The inner layer consists of axons (white matter) plus basal ganglia, which control motor coordination and steadiness.

Supporting roles

Other main parts of the brain are the cerebellum and the brain stem:
• The *cerebellum* lies beneath the cerebrum, at the base of the brain. It coordinates muscle movements, controls posture, and maintains equilibrium.
• The *brain stem* includes the midbrain, pons, and medulla oblongata. It houses cell bodies for most of the cranial nerves. Along with the thalamus and hypothalamus, it makes up a nerve network called the *reticular formation*, which acts as an arousal mechanism.

Two-way conduction system

The spinal cord extends downward from the brain to the second lumbar vertebrae. The spinal cord functions as a two-way conduction pathway between the brain stem and the peripheral nervous system.

Assessment

To plan nutritional therapy for a patient with neurologic disease, first perform a nutrition-focused assessment that includes a health history, a physical examination, and diagnostic test findings.

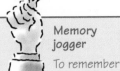

Memory jogger

To remember the basic areas of the brain, think **N**erves **C**an **C**ontrol **B**ody **R**eactions:

Neurons

Cerebrum

Cerebellum

Brain stem

Reticular formation.

Health history

Obtain a history to assess the patient's neurologic status. Focus the health history on the patient's eating habits, weight, and past illnesses and preexisting conditions. Gather information about the patient's:

- dietary intake
- knowledge of healthy eating habits
- willingness to change eating habits, if needed
- ability to buy and prepare healthy foods
- frequency of eating out
- physical activity and exercise
- religious and ethnic influences on food choices
- food allergies and intolerances
- use of alcohol, caffeine, tobacco, and recreational drugs
- use of nutritional supplements
- current and past medication use
- medical history
- family history of neurologic disease.

Physical examination

Focus the physical examination on nutrition-related aspects, such as the patient's weight and height and his ability to feed himself and swallow. Evaluate your patient's vital signs and mental status. These observations will provide clues about neurologic dysfunction.

Observing the patient's behavior can give you clues about his mental status. Does he have trouble concentrating, have memory loss, or seem disoriented?

Calcium and glucose are two important lab tests for neurologic disease.

Diagnostic tests

To evaluate a patient for neurologic disease, the doctor may order various laboratory and diagnostic tests, including:

- calcium levels
- glucose levels
- EEG
- computed tomography scan
- magnetic resonance imaging.

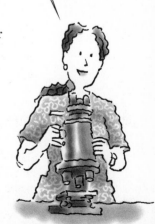

Alzheimer's disease

Alzheimer's disease, also referred to as *primary degenerative dementia*, is a progressive degenerative disorder of the cerebral cortex. Cortical degeneration is most marked in the frontal lobes, but atrophy occurs in all areas of the cortex. It accounts for more than half of all cases of dementia. An estimated 5% of people over age 65 have a severe form of the disease, and 12% suffer from mild to moderate dementia.

Because this is a primary progressive dementia, the prognosis is poor. The average duration of illness before death is 8 years.

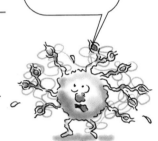

Neurofibrillary tangles cause a mess of symptoms in a patient with Alzheimer's.

Pathophysiology

The cause of Alzheimer's disease is unknown, but several factors are thought to be implicated in the disease, including:
• neurochemical factors, such as deficiencies in the neurotransmitters acetylcholine, somatostatin, substance P, and norepinephrine
• environmental factors
• genetic factors.

Genetic studies show that an autosomal dominant form of Alzheimer's disease is associated with early onset and death. A family history of Alzheimer's disease and the presence of Down syndrome are two known risk factors.

The brain tissue issue

The brain tissue of patients with Alzheimer's disease has three distinguishing features:
• neurofibrillary tangles, formed out of proteins, in neurons
• neuritic plaques
• granulovascular degeneration of neurons.

Degeneration of de neurophil

The disease causes degeneration of neurophils (dense complexes of interwoven cytoplasmic processes between nerve cells and neuroglial cells), especially in the frontal, parietal, and occipital lobes. It also causes enlargement of the ventricles (cavities within the brain filled with CSF).

Early cerebral changes include formation of microscopic plaques, consisting of a core surrounded by fibrous tissues. Later on, atrophy of the cerebral cortex becomes strikingly evident.

Plaque attack

If a patient has a large number of neuritic plaques, his dementia will be more severe. The plaques contain amyloid, which may exert neurotoxic effects. Evidence suggests that plaques play an important part in bringing about the death of neurons.

Acetylcholine shortage

Problems with neurotransmitters and the enzymes associated with their metabolism may play a role in the disease. The severity of dementia is directly related to reduction of the amount of the neurotransmitter acetylcholine.

On autopsy, the brains of Alzheimer's patients may contain as little as 10% of the normal amount of acetylcholine and are typically atrophic, weighing less than 1,000 g. The weight of a normal brain is commonly about 1,380 g.

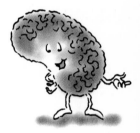

What's a brain got to do to get a little acetylcholine around here?

What to look for

Alzheimer's disease has an insidious onset. Initially the patient undergoes almost imperceptible changes. These changes may include forgetfulness, recent memory loss, difficulty learning and retaining new information, inability to concentrate, and deterioration in personal hygiene and appearance. As the disease progresses, signs and symptoms indicate a degenerative disorder of the frontal lobe. They may include:
- difficulty with abstract thinking and activities that require judgment
- progressive difficulty with communicating
- severe deterioration of memory, language, and motor function progressing to coordination loss and an inability to speak and write
- irritability, mood swings, hostility, and combativeness.

Neurologic examination commonly reveals an impaired sense of smell (usually an early symptom), an inability to recognize and understand the form and nature of objects by touching them, gait disorders, and tremors.

In the final stages, urinary or fecal incontinence, twitching, and seizures commonly occur.

Treatment

Therapy consists of the anticholinesterase drugs galantamine, donepezil, or rivastigmine to help improve symptoms. Tacrine, once commonly prescribed, is now rarely used due to the severity of side effects and numerous drug interactions. Memantine, an N-methyl D-aspartate antagonist, is prescribed to treat symptoms of moderate to severe Alzheimer's disease. Vitamin E may help protect brain cells from damage. Other drugs can be used, as needed, to control behavioral symptoms, such as anxiety, agitation, sleep disturbances, and depression.

Nutritional therapy

Although there's no evidence that Alzheimer's disease changes nutritional requirements, it does have significant effects on the patient's nutritional status. Initially, the patient may have difficulty purchasing and cooking food. He may forget to eat or may forget he has eaten and eat again. Mood swings may cause fluctuations in appetite. Food preferences change with alterations in the patient's sense of smell. Agitation may increase calorie requirements by as much as 1,600 cal/day.

All choked up

The patient with Alzheimer's disease may hoard food or may forget to chew food thoroughly, placing him at risk for choking. Therefore, mealtime should be closely supervised. Food temperatures should be monitored to prevent burns.

Follow a routine

Meals should be served at the same time each day in familiar surroundings. Distractions should be kept to a minimum. It may be necessary to offer one food at a time because a whole plate or tray of food can be overwhelming. (See *Sticking to the patient's personal routine.*)

Consistency counts

It may be necessary to modify food consistency to prevent choking. Food should be cut into small pieces and the patient reminded to chew, as necessary. Easy-to-consume snacks, such as finger foods, should be offered between meals. When the patient can no longer take in food orally, tube feedings may be initiated. However, this choice needs to be discussed with the family.

Epilepsy

Also known as *seizure disorder*, epilepsy is a brain condition that's characterized by recurrent seizures. Seizures are paroxysmal events associated with abnormal electrical discharges of neurons in the brain. The discharge may trigger a convulsive movement, an interruption of sensation, an alteration in level of consciousness, or a combination of these symptoms. In most cases, epilepsy doesn't affect intelligence.

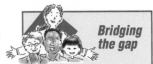

Bridging the gap

Sticking to the patient's personal routine

Sticking to a routine is important when caring for the patient with Alzheimer's disease. However, make sure it's as close to the patient's *personal* routine as possible. Be aware that certain beliefs may play a part in that routine.

Religion tends to have a great impact on eating habits, even greater than nationality and culture. Orthodox Jews, for example, eat Kosher foods, and use separate dishes and utensils for meat and dairy. Question the family about the patient's religious practices surrounding food. Remember, religious practices can vary significantly, even among denominations of the same faith.

Under control

More than 2.7 million Americans are living with epilepsy. The condition appears most commonly in early childhood, early adolescence, and advanced age. About 80% of patients have good seizure control with strict adherence to prescribed treatment.

Pathophysiology

In about half the cases of epilepsy, the cause is unknown and the patient has no other neurologic abnormality. In other cases, however, possible causes of epilepsy include:
- birth trauma (inadequate blood supply to the brain)
- anoxia (after respiratory or cardiac arrest)
- infectious diseases (meningitis, encephalitis, or brain abscess)
- ingestion of toxins (mercury, lead, or carbon monoxide)
- brain tumor
- fever
- head trauma or injury.

Hyperactivity

This is what happens during a seizure:

The electronic balance of the neuronal level is altered, causing the neuronal membrane to become susceptible to activation.

Increased permeability of the cytoplasmic membranes helps hypersensitive neurons fire abnormally. Abnormal firing may be activated by hyperthermia, hypoglycemia, hyponatremia, hypoxia, or repeated sensory stimulation.

Once the intensity of a seizure discharge has progressed sufficiently, it spreads to adjacent brain areas. The midbrain, thalamus, and cerebral cortex are most likely to become epileptogenic.

Excitement feeds back from the primary focus and to other parts of the brain.

The discharges become less frequent until they stop.

Getting complicated

Depending on the type of seizure, injury may result from a fall at the onset of a seizure or afterward, when the patient is confused. Injury may also result from the rapid, jerking movements that occur during or after a seizure. Anoxia can occur due to airway occlusion by the tongue, aspiration of vomit, or traumatic injury. A continuous seizure state known as *status epilepticus* can cause respiratory distress and even death.

What to look for

Signs and symptoms of epilepsy vary depending on the type and cause of the seizure.

Complex partial seizure

Signs and symptoms of a complex partial seizure are variable but usually include purposeless behavior, a glassy stare, aimless wandering, and lip-smacking. An aura may occur first, and seizures may last a few seconds to 20 minutes. Afterward, mental confusion may last for several minutes.

Absence seizure

Absence seizure occurs most often in children. It usually begins with a brief change in the level of consciousness, signaled by blinking or rolling of the eyes, a blank stare, and slight mouth movements. The patient retains his posture and continues preseizure activity without difficulty. Seizures last from 1 to 10 seconds, and impairment is so brief that the patient may be unaware of it. However, if not properly treated, these seizures can recur up to 100 times per day and progress to a generalized tonic-clonic seizure.

Generalized tonic-clonic seizure

Typically, a generalized tonic-clonic seizure begins when the patient's body stiffens (tonic phase). It then alternates between episodes of muscle spasm and relaxation (clonic phase). The patient may fall to the ground and lose consciousness. Tongue biting, incontinence, labored breathing, apnea, and cyanosis may also occur.

The seizure stops in 2 to 5 minutes, when abnormal electrical conduction of the neurons is completed. Afterward, the patient regains consciousness but is somewhat confused. He may have difficulty talking and may have drowsiness, fatigue, headache, muscle soreness, and arm or leg weakness. He may fall into a deep sleep afterward.

Treatment

Common first-line antiepileptic medications include carbamazepine, ethosuximide, oxcarbazepine, phenytoin, and valproic acid. Medications that can be added to or replace first-line medications include felbamate, gabapentin, lamotrigine, levetiracetam, tiagabine, topiramate, and zonisamide. Other medications used to treat epilepsy include benzodiazepines, phenobarbital, and primidone.

Distress call

Some drugs used to treat epilepsy cause GI distress. Encourage the patient to take the drug with food to minimize distress, if appropriate.

Other treatments for epilepsy may include surgery to remove a focal lesion or correct the underlying problem or insertion of a vagal nerve stimulator.

Medication meddler

If the patient taking phenytoin requires enteral feedings, separate dosing and feeding times as much as possible and by no less than an hour. Enteral feedings may interfere with the absorption of oral suspension.

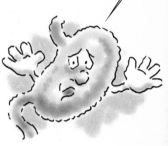

Some drugs used to treat epilepsy cause GI distress.

Nutritional therapy

Most patients with epilepsy don't require dietary changes. However, those patients who don't attain seizure control through use of antiseizure medications are sometimes prescribed ketogenic diets in conjunction with their medications. The diet is most effective when used for children.

Children selected for ketogenic therapy typically experience at least two seizures per week despite receiving two antiseizure medications. Research has shown that elevated blood ketone levels in these children reduce the incidence of seizure activity, sometimes to the point that antiseizure medications are no longer needed.

Change in the popularity poll

Initially studied in the 1920s, the ketogenic diet was used to treat intractable seizures. As different seizure medications were developed, fewer people were encouraged to follow this diet. Recently, however, there has been a resurgence of its use.

What? High fat, low carb, and low protein?

This high-fat, low-carbohydrate, low-protein diet causes ketosis as the body is forced to use fatty acids instead of glucose for energy. This reaction causes mild starvation and dehydration. In addition, the diet places the patient at risk for hypoglycemia.

A dietitian uses the patient's age and weight to calculate the caloric needs. The patient's calorie allotment for the diet is restricted and based on the patient's age and activity level. When the patient begins the diet, he's usually started at a ratio of 4 parts fat to 1 part carbohydrate and protein. Children under age 15 months or obese children may be started on a 3:1 ratio.

On the way to ketosis

When a patient requires a ketogenic diet to control seizures, a dietitian uses age and weight to determine caloric needs. Then she uses formulas to determine fat, protein, and carbohydrate needs. When the individual diet plan is formulated, the patient prepares for admission to the hospital to initiate treatment. The day before hospitalization, he consumes a low-carbohydrate diet and, after dinner, fasts with the exception of water. The typical postadmission treatment plan is outlined here.

Day 1
- Patient continues to fast with the exception of fluids.
- Oral intake is increased to 3 to 4 times the maintenance level; patient consumes water or diet, caffeine-free soda.
- Family meets with the dietitian.
- Baseline laboratory tests such as serum antiseizure medication level, lipoprotein level, and electrolyte levels are obtained.
- Baseline EEG is obtained.
- Anti-seizure medication doses are decreased because levels may rise during the fasting period.
- I.V. therapy is initiated.
- Parent or other family member is instructed to keep a seizure diary and an accurate record of the patient's intake.

Your responsibilities
- Maintain strict intake and output.
- Monitor urine for ketones after every void.
- Monitor blood glucose levels every 4 to 6 hours as ordered.
- Weigh the patient after the first void in the morning.
- Monitor vital signs every 4 hours.
- Measure the child's head circumference, if age appropriate.
- Instruct the family about checking urine for ketones and monitoring blood glucose levels.
- Explain to the patient and family that the patient can't use toothpaste or mouthwash with sugar or carbohydrate in them.

Day 2
- Dietitian develops meal plans.
- Patient receives I.V. normal saline solution, if needed.
- Family begins learning how to plan and prepare meals.
- Urine ketone levels become elevated (4+ is target value).
- Laboratory tests such as serum electrolytes and antiseizure medication levels are obtained.

Your responsibilities
- Monitor blood glucose and urine ketone levels.
- Monitor weight after first morning void.
- Monitor vital signs.

Day 3
- Patient is in ketosis.
- Food is reintroduced using one-third strength meals.
- Family continues learning dietary planning and food preparation.
- Serum antiseizure medication levels and electrolyte levels are obtained.

Your responsibilities
- Monitor blood glucose and urine ketone levels.
- Monitor weight after first morning void.
- Monitor vital signs.
- Have parents perform a return demonstration of blood glucose and ketone testing.

Day 4
- Meals are progressed to two-thirds strength.
- Family education regarding meal planning and preparation continues.
- Serum antiseizure medication levels and electrolyte levels are obtained.

Your responsibilities
- Monitor weight, vital signs, and blood and ketone levels.
- Reinforce family education.

Day 5
- Patient begins full-strength diet.
- Serum antiseizure medication levels and electrolyte levels are obtained.
- If the patient's condition is stable and the family understands dietary teaching, the patient is discharged from the facility.

Your responsibilities
- Monitor weight and vital signs.
- Review discharge teaching.

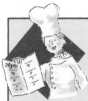

Menu maven

Serving up a ketogenic diet

Meal preparation for the patient receiving a ketogenic diet can be difficult. The patient's family must be educated about the type and amount of food allowed at each meal because any deviation can easily prevent ketosis. The menu below shows the types of food consumed on the diet. The amount of food consumed is highly individualized.

Breakfast
- Scrambled eggs with butter
- Diluted cream
- Orange juice

Lunch
- Spaghetti squash with butter and Parmesan cheese
- Lettuce leaf with mayonnaise
- Orange diet soda mixed with whipped cream

Dinner
- Hot dog slices with sugar-free ketchup
- Asparagus with butter
- Chopped lettuce with mayonnaise

Snack
- Sugar-free vanilla cream ice pop

The brink of drink

Fluid intake is restricted to 75% of the patient's typical intake. As a rule, the patient should consume no more milliliters of fluid per day than the number of calories prescribed in the diet. For example, if the patient is prescribed a 1,500-calorie diet, he should consume no more than 1,500 ml of fluid per day. Fluid intake should be spread over the course of the day and no more than 120 ml should be consumed in a 2-hour period. Urine specific gravity is maintained between 1.020 and 1.025. Beverages containing aspartame or caffeine must be avoided because they inhibit ketosis.

For a patient with epilepsy, fluid intake is restricted to 75% of the patient's typical intake.

That means one of us has got to go.

Don't get caught short

A dietitian calculates the patient's protein allowance, making sure that he consumes the RDA. The diet is supplemented daily with calcium; a sugar-free, lactose-free multivitamin; and fluoride, if indicated. (See *On the way to ketosis.*)

Family education is the key to success. The patient's family is taught meal planning and preparation and blood glucose monitoring during the patient's hospitalization. (See *Serving up a ketogenic diet.*)

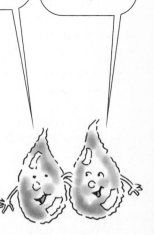

Parkinson's disease

Parkinson's disease produces progressive muscle rigidity, loss of muscle movement (akinesia), and involuntary tremors. The patient's condition may deteriorate for about 10 years until death finally ensues.

Parkinson's disease is one of the most common crippling diseases in the United States. It affects men and women equally and usually occurs in middle age or later, striking 1 in every 100 people over age 60. (See *Young-onset Parkinson's disease.*)

Pathophysiology

In most cases, the cause of Parkinson's disease is unknown. However, some cases result from exposure to toxins, such as manganese dust and carbon monoxide, that destroy cells in the substantia nigra of the brain.

Dopamine pathway defect...

Parkinson's disease affects the extrapyramidal system of the brain, which influences the initiation, modulation, and completion of movement. The extrapyramidal system includes the corpus striatum, subthalmic nucleus, substantia nigra, and red nucleus.

In Parkinson's disease, a dopamine deficiency occurs in the basal ganglia, the dopamine-releasing pathway that connects the substantia nigra to the corpus striatum.

...causes neurotransmitter imbalance

Reduction of dopamine in the corpus striatum upsets the normal balance between the inhibitory dopamine and excitatory acetylcholine neurotransmitters. This prevents affected brain cells from performing their normal inhibitory function within the CNS and causes most parkinsonian symptoms.

What to look for

Important signs of Parkinson's disease include:
• muscle rigidity
• akinesia
• unilateral pill-rolling tremor.

Muscle rigidity results in resistance to passive muscle stretching, which may be uniform (lead-pipe rigidity) or jerky (cogwheel rigidity).

Akinesia causes a masklike facial expression and gait and movement disturbances. The patient walks with his body bent forward, takes a long time initiating movement when performing a purposeful action, pivots with difficulty, and easily loses his balance.

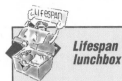

Lifespan lunchbox

Young-onset Parkinson's disease

Young-onset Parkinson's disease is the appearance of parkinsonian symptoms before age 40. Although young patients experience all the typical symptoms, dystonic spasms are more common and may appear before the onset of other characteristic symptoms of Parkinson's disease. Younger patients are also less likely to experience tremors than people who develop Parkinson's disease after age 60. Levodopa is effective in treating symptoms in younger patients; however, younger patients are more likely to develop dyskinesia while taking this drug.

Pill-rolling tremor is insidious. It begins in the fingers, increases during stress or anxiety, and decreases with purposeful movement and sleep.

Supplemental symptoms

Other signs and symptoms of Parkinson's disease include:
- high-pitched, monotone voice
- drooling
- dysarthria (impaired speech due to disturbance in muscle control)
- dysphagia (difficulty swallowing)
- fatigue.

Compiling the complications

Common complications of Parkinson's disease include injury from falls, food aspiration due to impaired voluntary movements, urinary tract infections, and skin breakdown due to increased immobility.

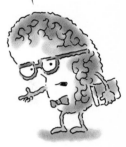

Dopamine reduction prevents my cells from doing their job and causes most parkinsonian symptoms.

Treatment

Because Parkinson's disease has no cure, treatment aims to relieve symptoms and keep the patient functional as long as possible. Treatment consists of drugs, physical therapy and, in severe cases that are unresponsive to drugs, stereotactic surgery or fetal cell transplantation (controversial).

A look at levodopa

Drug therapy usually includes levodopa, a dopamine replacement that's most effective during the early stages of treatment. It's given in increasing doses until symptoms are relieved or adverse effects develop. Because adverse effects can be serious, levodopa is frequently given along with carbidopa to halt peripheral dopamine synthesis. Unfortunately, levodopa doesn't prevent the progressive brain changes found in Parkinson's disease.

Other drugs that can be used include anticholinergics, antihistamines, amantadine, entacapone, selegiline, and catechol-O-methyl transferase inhibitors.

Is neurosurgery next?

When drug therapy fails, stereotactic neurosurgery is sometimes effective. In this procedure, electrical coagulation, freezing, radioactivity, or ultrasound destroys the ventrolateral nucleus of the thalamus to prevent involuntary movement. Such neurosurgery is most effective in comparatively young, otherwise healthy people

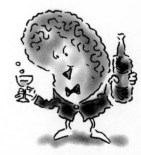

Here's to levodopa and carbidopa. They make a beautiful pair!

with unilateral tremor or muscle rigidity. Like drug therapy, neurosurgery is a palliative measure that can only relieve symptoms.

Other treatments include brain stimulator implantation, fetal cell transplantation (controversial), and neurotransplantation.

Exercise expectations

The patient with Parkinson's disease should be encouraged to exercise at least three times per week while he's able. His exercise regimen should include aerobic, strengthening, and stretching exercises.

Easy PT

Physical therapy helps maintain the patient's normal muscle tone and function. It includes active and passive range-of-motion exercises, routine daily activities, walking, and baths and massage to help relax muscles.

Nutritional therapy

Constipation, a common complication of Parkinson's disease, can interfere with the uptake of drugs such as levodopa. Patients should be encouraged to consume a high-fiber diet. High-fiber foods should be gradually substituted for refined, low-fiber foods to avoid symptoms of intolerance (gas, diarrhea, and cramping).

Coffee, tea, or…lemon water?

The patient should also increase his fluid intake to at least 8 to 10 glasses daily. Encourage the patient to drink hot coffee, tea, or lemon water to stimulate peristalsis. Encourage the intake of prunes or prune juice, which have laxative effects.

Vivacious vitamin D

The gait disturbance associated with Parkinson's disease places the patient at risk for falls. This, combined with inadequate intake of vitamin D and calcium, places the patient at increased risk for fractures. Consuming adequate amounts of vitamin D helps promote calcium absorption and prevent bone density loss.

Be smart about B_6

Excessive intake of pyridoxine (vitamin B_6) can reduce the effectiveness of levodopa. If the patient takes over-the-counter supplements, discuss the interaction. Encourage the patient to limit his intake of foods fortified with vitamin B_6.

Levodopa, an amino acid, competes for absorption with other amino acids found in dietary protein. Absorption of levodopa may be reduced, lessening the drug's effectiveness. Excess protein in-

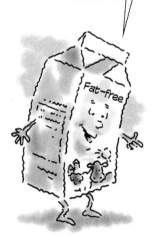

Ensuring adequate amounts of vitamin D helps to promote calcium absorption and prevent bone density loss.

take should be avoided and the majority of the daily allowance of protein should be consumed during the evening meal. (See *Ineffective mix*.)

Difficult going down

Eating, and especially swallowing, may be difficult for the patient with Parkinson's disease. A dietitian can suggest meal choices that are easier to swallow, such as pudding, custard, scrambled eggs, hot cereals, and yogurt.

Slowing down

Patients with Parkinson's disease may eat very slowly. Using insulated dishes or a warming tray helps keep food warm. Distractions can cause the elderly patient with Parkinson's disease to lose focus while eating. If interrupted during eating, patients may have trouble starting again. It's best to plan uninterrupted mealtimes. Because hand coordination becomes poor, plate guards and special eating utensils may be helpful. Soft textured foods may be necessary for those who have difficulty chewing.

Parkinson's disease also slows gastric motility, prolonging digestion. Food takes less time to digest when consumed in small amounts. Encourage the patient to consume small, frequent meals instead of consuming three larger meals per day.

Weighing in on weight loss

Weight loss can be a problem for patients with Parkinson's disease. Patients sometimes become so diligent about limiting protein and fat intake that they deprive themselves of necessary calories. Encouraging nutrition supplements can combat calorie deprivation.

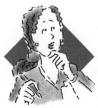

Quick quiz

1. Which characteristic increases the likelihood of a patient with Alzheimer's disease experiencing weight loss?
- A. A slow shuffling gait
- B. Loss of fine motor coordination
- C. Agitation
- D. Lethargy

Answer: C. Agitation increases caloric needs, leading to weight loss.

Ineffective mix

Unlike most drugs, which are absorbed in the stomach, carbidopa-levodopa (Sinemet) is absorbed in the small bowel. Any condition that delays stomach emptying can reduce the absorption of carbidopa-levodopa. Some foods that are high in protein compete with the drug for entry into the brain. When less carbidopa-levodopa enters the brain, the exacerbation of parkinsonian symptoms occurs.

To help maintain adequate protein intake and drug absorption, the patient should take these precautions:
• Restrict protein intake if typical intake is higher than the recommended daily allowance.
• Eat small amounts of protein divided evenly throughout the day or restrict protein intake to the evening meal to get the full effects of medication during the day.

2. How does the ketogenic diet control seizures?
   A.   By forcing ketone production
   B.   By limiting the number of circulating ketones
   C.   By increasing the amount of dopamine available to the brain
   D.   By increasing acetylcholine levels

Answer: A. The ketogenic diet induces mild starvation and dehydration, forcing the body to produce ketones, which have naturally occurring seizure-suppressing properties.

3. The patient prescribed a ketogenic diet should avoid which of the following foods?
   A.   Butter
   B.   Oatmeal cookie
   C.   Eggs
   D.   Mayonnaise

Answer: B. The ketogenic diet is high in fat and protein and low in carbohydrates. Foods that contain sugar, such as an oatmeal cookie, should be avoided. A small deviation in the diet can prevent ketosis.

4. Why might a doctor suggest that a patient with Parkinson's disease limit protein intake to one meal per day?
   A.   Protein competes with levodopa for entry into the brain.
   B.   Protein potentiates the effect of levodopa.
   C.   Protein delays gastric emptying.
   D.   Protein induces ketosis when consumed with levodopa.

Answer: A. Protein and levodopa compete for entry into the brain. The less levodopa that gets to the brain, the less symptom control the patient receives. Consuming protein during the last meal of the day allows adequate protein intake while maintaining adequate drug levels.

Scoring

☆☆☆   If you answered all four questions correctly, congratulations! You've got a head for this kind of information.

☆☆   If you answered three questions correctly, good job! Your neuro-logic is right on track!

☆   If you answered fewer than three questions correctly, that's okay. Reading about neurologic disorders can be a real brain drain. Review the chapter and try again.

Diabetes mellitus

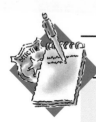

Just the facts

Nutrition is an important factor in the development and treatment of diabetes mellitus. In this chapter, you'll learn:

♦ the relationship between glucose metabolism and dietary intake

♦ the role of medications, exercise, and diet in blood glucose control

♦ nutrition therapy guidelines for patients with diabetes.

A look at diabetes mellitus

Diabetes mellitus is a chronic disease of insulin deficiency or resistance in which disturbances in carbohydrate, protein, and fat metabolism lead to hyperglycemia (increased blood glucose level). It affects 6.3% of the U.S. population, or roughly 18 million people. Half of those affected are undiagnosed.

Squeezing the dollar

Diabetes mellitus and its complications account for a larger portion of U.S. health care spending than any other single disease. Diabetes is the third leading cause of blindness and the most common cause of limb loss (excluding trauma) in the United States. Having diabetes doubles a person's risk of developing heart disease.

However, some experts estimate that nearly 99% of diabetes outcomes depend on patient self-care. So teaching your patients good self-care skills gives them an excellent chance of avoiding diabetes complications.

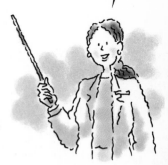

Your biggest impact on a patient with diabetes may be teaching self-care skills.

Type writers

In 1997, the American Diabetes Association (ADA) revised the diabetes classification system and, in 2003, it made changes to the diagnostic criteria for impaired fasting glucose. Currently, there are four main types of diabetes:
- type 1
- type 2
- gestational (diabetes during pregnancy)
- other (includes diabetes caused by genetic defects in insulin action, genetic defects of beta cell function, and other genetic syndromes; pancreatic or endocrine disease; drug or chemical causes; infections; and immune-mediated causes).

Diagnosing diabetes

Diabetes is diagnosed in anyone with a fasting plasma glucose level of 126 mg/dl (SI, 7 mmol/L) or higher on two different days. Diabetes is also diagnosed if the patient has a glucose reading of either:
- 200 mg/dl (SI, 11.1 mmol/L) or higher 2 hours after receiving solution in a glucose tolerance test
- 200 mg/dl or higher on any plasma glucose test on two different days (taken at any time of day regardless of the last meal) and symptoms of diabetes.

Three's company

To aid evaluation and check for complications, three other tests also may be done:
- Glycosylated hemoglobin (HbA_{1c}) tests monitor long-term effectiveness of therapy in a patient previously diagnosed with diabetes. These tests show variants in hemoglobin levels that reflect average blood glucose levels over the previous 2 to 3 months.
- Ophthalmologic examination may show diabetic retinopathy.
- Urinalysis determines presence of acetone in the urine.

Caught in the middle

Some people have *prediabetes*, an intermediate state between normal glucose metabolism and diabetes. Prediabetes increases the risk of developing diabetes, heart attack, and stroke. About 41 million Americans ages 40 to 74 have prediabetes.

The two forms of prediabetes are:
- *impaired fasting glucose*, diagnosed in patients with fasting plasma glucose levels of 100 to 125 mg/dl (SI, 5.6 to 6.9 mmol/L)
- *impaired glucose tolerance*, in which oral glucose tolerance test results are above normal but not high enough for a diabetes

Diabetes screening guidelines

Use these guidelines to screen for prediabetes and diabetes in asymptomatic patients:

• Adults should be tested for prediabetes and diabetes every 3 years starting at age 45, especially patients with a body mass index of 5 kg/m^2 or higher.

• People at increased risk for diabetes may need to be tested earlier or more often (such as once per year). Higher-risk groups include those with sedentary lifestyles, presence of a first-degree relative with diabetes, high-risk ethnic groups (such as Blacks, Hispanics, Native Americans, Asian Americans, and Pacific Islanders), women with gestational diabetes, women who have delivered a baby greater than 9 lb, women with polycystic ovary disease, and anyone with hypertension. Risk factors also include high-density lipoprotein cholesterol level less than 35 mg/dl (SI,
0.90 mmol/L) or a triglyceride level greater than 250 mg/dl (2.82 mmol/L) ; impaired glucose tolerance or impaired fasting glucose on prior testing; clinical conditions linked with insulin resistance; or a history of vascular disease.

diagnosis—140 to 199 mg/dl (SI, 7.8 to 11.0 mmol/L), 2 hours after the patient ingests 75 g of glucose.

Sugar, get yourself screened

Guidelines are available to screen for diabetes in patients who are asymptomatic. (See *Diabetes screening guidelines*.)

Type 1 and type 2 diabetes

Type 1 and type 2 diabetes are the most common forms of diabetes mellitus. Type 1, which accounts for approximately 5% to 10% of diabetes cases, can occur at any age. Usually, though, it's detected before age 30 in people of normal or below-normal weight. The cause isn't known, although experts suspect that multiple factors, including genetic susceptibility, are involved.

Type 2 diabetes is the most common diabetes form in adults, accounting for more than 90% of diabetes cases in the United States. It's associated with multiple factors, including a family history of the disease, advancing age, obesity, and lack of exercise. Type 2 diabetes is more common in Blacks, Hispanics, Asian Americans, Pacific Islanders, and Native Americans. (See *Diabetes in Native Americans*, page 336.)

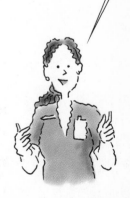

Diabetes is hard to typecast. Types 1 and 2 can both occur at any age.

Breaking the mold

Type 2 diabetes doesn't always fit into set patterns. For example, some patients have an ideal weight and no family history of the disease. Type 2 diabetes can also occur in children. In fact, childhood type 2 diabetes is an emerging epidemic linked to poor eating habits and a sedentary lifestyle.

Pathophysiology

Normally, insulin allows glucose to travel into cells where it's used for energy and stored as glycogen. Insulin also stimulates protein synthesis and free fatty acid storage in adipose tissue. When insulin is deficient, tissues can't access essential nutrients for fuel and storage.

Diabetes mellitus results from insulin deficiency, although the pathophysiology differs with the type of diabetes.

What goes wrong in type 1

In type 1 diabetes, suppression or destruction of the pancreatic beta cells (which produce insulin) impairs insulin production, preventing normal food metabolism. As a result, the blood glucose level rises and cells can't use glucose for energy. Eventually, glucose spills into the urine.

Total lack of insulin leads to buildup of ketone bodies (ketosis). Unless treated, ketosis reduces blood pH, resulting in diabetic ketoacidosis, a life-threatening form of metabolic acidosis.

Attack on beta cells

Type 1 diabetes is subdivided into *idiopathic diabetes* (which has an unknown cause) and *immune-mediated diabetes*. In immune-mediated diabetes, the body's immune system destroys the beta cells. This causes an inflammatory response in the pancreas called *insulitis*.

By the time type 1 diabetes becomes apparent, 80% of beta cells are gone. Some experts believe the beta cells aren't destroyed by the antibodies but are disabled—and might be reactivated later. Islet cell antibodies may be present long before symptoms appear. These immune markers also precede evidence of beta cell deficiency. Autoantibodies against insulin have also been noted.

What goes wrong in type 2

Experts have identified three etiologies for type 2 diabetes:

 resistance to insulin action in target tissues

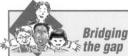

Bridging the gap

Diabetes in Native Americans

In Native Americans, type 2 diabetes may appear during the teens or early twenties, leading to complications and a higher mortality rate at younger ages. The greatest occurrence of diabetes occurs among Pimas (Arizona), Senecas (Oklahoma), and Cherokees (North Carolina); Navajos, Hopis, and Apaches have the lowest rates of occurrence.

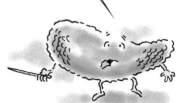

Even though the patho differs from type to type, diabetes mellitus essentially results from insulin deficiency.

abnormal insulin secretion

inappropriate hepatic gluconeogenesis (carbohydrate formation from non-carbohydrate molecules).

Insulin resistance and abnormal insulin secretion eventually lead to impaired glucose tolerance. The pancreas simply can't produce enough insulin to drive blood glucose and other nutrients into body tissues and shut off the liver's glucose production.

Complications

Research shows that glucose readings don't have to be as high as previously thought for complications to develop. Two acute diabetes complications—diabetic ketoacidosis (DKA) and hyperosmolar hyperglycemic nonketotic syndrome (HHNS)—can lead to shock, coma, and even death. Hypoglycemia (low blood sugar) can also occur.

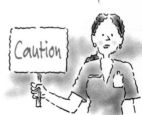

Diabetes complications can lead to shock, coma, and even death.

DKA

DKA occurs most often with type 1 diabetes—and sometimes is the first sign of the disease. The condition is triggered by extremely high blood glucose levels. Ketone buildup causes metabolic acidosis, and severe hyperglycemia leads to dehydration. Although life-threatening, DKA is reversible.

HHNS

HHNS is most common in patients with type 2 diabetes, although it can occur in anyone whose insulin tolerance is stressed and in patients who have undergone certain therapeutic procedures (such as peritoneal dialysis, hemodialysis, tube feedings, or total parenteral nutrition).

As with DKA, HHNS is triggered by insulin deficiency. However, HHNS doesn't involve ketosis. Nonetheless, coma can occur if extremely high blood glucose levels cause dehydration of brain tissues.

Hypoglycemia

Acute hypoglycemia may occur if a diabetic patient:
• eats too little
• exercises too much
• drinks alcohol without eating enough carbohydrates
• takes too much antidiabetic medication
• doesn't prepare or inject insulin properly.

Signs and symptoms include weakness, confusion, syncope, diaphoresis (profuse sweating), and heart palpitations. Untreated, hypoglycemia can cause seizures, brain damage, coma, and death.

Long-term complications

Patients with diabetes mellitus are at higher risk for chronic complications affecting virtually all body systems. The most common complications are cardiovascular disease such as atherosclerosis, peripheral vascular disease, retinopathy, nephropathy (kidney disease), diabetic dermopathy (skin disease), and peripheral and autonomic neuropathy.

In addition, because hyperglycemia impairs resistance to infection, diabetes may cause skin and urinary tract infections as well as vaginitis. Glucose content of the skin and urine encourages bacterial growth.

The paths of neuropathies

Peripheral neuropathy usually affects the hands and feet and may cause numbness or pain. Autonomic neuropathy may manifest in several ways, including gastroparesis (leading to delayed gastric emptying and nausea and fullness after meals), nocturnal diarrhea, impotence, and postural hypotension.

What to look for

The body eliminates excess glucose in urine. As it does so, it excretes a large volume of water, causing the patient with hyperglycemia to become dehydrated and extremely thirsty. Although he may be consuming adequate calories, glucose isn't being absorbed or used properly, so he becomes very hungry and may lose weight.

Patients with type 1 diabetes usually report rapid symptom onset, including muscle wasting and subcutaneous fat loss. With type 2 diabetes, symptoms usually are vague, longstanding, and of gradual onset. Typically, the patient reports a family history of diabetes, gestational diabetes, delivery of a baby weighing more than 9 lb (4 kg), severe viral infection, or use of drugs that increase blood glucose levels. Obesity, especially in the abdominal area, also is a common finding.

Trying triad

With either type 1 or type 2 diabetes, as the body tries to eliminate excess glucose and ketones, the patient may experience the classic symptom triad of:

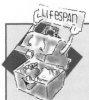

Lifespan lunchbox

Diabetes symptoms in elderly patients

In older adults, two of the classic symptoms of diabetes—polydipsia and polyuria—may be absent. Nonspecific complaints may be the only clues to the disease. Older adults and their caregivers may report appetite loss, weight loss, unexplained fatigue, slow wound healing, mental status changes, incontinence, and decreased vision. Constipation or abdominal bloating may result from gastric hypotonicity. Recurrent bacterial or fungal infections of the skin, urinary tract infections, and pruritus vulvae (in women) may also occur.

Memory jogger

The three **Ps** of the classic symptom triad may help you identify a patient with type 1 or type 2 diabetes mellitus:

Polydipsia

Polyphagia

Polyuria.

polyuria—excessive urination

polydipsia—excessive thirst

polyphagia—excessive eating. (See *Diabetes symptoms in elderly patients.*)

Beyond the triad

Other signs and symptoms of diabetes may include:
- weakness and fatigue
- irritability
- vision changes
- muscle wasting
- weight loss
- dry, itchy skin or cool skin
- dry mucous membranes
- slow peripheral pulses
- decreased reflexes
- poor wound healing
- vaginal discomfort.

In addition, patients with DKA may have a fruity breath odor from increased acetone production.

Treatment

Diabetes treatment should include the patient, family, and an interdisciplinary health care team. Treatment varies with the diabetes type and any coexisting medical problems. For type 1 and type 2 diabetes, the goal is to normalize blood glucose levels and decrease complications. Treatment emphasizes lifestyle changes involving diet and exercise. Some patients also require medication.

In type 1 diabetes, lack of insulin production by the pancreas may make the blood glucose level particularly hard to control, so food intake and exercise patterns must be consistent.

Medication

All patients with type 1 diabetes receive drug therapy. With type 2 diabetes, the need for medication depends on individual factors.

Drug therapy for type 1

The patient with type 1 diabetes must receive insulin by subcutaneous or I.V. injection to survive. The Food and Drug Administration has also recently approved an inhaled insulin product. (See *Inhaled insulin therapy.*) Treatment requires a strict regimen that includes daily insulin injections along with a carefully calculated diet, planned physical activity, and home blood glucose testing several times per day.

Types for type 1

Current forms of insulin replacement include single-dose, mixed-dose, split-mixed dose, and multiple-dose regimens. Patients on multiple-dose regimens may use an insulin pump, which can administer variable rates throughout the day.

Insulin may be rapid-acting (Lispro), short-acting (Regular), intermediate-acting (NPH), long-acting (Ultralente), or a combination of rapid-acting and intermediate-acting. It may be standard or purified, derived from beef, pork, or human sources. Today, purified human insulin is commonly used.

In addition to insulin

The insulin dosage must be balanced with food intake and daily activities. Blood glucose levels must be monitored closely. Patients who don't use an insulin pump must inject insulin at least twice per day to achieve adequate glucose control overnight without causing daytime drowsiness.

Drug therapy for type 2

For many patients with type 2 diabetes, dietary regulation and adequate exercise may sufficiently control the blood glucose level. Otherwise, the patient may require insulin or, more commonly, oral antidiabetic agents. These agents include:
- sulfonylureas, such as glipizide (Glucotrol), glyburide (Micronase, Glynase, and DiaBeta), and glimepiride (Amaryl), which increase insulin secretion and enhance insulin action on the liver and peripheral tissues
- metformin (Glucophage), a biguanide that decrease glucose production by the liver and improves glucose uptake

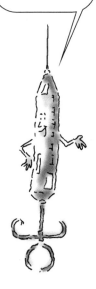

Patients with type 1 diabetes require insulin injections for glucose control.

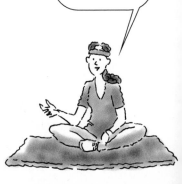

For patients with type 2, diet and exercise may be all the therapy that's necessary.

- alpha-glucosidase inhibitors (starch blockers), such as acarbose (Precose) or miglitol (Glyset), which slow digestion and absorption of starches and sugars, thus countering the rapid blood glucose rise that follows eating
- thiazolidinediones, insulin sensitizers, such as rosiglitazone (Avandia) or pioglitazone (Actos), that increase glucose uptake in tissues and lower serum glucose levels in patients with insulin resistance
- meglitinides, repaglinide (Prandin), and nateglinide (Starlix), which are taken before meals to stimulate the release of insulin, act very quickly, and may cause hypoglycemia.

Some patients receive combinations of these drugs—for instance, metformin with sulfonylureas.

Two injectable drugs have recently been approved for the adjunctive treatment of diabetes in patients who haven't achieved their target HbA_{1c} goals:

- Pramlintide (Symlin) is a synthetic form of the hormone amylin, which is manufactured along with insulin by the beta cells of the pancreas. It's administered with meals and may improve HbA_{1c} levels in patients with type 1 diabetes and patients with type 2 diabetes who are on insulin therapy. Patients taking pramlintide must be monitored for insulin-induced hypoglycemia.
- Exenatide (Byetta), the first of a new class of drugs called *incretin mimetics*, is injected at mealtimes to increase insulin secretion in patients with type 2 diabetes taking metformin, a sulfonylurea, or a combination of metformin and a sulfonylurea. Monitor patients for hypoglycemia, especially those taking a sulfonylurea.

Dietary approaches

Treatment of diabetes requires a diet planned to meet a patient's nutritional needs, control his blood glucose level, and help him reach and maintain an appropriate weight. Obesity increases the body's need for insulin to compensate for the extra glucose consumed with a higher food intake. So even a moderate weight loss (for example, 10 to 20 lb [4.5 to 9 kg]) can lower blood glucose levels and counter insulin resistance. For more details on dietary approaches, see "Nutrition therapy for diabetes," page 346.

Exercise

In type 1 diabetes, exercise doesn't improve glycemic control. However, it yields cardiovascular and other important benefits.

In patients with type 2 diabetes, exercise helps control blood glucose levels. The muscles use more glucose during vigorous physical activity. Exercise improves glucose tolerance and makes body cells more sensitive to insulin, allowing them to use avail-

Inhaled insulin therapy

In January 2006, the FDA approved Exubera, a rapid-acting dry powder form of recombinant human insulin. Inhaled using a handheld device, the drug rapidly passes into the bloodstream, regulating blood glucose levels. It should be taken before meals.

For patients with type 1 diabetes, Exubera is used in combination with long-acting insulin. For patients with type 2 diabetes, Exubera may be used alone as an alternative to rapid-acting insulin or along with oral antidiabetic agents or with long-acting insulin.

Adverse effects of Exubera include hypoglycemia, cough, sore throat, and dry mouth.

Baseline pulmonary function testing should be done before starting the drug, after 6 months of treatment, and annually thereafter.

Exubera is contraindicated in patients who smoke or have quit smoking within the past 6 months and shouldn't be used by patients with a history of chronic lung disease.

able insulin stores more efficiently. Also, exercise helps the patient reach and maintain a healthy weight and can delay or even help prevent cardiovascular disease—the leading cause of death among diabetic patients.

Advise the patient to warm up before exercise and cool down afterward. Instruct him to exercise 5 days per week for optimal glycemic control. Stress that even a short period of physical activity—30 minutes at a time—provides benefits.

Exercise-induced hypoglycemia

If your patient takes insulin or oral antidiabetics, caution him about the possibility of exercise-induced hypoglycemia. During exercise, blood insulin levels can rise from increased insulin sensitivity or mobilization from subcutaneous deposits.

For planned exercise, the patient may need to decrease the insulin dosage. Moderate exercise increases the muscles' glucose uptake by 2 to 3 mg/kg of body weight/minute above resting levels. Higher-intensity activity can raise glucose uptake as much as 6 mg/kg of body weight/minute. (See *Exercise tips for patients with diabetes.*)

Exercise agonies

If your patient has diabetic retinopathy, tell him that strenuous exercise may lead to retinal hemorrhage or detachment. If he has neuropathy, advise him that exercise may cause foot injury.

Self-monitoring

Because blood glucose changes may cause misleading signs and symptoms—or none at all—a patient with diabetes must monitor his blood glucose levels closely to determine if he needs to adjust his medication, diet, or exercise. Self-monitoring allows the patient to determine metabolic status quickly. It's especially useful for those on a tight-control regimen.

Custom-made monitoring

Test method, timing, and frequency are tailored to a patient's needs. Generally, blood should be tested before meals and at bedtime. More frequent monitoring may be necessary:
• during stress, illness, or surgery
• during pregnancy
• after a change in the medication dosage, meal plan, or activity level
• when a patient starts a new medication.

Advise a patient to record blood glucose values in a log, noting any changes in diet, medication, or activity level as well as stress,

Exercise tips for patients with diabetes

Exercise frequency and intensity should be tailored to the patient's needs. The lists below are exercise tips for type 1 and type 2 diabetes.

Type 1 tips
• Exercise decreases blood glucose levels, which can lead to hypoglycemia. Eat a light carbohydrate snack about 30 minutes before exercising and carry fast-acting carbohydrates or glucose tablets to take in case hypoglycemia occurs.
• Consume an additional 10 to 15 g of carbohydrates for each hour of moderate exercise and an extra 20 to 30 g for each hour of vigorous exercise.
• Time exercise sessions so they don't coincide with peak insulin effects.
• Exercise within 2 hours of eating to help prevent hypoglycemia.
• Check the blood glucose level before and after exercise. With poorly controlled type 1 diabetes, exercise may actually worsen hyperglycemia. Avoid exercise if the fasting glucose level exceeds 300 mg/dl (SI, 16.65 mmol/L) (or 250 mg/dl [SI, 13.88 mmol/L] when ketosis is present).

Type 2 tips
• Exercise for 20 to 45 minutes at least three times per week.
• If taking an oral antidiabetic or insulin, exercise within 2 hours of eating.
• Stop exercising if hypoglycemia signs or symptoms occur.

illness, or insulin reactions. Emphasize that a blood glucose level above 240 mg/dl (SI, 13.32 mmol/L) may be dangerous. If a patient's level is that high, instruct him to check his urine for ketones and to call the practitioner for further instructions.

Monitoring long-term glucose control

The practitioner may order an HbA_{1c} test every 12 weeks to determine long-term blood glucose control. Test results reveal average blood glucose levels over a 3-month period. After a patient has achieved treatment goals, testing may be done twice per year.

Ur-ine for something

Although urine glucose testing is used less commonly than in the past, it can detect ketone bodies — particularly important for the ketosis-prone patient.

Also, diabetic patients should have their urine tested for albumin every year to screen for kidney disease. If albumin is detected, the dietary protein allowance may need to be decreased. Although research isn't conclusive on how much protein is optimal for these patients, some experts recommend 0.6 to 0.8 g/kg of body weight.

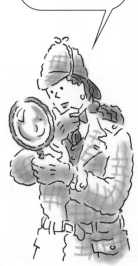

Diabetic patients must stay focused on blood glucose levels in case medication, diet, or exercise adjustments are needed.

Treatment of acute complications

Meticulous control of blood glucose levels is crucial in preventing both acute and chronic diabetes complications. Make sure your patient knows what to do in case an acute complication occurs.

Treating hypoglycemia

If the blood glucose level drops below 20 mg/dl (SI, 1.11 mmol/L), brain damage can occur if glucose isn't administered within minutes. If the blood glucose level is less than 80 mg/dl (SI, 4.44 mmol/L), scheduled insulin shouldn't be given until the level rises from carbohydrate consumption.

If the patient is unconscious, a glucagon injection raises the blood glucose level rapidly. In a conscious patient, a glucose-containing product should be squeezed into the mouth. Alternatives include:
- placing honey on the tongue
- squeezing cake-decorating icing between the gum and cheek
- giving fruit juice, a nondiet soft drink, or water with 3 tsp of added sugar
- giving grape jelly, six jelly beans, or 10 gum drops. (See *Hypoglycemia in young children.*)

Advise your patient with diabetes to carry me around in a chocolate bar. I act fast and taste sweet!

Rule of 15, really?

Many clinicians recommend that diabetic patients use the Rule of 15 to treat hypoglycemia. (See *Rule of 15.*)

Instruct a diabetic patient to carry fast-acting carbohydrates (such as chocolate bars or jelly beans) at all times. Make sure others in the patient's household know how to treat hypoglycemia because a patient who becomes unconscious or confused needs help administering treatment.

Treating DKA and HHNS

Emergency treatment for DKA or HHNS may include insulin and I.V. fluid administration, along with correction of electrolyte imbalances.

Preventing long-term complications

Preventing long-term diabetic complications requires stringent glycemic monitoring and control, along with measures to prevent specific complications. If the patient smokes, urge him to stop.

Don't get disheartened

Because diabetes mellitus increases the risk of heart disease, the patient should eat a heart-healthy diet (see chapter 13, Cardiovas-

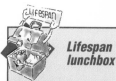

Lifespan lunchbox

Rule of 15

To treat hypoglycemia, teach your patient the Rule of 15:

• If the blood glucose level is below 70 mg/dl (SI, 3.89 mmol/L), eat 15 g of an easily absorbable carbohydrate. If the level is below 50 mg/dl (SI, 2.78 mmol/L), ingest 30 g of carbohydrate instead of 15 g.

• Wait 15 minutes and then recheck the blood glucose level.

• If the level hasn't risen, repeat the process of eating 15 g (or 30 g) of carbohydrate and rechecking the level after 15 minutes, until the blood glucose level registers above 70 mg/dl.

• Then eat a meal containing carbohydrate, protein, and fat.

Sugar therapy

Examples of 15 g of easily absorbable carbohydrate include:

• three glucose tablets

• six or seven hard candies

• 1 tbsp sugar

• 2 tbsp raisins

• 6 oz (177 ml) of a nondiet soft drink

• 4 oz (118 ml) of fruit juice.

　　Low-fat and no-fat carbohydrates work faster because they're broken down more easily.

Hypoglycemia in young children

Many children under age 7 experience hypoglycemic unawareness due to immature counterregulatory mechanisms (hormonal and neural responses). These young children don't have the cognitive ability to identify the symptoms of hypoglycemia or take action to treat symptoms. As a result, they're at great risk for hypoglycemia and its complications.

　　When choosing target blood glucose goals in this age-group, the risk of hypoglycemia must be taken into account. For children with type 1 diabetes who are younger than age 6, the plasma blood glucose goal range is 100 to 180 mg/dl before meals and 110 to 200 mg/dl at bedtime and overnight.

cular disorders), control blood pressure and cholesterol levels, maintain a normal weight, and exercise regularly.

Visualize yearly eye exams

To safeguard vision, advise the patient to get annual eye examinations to detect retinopathy-related damage before symptoms appear. Taking measures to control blood glucose and blood pressure levels can decrease the risk and progression of diabetic retinopathy.

Dental do's

To minimize dental complications, such as gum disease and abscesses, instruct the patient to have regular dental checkups and follow good home care. Tell him to brush his teeth after every meal, floss daily, and report bleeding, pain, or soreness in the gums and teeth immediately.

Keeping a clean bill of health for the kidneys

To help prevent kidney disease, advise the patient to keep blood pressure and blood glucose levels under control and get prompt treatment for urinary tract infections.

Saving skin

Because skin breaks increase the infection risk, tell the patient to check his skin daily for cuts and irritated areas. Tell him to bathe daily with warm water and a mild soap and to apply a lanolin-based lotion afterward to prevent dryness. Advise him to pat the skin dry thoroughly, especially between the toes and in skinfolds. Instruct him to wear cotton underwear to let moisture evaporate and help prevent skin breakdown.

Solid footing

Proper foot care can improve blood circulation to the feet, helping to prevent gangrene and infection. Tell the patient to avoid foot injury and temperature extremes. Instruct him to wash his feet daily with warm water and mild soap and to dry them thoroughly. Advise him to trim toenails to match the shape of the toes—but not too short. Instruct the patient to wear only soft, clean, absorbent socks of a natural fabric or stockings and avoid tight-fitting shoes.

Emphasize the need to examine his feet daily for cuts, scrapes, cracks, bruises, corns, calluses, swelling, and redness—and to call the practitioner if these appear.

Other treatments

The practitioner may recommend pancreas transplantation for certain patients with type 1 diabetes. This procedure may eliminate the need for exogenous insulin, frequent daily blood glucose level measurement, and certain dietary restrictions. It also may prevent episodes of acute hypoglycemia and hyperglycemia. However, pancreas transplantation is only partially successful in reversing long-term neurologic and renal complications.

Experimental explorations

Experimental approaches to treating or curing diabetes include:
- islet cell transplantation
- artificial pancreas implantation
- genetic manipulation (transplanting a fat or muscle cell with a human insulin gene into a patient with type 1 diabetes).

Nutrition therapy for diabetes

The cornerstone of diabetes treatment, a proper diet is essential for effective control of the blood glucose level. A patient must carefully regulate consumption of carbohydrates, fats, and proteins through a personal meal plan based on food preferences, health concerns, and drug therapy. If he's overweight, weight reduction is a primary goal. To assess the effectiveness of nutrition therapy, blood glucose levels, lipid levels, and weight must be monitored regularly.

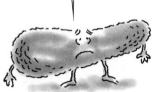

Pancreas transplantation is only partially successful in reversing long-term neurologic and renal complications.

Dear diary

Whether your patient has type 1 or type 2 diabetes, encourage him to keep a food diary (including specific foods and portions eaten) to determine whether and where he needs to make dietary changes. Keeping a food record can yield a wealth of information about the patient's intake.

Nutrition in type 1 diabetes

Most patients with type 1 diabetes are of normal weight and should consume enough calories to maintain weight. Eating a consistent amount of carbohydrates is crucial. Carbohydrate goals should be established for each meal and snack, and the patient should try to achieve the goal set for each meal. For instance, if he should consume 60 g of carbohydrate at breakfast, lunch, and dinner and a 30-g carbohydrate snack at bedtime, urge him to make daily food choices that match these goals.

Let's talk percentages

About 10% to 20% of total calories should come from protein. Total fat intake depends on the patient's weight, blood cholesterol levels, and preferences. If he's overweight and has high cholesterol, the doctor may recommend that 20% or 25% of calories come from fat, with no more than 10% from saturated fat.

Guidelines galore

Also provide the following nutritional guidelines:
• Limit cholesterol intake to 300 mg/day to reduce the risk of heart disease.
• Don't be afraid of sugar—but use it cautiously. No longer taboo for diabetic patients, sugar can be substituted for other carbohydrates as long as the overall diet is healthy.
• Restrict sodium intake to 2 to 4 g/day to help control blood pressure and maintain cardiovascular health.
• Eat a variety of lean protein foods, such as lean meat, fish, poultry, tofu, egg whites, and low-fat dairy products (see *Dealing out protein*).
• Limit starches—especially quickly absorbable starches, such as those in potatoes and white and processed flours. Get most starches from beans and whole unprocessed grains. Replace some starch with low-fat protein and monounsaturated fats.
• Eat 20 to 35 g of fiber daily to help prevent constipation and reduce cholesterol levels.
• Consume plenty of fresh vegetables and fruits—but not fruit juices, which are high in sugar.
• Restrict alcohol to two drinks per day, and only if the blood glucose level is well controlled. To avoid hypoglycemia, always ingest

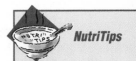

NutriTips

Dealing out protein

To help your patient track the amount of protein he's getting, inform him that one meat serving (3 oz [85 g]) is about the size of a deck of playing cards. Likewise, he can track cheese intake by thinking of one cheese serving as one individually wrapped slice or one cube about the size of a die.

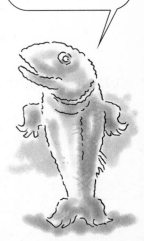

Recommend a variety of lean protein foods, such as lean meat, poultry, tofu, egg whites and, well, (gulp!) me.

food along with alcohol. Also, don't reduce food intake to compensate for alcohol calories. (A patient who is pregnant or has a history of alcohol abuse should abstain from alcohol completely.)

• Coordinate meal timing with the insulin schedule and insulin type. For example, if the patient is taking a fast-acting insulin (such as Lispro) to provide coverage before meals, he should eat within 15 minutes of the injection to avoid hypoglycemia.

Nutrition in type 2 diabetes

For a patient with type 2 diabetes, the goal of nutrition therapy is to maintain adequate nutrition while achieving or maintaining a reasonable weight and normal levels of blood glucose and cholesterol.

If the patient is overweight, the diet should promote weight loss. Research shows that even a minimal weight loss — 10 or 15 lb (4.5 or 7 kg) — can improve glycemic control. Typically, the practitioner recommends therapeutic lifestyle changes, including:

• moderate calorie restriction (for example, 500 fewer average daily intake)
• reduction in total fat intake, especially saturated fat
• increased physical activity.

Rules to eat by

Provide the following nutritional guidelines for a patient with type 2 diabetes:

• Get about 50% of total daily calories from complex carbohydrates, including grains, whole grain bread, beans and other legumes, and vegetables and fruits (but not fruit juices).
• Allow roughly 12% to 20% of daily calories to come from protein (less if kidney disease is present).
• Eat a variety of lean protein foods, such as lean meat, fish, poultry, tofu, egg whites, and low-fat dairy products.
• Limit total fat intake to less than 30% of daily calories, with less than 10% of calories coming from saturated fats. If the low-density lipoprotein level is above normal, limit saturated fat to 7% of calories and restrict dietary cholesterol to less than 200 mg/day.
• Cut back on concentrated simple sugars, such as sucrose, honey, fruit juices, or corn syrup. (See *Softening the blow of soft drinks.*)
• Be stingy with starches. Get most starch from beans and whole unprocessed grains (rather than potatoes or white or processed flours). Replace some starch with low-fat protein and monounsaturated fats.
• Substitute any alcohol intake for fat calories, with one alcoholic beverage replacing two fat exchanges. (However, alcohol should be avoided if the patient is trying to lose weight, has a high triglyceride level, is pregnant, or has a history of alcohol abuse.)

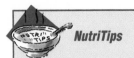
NutriTips

Softening the blow of soft drinks

A good way for a diabetic patient to cut back on calories is to cut down on nondiet soft drinks. On average, a 12-oz (355-ml) can of nondiet soft drink provides about 150 calories. So drinking just a few cans per day adds hundreds of extra calories.

Encourage your patient to turn to low-calorie or no-calorie alternatives, such as diet soft drinks, sugar-free punch, and water.

Think small and think often

Proper meal timing can help prevent extreme blood glucose levels. Many type 2 diabetics achieve good glycemic control by eating smaller food portions more often—five to six small meals daily instead of three larger ones—or small meals combined with high-protein or complex carbohydrate snacks throughout the day. This practice offers several advantages:

• The body processes smaller amounts of glucose more easily than larger amounts.

• Eating before hunger sets in usually leads to better food choices than eating in a ravenous rush.

Type 2 diabetic patients who take insulin should coordinate meals with the type and timing of insulin administration. Patients on oral antidiabetics should avoid skipping meals but don't need the tight schedule required by those on insulin. For better results, though, these patients should adhere to a consistent pattern, eating meals of approximately the same composition at about the same time each day.

Meal planning

Options for helping a patient plan better meals include exchange lists, carbohydrate counting, and the menu approach (see *Sample menu for a diabetic patient*, page 350). The patient should work with a dietitian and a health care provider to determine which type of meal planning best fits his condition and preferences.

Exchange lists

Exchange lists serve as the basis for a meal-planning system devised by the ADA and the American Dietetic Association. The lists simplify meal planning, eliminate the need for daily calculations, and ensure a consistent intake. However, not all patients may want to follow such structured meal planning, and some may not be able to understand how to use the exchange lists.

Categories, names of...

The system groups foods into three main categories—carbohydrates, meat and meat substitutes, and fats. Within each category, subgroups form the exchange lists. Each serving within a list contains about the same amount of calories, carbohydrate, protein, and fat. Combination lists (which include courses, frozen courses, soups, and fast foods) are included so the patient can incorporate mixed food items into the meal plan.

Using these lists, the patient can exchange or trade foods with others in the same main category to fulfill the basic food plan while maintaining proper caloric intake and nutrient balance. The number

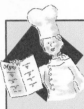

Menu maven

Sample menu for a diabetic patient

This sample menu shows one day's meals and snacks for a diabetic patient. Foods with 5 g of carbohydrate and 25 calories or less per serving are considered "free." This means they can be added to the meal plan in limited amounts and don't have to be counted.

Breakfast
- 2 slices whole wheat toast
- 1 tsp olive oil or light margarine
- ¼ cup egg substitute or egg white omelet
- ½ cup cooked oatmeal
- ½ cup apple or orange juice
- 1 cup coffee

Morning snack
- 6 low-salt crackers with 2 tbsp of peanut butter

Lunch
- Turkey (2 oz [57 g]) sandwich made with 2 slices of whole wheat bread, 1 oz (28 g) low-fat cheese, 1 tsp light mayonnaise, tomato slices, and lettuce
- 1 apple (the size of a tennis ball)
- 1-oz (28-g) bag of baked chips
- 1 can diet soft drink or water

Afternoon snack
- Carrot sticks

Dinner
- 2 cups cooked whole wheat spaghetti
- 1 cup spaghetti sauce
- 2 oz (57 g) lean ground beef
- 1 cup salad with 1 tomato
- 1 slice garlic bread with ½ tsp margarine
- 8 oz (237 ml) water or diet soft drink

Bedtime snack
- ¼ cup low-fat cottage cheese
- ½ cup canned fruit in its own juice

of servings he can eat from each list depends on calorie content and diet composition. Portions must be kept to the specified sizes.

Foods and beverages that supply less than 5 g of carbohydrate or less than 20 calories per serving are considered "free." Unless a portion size is specified, the patient can eat free items as desired. (See *Understanding exchange lists*.)

Carbohydrate counting

Carbohydrate counting emphasizes eating a consistent amount of carbohydrates rather than restricting the *type* of carbohydrate. It lets the patient swap an occasional high-sugar food for other carbohydrate-containing foods. The system is based on two concepts:
- The amount of carbohydrate consumed determines the blood glucose level after a meal or snack. (Carbohydrate is the main nutrient affecting blood sugar. Within an hour or two of consumption, most carbohydrate changes to blood glucose.)
- Eating equal amounts of sugar or starch raises the blood glucose level by roughly the same amount.

It's all in the label

Carbohydrate information on food labels has simplified carbohydrate counting. The system is easier to learn than the exchange lists system, gives the patient more flexible food choices, and pro-

> Carbohydrate counting emphasizes the amount of carb intake rather than the type of carbs.

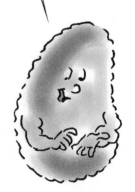

Understanding exchange lists

Some diabetic patients may wish to plan meals using the exchange lists system of the American Diabetes Association and the American Dietetic Association. The system centers on three main food categories—carbohydrates, meat and meat substitutes, and fats.

Carbohydrate group

The carbohydrate group includes:
• starch, with exchange lists that include bread; cereal and grains; starchy vegetables; crackers and snacks; dried beans, peas, and lentils; and starchy foods prepared with fat
• fruit, with exchange lists that include fruit and fruit juice
• milk, with exchange lists that include fat-free and very-low-fat milk, low-fat milk, and whole milk
• other carbohydrates—for example, brownies, cakes, cookies, doughnuts, ice cream, jam, potato chips, sherbet, and yogurt.

Depending on the specific food, an exchange from the carbohydrate group provides:
• 12 to 15 g carbohydrate
• 3 to 8 g protein
• 0 to 8 g fat
• 25 to 150 calories.

Meat and meat-substitute group

The meat and meat-substitute group includes:
• very lean meats
• lean meats
• medium-fat meats
• high-fat meats.

An exchange from this group provides:
• 0 g carbohydrate
• 7 g protein
• 0 to 8 g fat
• 35 to 100 calories.

Fat group

The fat group includes monounsaturated fats, polyunsaturated fats, and saturated fats. An exchange from this group provides:
• 0 g carbohydrate
• 0 g protein
• 5 g fat
• 45 calories.

Free foods

A free food is a food or beverage that provides fewer than 20 calories or 5 g of carbohydrate per serving. Examples include:
• fat-free cream cheese, mayonnaise, and margarine
• sugar-free candy, gelatin, and gum
• bouillon
• broth
• mineral water
• coffee
• ketchup
• mustard
• seasonings (such as garlic and herbs).

Foods with a specified serving size should be spread throughout the day to avoid increased blood glucose levels. If the serving size isn't specified, the food can be eaten as often as desired.

vides a better estimate of how much the blood glucose level will rise after a meal or snack. Also, if the patient takes insulin, carbohydrate counting can be helpful in determining insulin dosages. (See *Carb counting for kids*, page 352.)

If your patient counts carbohydrates, emphasize the importance of keeping accurate food logs and recording blood glucose levels before and after eating.

Menu approach

In the menu approach, the patient and dietitian collaborate to develop menus tailored to the patient's needs and preferences. As the patient desires, menus may be relatively flexible or more rigid, dictating specific foods and the amounts that the patient must eat at specific times.

The menu approach is best for patients who have fairly regimented eating habits or who want to be told exactly what and how much to eat. It isn't ideal for those who want or need flexibility.

Adjusting diet to exercise, illness, and stress

Patients with diabetes may need to adjust their diet for exercise, illness, and stress.

Exercise adjustments

Instruct the patient to check blood glucose levels before, during, and after exercise. If the pre-exercise level exceeds 100 mg/dl, he should base dietary adjustments on the anticipated duration and intensity of exercise:
- For short-duration, low-intensity exercise, no extra carbohydrate is needed.
- For longer-lasting, higher-intensity exercise, he should consume an additional 15 to 30 g of carbohydrate for every 30 to 60 minutes of exercise.

Illness adjustments

Illnesses as minor as a cold may cause hyperglycemia. During illness, glucagon and epinephrine secretion increase, contributing to higher blood glucose levels. As a result, intracellular glucose, fluid, and electrolytes may be lost, leading to dehydration, electrolyte imbalance, and nutrient loss. To prevent these problems, the patient needs to adjust food intake.

Review these sick-day guidelines with the patient:
- Maintain adequate food intake. Don't skip meals.
- As a general rule, consume 15 g of carbohydrate every 1 to 2 hours. If you can't tolerate solid food, drink liquids containing carbohydrates (such as nondiet cola, milk, fruit juice, or tomato juice), or eat gelatin or sherbet. (See *Serving up an adequate diet to an ill diabetic patient.*)
- Keep taking insulin, if prescribed, but adjust the dosage as needed.
- Increase fluid intake if vomiting, diarrhea, or fever occurs.
- Monitor blood glucose levels often—every 4 to 6 hours until symptoms subside. If the level exceeds 240 mg/dl for more than 24 hours, call the practitioner right away. Also monitor urine ketones if advised by the practitioner.
- Call the practitioner if the illness lasts more than 2 days.

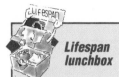

Lifespan lunchbox

Carb counting for kids

Carbohydrate counting can be particularly effective in helping children stick to their recommended diet while meeting caloric needs. In addition to allowing more flexibility in food choices, this meal planning approach provides extra calories in the form of fat and protein—which most active, growing children need.

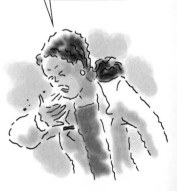

Achoo! Illnesses as minor as a cold may cause hyperglycemia in patients with diabetes.

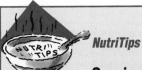

NutriTips

Serving up an adequate diet to an ill diabetic patient

When illness strikes, the appetite may go AWOL. For a diabetic patient, though, skipping meals can be especially dangerous. To help your diabetic patient consume adequate carbohydrates during illness, urge him to substitute liquids for solid foods if his appetite is poor. Advise him to choose among the high-carbohydrate foods listed below.

Food	Serving (cup)	Carbohydrate (g)
Milk	1	12
Apple juice	½	15
Grape juice	⅓	15
Orange juice	½	15
Pineapple juice	½	15
Prune juice	⅓	15
Tomato juice	½	5
Nondiet cola	½	13
Nondiet ginger ale	¾	16
Regular gelatin	½	20
Sherbet	½	30

Stress adjustments

As with illness, the hormonal changes that occur in response to pronounced stress can affect glycemic control. Recommend that the patient learn effective stress-management techniques, especially if he takes insulin.

Adjusting to eating out

If the patient eats out often, make sure he understands his meal-planning system. Advise him to choose restaurants with an appropriate food selection. Instruct him to plan ahead so that he can adjust his food intake before and after a meal out according to his overall dietary allowances.

Also provide the following guidelines:
• Eat only small portions, even if the restaurant serves large ones.
• Use oil and vinegar (or fresh lemon juice) instead of regular salad dressing, or ask for dressing on the side.
• Order roasted, broiled, baked, or grilled meat, fish, or poultry instead of fried, sautéed, or breaded entrées.
• Avoid sweetened juices, fried vegetables, creamed or thick soups, stews, and casseroles.
• Order potatoes, rice, and noodles plain, steamed, baked, or boiled—not fried.
• Choose fresh fruit rather than pastry for dessert.

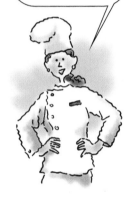

Order roasted, broiled, baked, or grilled meat, fish, or poultry instead of fried, sautéed, or breaded entrées.

Making travel adjustments

Advise the patient to talk to the dietitian when planning a trip. Instruct him to find out which foods will be available at his destination and on the way there. If he plans to fly, he can order a diabetic diet from the airline.

Here are some other travel guidelines to relay:
• Always carry appropriate snacks and quick-acting carbohydrates.
• Plan for any time-zone changes.
• Wear medical identification jewelry.
• If you take medication, have the practitioner write a letter covering the prescription and insulin syringes.
• Make sure travel companions know signs, symptoms, and treatment for hypoglycemia and other acute diabetes complications.

Other forms of diabetes

Besides type 1 and type 2 diabetes, the two other major categories of diabetes mellitus are:
• gestational diabetes (diabetes during pregnancy)
• other specific types of diabetes—a group of disorders marked by altered glucose metabolism.

Gestational diabetes

Gestational diabetes develops in about 4% of pregnancies, affecting approximately 135,000 pregnant women in the United States each year. Although the disorder usually disappears once the pregnancy ends, 5% to 10% of women with gestational diabetes are found to have type 2 diabetes. Also, women who have had gestational diabetes have a 20% to 50% chance of developing type 2 diabetes within 5 to 10 years.

Gestational diabetes may lead to congenital malformations, increased birth weight, and a higher risk of prenatal mortality. Strict metabolic control may reduce these risks.

Gestational diabetes is more common in Blacks, Hispanics, Native Americans, and people with a family history of diabetes. Obesity also increases the risk.

Managing gestational diabetes

Medical care for a patient with gestational diabetes promotes a healthy pregnancy and delivery for mother and child. Initially, the disorder is managed by diet and then, if necessary, by insulin therapy. About 6 weeks after delivery, the patient should be reevaluated for diabetes.

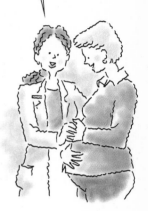

Medical care for gestational diabetes promotes a healthy pregnancy and delivery for mother and child.

Other specific types of diabetes

Other specific types of diabetes account for 1% to 5% of diagnosed diabetes cases. They include eight specific causes of altered glucose metabolism:
- genetic defects of beta cells
- genetic defects in insulin action
- certain pancreatic diseases (such as pancreatitis and cystic fibrosis) or pancreas injury or removal
- certain endocrine diseases, such as Cushing's syndrome, hyperthyroidism, and polycystic ovarian syndrome
- infections, such as measles in a fetus or newborn (congenital rubella) and cytomegalovirus
- certain rare immune disorders
- other genetic syndromes, such as Down syndrome, Klinefelter's syndrome, and Huntington's disease
- drug- or chemical-induced injury to the pancreas (drugs that can cause diabetes include glucocorticoids, thyroid hormone, diazoxide, beta-adrenergic agonists, thiazides, and phenytoin).

Managing other specific types of diabetes

Depending on the body's ability to produce insulin and the degree to which insulin resistance plays a role in altered metabolism, some patients may require exogenous insulin.

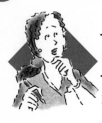

Quick quiz

1. What's a long-term complication of diabetes?
   A.   Retinal detachment
   B.   Skeletal deformities
   C.   Heart disease
   D.   Deafness

Answer: C. Heart disease is a long-term complication of diabetes.

2. Diabetes meal planning should include:
   A.   a minimal amount of carbohydrates.
   B.   no meat.
   C.   salty snacks for fluid volume management.
   D.   a balance of carbohydrates, proteins, and fats.

Answer: D. The patient with diabetes must carefully regulate consumption of carbohydrates, fats, and proteins.

3. A good way for a patient with type 2 diabetes to reduce calories is to:
   A.   cut out all carbohydrates.
   B.   eliminate high-carbohydrate beverages, such as regular soft drinks and juices.
   C.   eat only vegetarian meals.
   D.   eat only one meal per day.

Answer: B. Because 12 oz of regular soft drink or juice provides approximately 150 calories, eliminating these beverages from the diet is a good way to reduce caloric intake.

Scoring

☆☆☆   If you answered all three questions correctly, awesome! You're hyperintelligent when it comes to hyperglycemia.

☆☆   If you answered two questions correctly, keep up the good work! There's no doubting your diabetic knowledge.

☆   If you answered fewer than two questions correctly, it seems your information level is low. Grab a cookie and a glass of orange juice, and dig in for a chapter review!

Human immunodeficiency virus

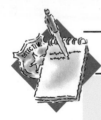

Just the facts

Human immunodeficiency virus (HIV) disease significantly alters the patient's nutritional status. In this chapter, you'll learn:

♦ pathophysiology and signs and symptoms of HIV disease

♦ treatments and nutritional therapy for HIV disease

♦ alternative treatment options.

Understanding HIV disease

Acquired immunodeficiency syndrome (AIDS) was first described by the Centers for Disease Control and Prevention (CDC) in 1981, after public health officials received a series of reports of pneumonia occurring in otherwise young, healthy men from Los Angeles. Previously, this type of pneumonia was seen only in immunosuppressed patients. It's now known that AIDS is the end-stage immune disorder caused by infection with the human immunodeficiency virus (HIV). The course of the disease is now commonly referred to as *human immunodeficiency virus disease*.

Immune impairer

HIV disease, characterized by progressive immune system impairment, destroys T cells and, therefore, the cell-mediated immune response. This immunodeficiency makes the patient more susceptible to infections and unusual cancers. (See *Facts about AIDS*, page 358.)

The CDC has established criteria for making a diagnosis of HIV disease. The course of HIV disease can vary, but it usually results in death from opportunistic infections. Most experts believe that virtually everyone infected with HIV eventually develops AIDS. (See *Classifying HIV infection*, page 359.)

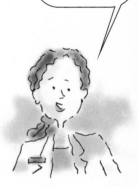

Most experts believe that everyone infected with HIV will develop AIDS.

Facts about AIDS

Acquired immunodeficiency syndrome (AIDS) was first described by the Centers for Disease Control and Prevention (CDC) in 1981. According to the CDC, 35 areas (33 states, Guam, and the U.S. Virgin Islands) have integrated HIV and AIDS surveillance programs. Current HIV and AIDS statistics based on these areas are listed here:

• Through 2004, an estimated 462,792 people were living with HIV or AIDS.

• Of the cases diagnosed in 2004, the largest number (17%) occurred in the 35 to 39 age-group.

• Blacks accounted for 50% of all cases diagnosed in 2004.

• In 2004, males accounted for 73% of all cases among adults and adolescents.

• Th estimated number of deaths among people with AIDS decreased 8% between 2000 and 2004.

Pathophysiology

HIV is an ribonucleic acid–based retrovirus that requires a human host to replicate. The average time between HIV infection and development of AIDS is 8 to 10 years.

HIV destroys CD4+ cells — also known as *helper T cells* — that regulate the normal immune response. The CD4+ antigen (cell surface marker) serves as a receptor for HIV and allows it to invade the cell. Afterward, the virus replicates within the CD4+ cell, causing cell death.

HIV can infect almost any cell that has the CD4+ antigen on its surface, including monocytes, macrophages, bone marrow progenitors, and glial, gut, and epithelial cells. The infection can cause dementia, wasting syndrome, and blood abnormalities.

Modes of transmission

HIV is transmitted three ways:

☝   through contact with infected blood or blood products during transfusion or transplantation (although routine testing of the blood supply since 1985 has greatly diminished the risk of contracting HIV this way) or by sharing a contaminated needle

✌   through contact with infected body fluids, such as semen and vaginal fluids, during unprotected sex (especially anal intercourse because it causes mucosal trauma)

🖐   across the placenta from an infected mother to a fetus or from an infected mother to an infant either through cervical or blood contact during delivery or through breast milk.

Although blood, semen, vaginal secretions, and breast milk are the body fluids that most readily transmit HIV, it has also been found in saliva, urine, tears, and feces. However, there's no evidence of transmission through these fluids.

Classifying HIV infection

The Centers for Disease Control and Prevention's revised guidelines for human immunodeficiency virus (HIV)–infected adolescents and adults categorizes patients on the basis of three ranges of CD4+ T-lymphocyte counts, along with three clinical conditions associated with HIV infection.

The classification system identifies where the patient lies in the progression of the disease and helps guide treatment.

Ranges of CD4+ T-lymphocytes
- Category 1: CD4+ cell count greater than or equal to 500 cells/mm^3
- Category 2: CD4+ cell count of 200 to 499 cells/mm^3
- Category 3: CD4+ cell count less than 200 cells/mm^3

Clinical categories
- Category A (conditions present in patients with documented HIV infection): Asymptomatic HIV infection; persistent, generalized lymph node enlargement; or history of acute HIV infection
- Category B (conditions present in patients with symptomatic HIV infection): Bacillary angiomatosis, oropharyngeal or persistent vulvovaginal candidiasis, fever or diarrhea lasting more than 1 month, idiopathic thrombocytopenic purpura, pelvic inflammatory disease (especially with a tuboovarian abscess), and peripheral neuropathy
- Category C (conditions present in patients with AIDS): Candidiasis of the bronchi, trachea, lungs, or esophagus; invasive cervical cancer; disseminated or extrapulmonary histoplasmosis; chronic, intestinal isosporiasis; Kaposi's sarcoma; Burkitt's lymphoma or its equivalent; primary brain lymphoma; disseminated or extrapulmonary *Mycobacterium avium* complex or *M. kansasii;* pulmonary or extrapulmonary *M. tuberculosis;* any other species of *Mycobacterium* (disseminated or extrapulmonary); *Pneumocystis carinii* pneumonia; recurrent pneumonia; progressive multifocal leukoencephalopathy; recurrent *Salmonella* septicemia; toxoplasmosis of the brain; wasting syndrome caused by HIV

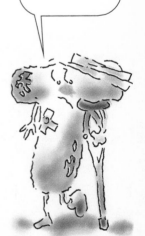

I regulate the normal immune response. When HIV invades me, it gets ugly fast.

What to look for

After initial exposure, the infected person may have no signs or symptoms, or he may have a flulike illness (primary infection) and then remain asymptomatic for years. As the syndrome progresses, he may have neurologic symptoms from HIV encephalopathy or symptoms of an opportunistic infection, such as *Pneumocystis carinii* pneumonia, cytomegalovirus, or cancer. Eventually, repeated opportunistic infections overwhelm the patient's weakened immune defenses, invading every body system. (See *HIV in children,* page 360.)

Treatment

Although HIV disease has no cure, several types of drugs are used to prolong life.

Teamwork works

Highly active antiretroviral therapy (HAART) reduces the number of HIV particles in the blood, increasing T-cell counts and improving the immunologic function. HAART protocols combine three or more antiretroviral drugs to produce the maximum benefit with the fewest adverse reactions. Combination therapy also helps to inhibit the production of mutant HIV strains resistant to particular drugs. Antiretroviral drugs fall into several categories:
• nucleoside reverse transcriptase inhibitors, such as abacavir (Ziagen), didanosine (Videx), emtricitabine (Emtriva), lamivudine (Epivir), stavudine (Zerit), zalcitabine (Hivid), and zidovudine (Retrovir)
• non-nucleoside reverse transcriptase inhibitors, such as delavirdine (Rescriptor), efavirenz (Sustiva), and nevirapine (Viramune)
• nucleotide analog reverse transcriptase inhibitor, this category includes tenofovir (Viread)
• protease inhibitors, such as amprenavir (Agenerase), atazanavir (Reyataz), fosamprenavir (Lexiva), indinavir (Crixivan), lopinavir (Kaletra), nelfinavir (Viracept), ritonavir (Norvir), and saquinavir (Fortovase)
• fusion inhibitors, such as enfuvirtide (Fuzeon).

The selection of an effective combination is a complex process. However, the use of combination therapy has reduced HIV in the blood of infected adults by 98%.

Anti-infective drugs, such as dapsone and rifabutin (Mycobutin), are used to prevent or combat opportunistic infections. Although many opportunistic infections respond to anti-infective drugs, infections tend to recur after treatment ends. Therefore, the patient usually requires lifelong prophylaxis.

Add-ons

Additional treatment may include:
• antineoplastic drugs, such as methotrexate (Trexall), to combat associated cancers
• immunomodulatory agents, such as interferon beta, to boost the immune system weakened by HIV disease and retroviral therapy
• human granulocyte colony-stimulating growth factor to stimulate neutrophil production (retroviral therapy causes anemia, so patients may receive epoetin alfa)
• supportive therapy, including fluid and electrolyte replacement, pain relief, and psychological support.

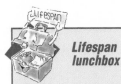

Lifespan lunchbox

HIV in children

In children, the incubation period of human immunodeficiency virus (HIV) averages only 17 months. Signs and symptoms resemble those for adults, except children are more likely to have a history of bacterial infections, such as otitis media, lymphoid interstitial pneumonia, and other types of pneumonia not caused by *Pneumocystis carinii*.

Combination drug therapy helps inhibit production of mutants like me!

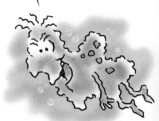

Nutritional assessment

HIV disease has an overwhelming effect on the patient's nutritional status. Early in the course of the disease, signs of malnutrition are subtle and often overlooked. The patient may be deficient in thiamine, riboflavin, vitamin B_6, vitamin B_{12}, folate, magnesium, zinc, and selenium. He may also experience minor weight loss. As the disease progresses, symptoms of malnutrition, such as fatigue, depression, diarrhea, and peripheral neuropathy, may be present and may worsen HIV symptoms.

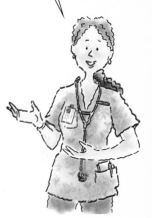

Combination drug therapy has reduced HIV in the blood of infected adults by 98%.

Weight-loss woes

As HIV disease worsens, the combined effects of drug therapy, opportunistic infection, cancer, and decreased nutritional intake cause profound weight loss. Some patients lose as much as 40% of their pre-HIV weight.

HIV wasting syndrome is diagnosed when involuntary weight loss reaches 10% or more of a patient's baseline body weight. This weight loss differs from weight loss due to dieting because there's a disproportionate loss of lean body mass compared with fat loss. (Lean body mass is defined as body mass minus stored fat and includes muscle, bone, connective tissue, body organs, and water.) HIV wasting decreases the patient's quality of life by causing depression, apathy, decreased functional capacity, and increased risk of opportunistic infection. If the patient's weight loss equals 40% of lean body mass, death typically ensues from factors such as malnutrition, reduced immune function, and organ dysfunction.

Combo therapy: not without problems

HAART therapy, combining three or more antiretroviral drugs, has greatly reduced the incidence of HIV wasting syndrome. However, some patients experience visceral fat accumulation, which results in hyperlipidemia and insulin resistance, placing the patients at risk for diabetes mellitus and heart disease.

Multifaceted malnutrition

The cause of malnutrition in patients with HIV disease is multifaceted:
• Metabolic rate is increased by fever, infection, cancer, and some medications, increasing nutrition and energy requirements.
• Malabsorption of nutrients may be caused by medications, low serum albumin levels, diarrhea, cancer, and infection.
• Oral intake is inadequate because of anxiety, depression, nausea, vomiting, impaired swallowing, impaired taste, fatigue, infection, shortness of breath, and mouth ulcers.

Nutritional therapy is required to help prevent and reverse malnutrition in the patient with HIV disease.

Health history

The first step in assessing the patient's nutritional status is completing a detailed health history. During the interview, ask the patient about weight loss. Ask him to compare his current weight with his typical weight to evaluate his weight loss pattern. Question the patient about other symptoms, such as nausea, anorexia, altered taste, diarrhea, mouth pain, difficulty chewing or swallowing, and fatigue.

Ask the patient about allergies, smoking, eating patterns, alcohol or drug use, food choices, and vitamin use. Ask about current medications (including over-the-counter medications and herbal preparations). Also ask the patient about his ability to prepare his medications.

A day in the life

Have the patient describe his typical day. This will give you important information about his routine activity level and eating habits. Ask him to recount what and how much he ate yesterday, how the food was cooked, and who cooked it. This information not only tells you about the patient's usual intake but also gives clues about food preferences, eating patterns, and even the patient's memory and mental status.

Ask the patient about his support system, which may include family, friends, and volunteers. Assess whether he has help with shopping and meal preparation. Socialization during meals may improve nutritional intake.

Physical examination

The second step in assessing the patient's nutritional status is performing the physical examination. In addition to observing the patient's body structure, do a head-to-toe assessment of his body systems.

Skin, hair, and nails

When assessing the patient's skin, hair, and nails, ask yourself these questions: Is his hair shiny and full? Is his skin free from blemishes and rashes? Is it warm and dry, with normal color for that particular patient? Are his nails firm with pink beds? Does the skin tent when pinched?

Eyes, nose, throat, and neck

Are the patient's eyes clear and shiny? Are the mucous membranes in his nose moist and pink? Is his tongue pink with papillae present? Are his gums moist and pink? Is his mouth free from ulcers or lesions? Is his neck free from masses that would impede swallowing?

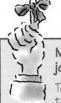

Memory jogger

To remember the four stages in assessing the nutritional status of a patient with HIV disease, think Hunger Ends After Lunch:

Health history

Examination

Anthropometric measurements

Laboratory studies.

Cardiovascular system

Is the patient's heart rhythm regular? Are his heart rate and blood pressure normal for his age? Are his extremities free from swelling? Are his jugular veins flat or distended?

GI system

Is the patient's appetite satisfactory? Are GI problems present? Are his elimination patterns regular? Is his abdomen free from abnormal masses on palpation?

Neurologic system

Is the patient alert and responsive? Are his reflexes normal? Is his behavior appropriate? Are his legs and feet free from paresthesia?

Anthropometric measurements

The third step in assessing nutritional status is taking anthropometric measurements. These measurements can help identify nutritional problems in the patient who's seriously underweight. These measurements include:
- height
- weight
- midarm circumference
- midarm muscle circumference
- skinfold thickness.

Midarm circumference, midarm muscle circumference, and skinfold thickness are used to evaluate muscle mass and subcutaneous fat, both of which reflect nutritional status.

Laboratory studies

The fourth step in assessing nutritional status is evaluating the patient's laboratory test results. Make sure to assess:
- *serum albumin, prealbumin, and retinol-binding protein levels* — Patients with HIV disease typically have low serum levels, indicating protein deficiency.
- *serum cholesterol* — Levels may be elevated from adverse effects of drug therapy.

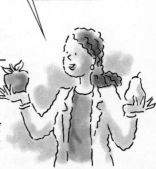

Nutritional therapy may help prevent or delay HIV wasting syndrome if initiated soon after diagnosis.

Nutritional therapy

When a patient is diagnosed with HIV disease, he should be referred to a dietitian for assessment and dietary teaching. Nutritional therapy may help prevent or delay HIV wasting syndrome if initiated soon after diagnosis. It should be initiated even if dietary intake appears adequate.

Aiming high

The goals of nutritional therapy aim to:
- provide a well-balanced, nutrient-rich diet
- preserve the patient's independence
- maintain the patient's quality of life
- slow disease progression.

Calorie high

Altered metabolism associated with HIV disease increases caloric needs. The recommended calorie intake for a patient with HIV disease is typically 35 to 45 cal/kg. These requirements increase in the presence of fever.

Protein provisions

Protein requirements also increase in patients with HIV disease. Daily protein intake should be increased to 1 to 2 g/kg. (See *Increasing dietary intake of protein.*)

Hold the fat

Patients who experience malabsorption may need to limit their fat intake. To make sure that calorie consumption is adequate, the patient may require supplemental medium chain triglycerides. Medium chain triglycerides, supplied in the form of oil, don't require lipase or bile for digestion and absorption, so people with impaired digestion or absorption are able to absorb them.

Vital facts about vitamins and minerals

It's recommended that patients with HIV take fat-soluble vitamins according to the Recommended Dietary Allowance (RDA). Water-soluble vitamins should be taken in amounts two to five times greater than the RDA. Patients should avoid large doses of iron and zinc because they can adversely affect immune function. Supplements of trace elements and antioxidants may also be prescribed.

Dealing with adversity

Patients with HIV disease may experience alterations in the sense of taste and problems with appetite and intake similar to patients with cancer. Patients should be encouraged to consume small, frequent meals despite a lack of appetite. Patients should be educated about techniques to improve taste when taste alterations occur. (See *When food doesn't taste good anymore,* page 366.)

Medications used to treat HIV disease can also affect nutrition. Many cause food-drug interactions and adverse effects that can impact appetite as well as drug absorption and elimination. Patients must be thoroughly educated about all aspects of their drug therapy. (See *Combating food-drug interactions,* pages 367 to 369.)

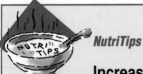

NutriTips

Increasing dietary intake of protein

The patient with human immunodeficiency virus disease typically needs to increase his intake of dietary protein. Use this list of tips to help him increase protein in his diet.

Food	Protein content	Suggestions for use
1 cup milk	8 g	• Add to soup, casseroles, fruit smoothies, pudding, cream sauces, milk shakes, and hot or cold cereal. • Substitute for other liquid in recipes.
¼ cup milk powder	7 g	• Add to milk to make double-strength milk. • Add to any food in which milk is added. • Mix with applesauce or other fruit purees. • Add to milkshakes.
2 tbsp peanut butter	4 to 9 g	• Spread on celery, apple slices, banana slices, crackers, bagels, bread, and muffins. • Mix with applesauce or yogurt.
1 oz (28 g) meat, chicken, or fish	12 to 19 g	• Add chunks to salads, casseroles, soup, noodles, and stir-fried vegetables.
1 cup kidney beans	15 g	• Add to salads, soups, or casseroles. • Use pureed chickpeas as a spread.
1 oz (28 g) hard cheese	7 g	• Melt into soups and casseroles. • Make cheese sauce for vegetables. • Add to salads and sandwiches.
1 cup yogurt	8 g	• Combine yogurt, fruit, and milk to make yogurt drinks. • Make vegetable dip containing yogurt, dill, and lemon juice. • Use as a topping for granola, cold cereal, pancakes, waffles, and French toast.
½ cup ice cream	2 to 4 g	• Make milkshakes. • Mix with fruit. • Use as a creamer for coffee and tea.

Stimulating appetite and combating fullness

Appetite stimulants are sometimes necessary to combat anorexia. Dronabinol (Marinol), cyproheptadine (Periactin), megestrol acetate (Megace), and mirtazapine (Remeron) are effective in some patients. Other drugs that may help include testosterone, growth hormones, and anabolic steroids.

Many patients also complain of feeling full and having heartburn after eating a small amount. Encouraging the patient to take the following precautions may help combat fullness and heartburn:

- Eat foods that are easily digested.
- Consume small meals throughout the day.
- Eat only half a portion at a time, wait 2 hours, and then eat the second half.
- Eat slowly.
- Wait at least ½ hour after meals before drinking fluids.
- Consume starches, which are easily digested, such as pasta, potatoes, rice, oatmeal, bread, fruit, and fruit juices.

Encourage the patient to avoid:

- drinking a lot of water or diet cola
- coffee, tea, or seltzer water
- fatty, fried foods
- spicy foods
- caffeine.

Ways to waste wasting

Several therapies are used to combat HIV wasting. The dietitian should suggest ways to increase calorie and protein intake. Antiemetics such as prochlorperazine (Compazine) should be prescribed if nausea is a problem. Antidiarrheal agents such as loperamide (Imodium) should be prescribed to control diarrhea. Increasing dietary fiber also helps combat diarrhea. Such anabolic steroids as nandrolone decanoate (Deca-Durabolin), oxandrolone (Oxandrin), or somatropin (Serostim) may also be prescribed to help build muscle mass.

Enteral nutrition

Enteral nutrition is sometimes necessary for patients who continue with malnutrition and HIV wasting despite other dietary interventions. Because some nutritional formulas cause diarrhea, the patient must be monitored closely. Three formulas — Advera Liquid Supplement, Immun-Aid Powdered Formula, and Impact Liquid — were developed for patients with altered immune function.

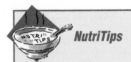 *NutriTips*

When food doesn't taste good anymore

As human immunodeficiency virus disease progresses, patients typically develop alterations in taste. Suggest these tips to help improve taste and increase intake:

- Marinate meat, chicken, or fish in sweet fruit juices, beer, Italian dressing, sweet wines, soy sauce, or sweet and sour sauce.
- Use seasonings, such as basil, oregano, and garlic.
- Add lemon juice, lime juice, or vinegar to food.
- Eat a tart apple or lemon wedge just before meals to stimulate saliva.
- Use mouthwash and brush your teeth at least twice per day with a soft toothbrush.
- Eat meat, chicken, fish, tofu, or beans cold, instead of hot.

Combating food-drug interactions

Some drugs used to treat HIV disease interact with food. Educate the patient about such interactions and the interventions needed to combat them.

Drug	Interaction	Patient education
Protease inhibitors		
amprenavir (Agenerase)	High-fat meals decrease drug absorption.	• Take drug with or without food but avoid high fat meals.
atazanavir (Reyataz)	Any food increases drug absorption.	• Take drug with, or immediately after, food. • Take with 8 oz of water.
fosamprenavir (Lexiva)	Food doesn't affect drug absorption.	• Take with or without food.
indinavir (Crixivan)	Any food especially high-fat, high-protein foods, substantially decreases drug absorption.	• Take drug on an empty stomach with water 1 hour before or 2 hours after a meal. • Take the drug with other liquids, such as fat-free milk, juice, coffee, or tea, if desired. • Meals high in fat, calories, and protein reduce the drug's absorption.
lopinavir (Kaletra)	Any food increases drug absorption.	• Take drug with meals.
nelfinavir (Viracept)	Any food increases drug absorption.	• Take drug with a meal or light snack. • Drink plenty of fluids but avoid grapefruit juice. • Monitor for adverse effects or altered plasma drug concentrations if grapefruit or grapefruit juice is consumed. Avoid these foods if an interaction is suspected.
ritonavir (Norvir)	Any food increases drug absorption.	• Take the drug with meals to improve absorption.
saquinavir (Fortovase)	Any food increases drug absorption.	• Take the drug within 2 hours of a meal. • Avoid consuming large amounts of grapefruit juice or grapefruit.
Nucleoside reverse transcriptase inhibitors		
abacavir (Ziagen)	Food doesn't affect drug absorption.	• Take with or without food.

(continued)

Combating food-drug interactions *(continued)*

Drug	Interaction	Patient education
Nucleoside reverse transcriptase inhibitors *(continued)*		
didanosine (Videx)	Any food substantially decreases drug absorption.	• Take the drug on an empty stomach, regardless of dosage form. Giving drug with meals can result in a 50% decrease in absorption. • Drink at least 1 oz (30 ml) of water with each dose.
emtricitabine (Emtriva)	Food doesn't affect drug absorption.	• Take with or without food.
lamivudine (Epivir)	Food doesn't affect drug absorption.	• Take with or without food.
stavudine (Zerit)	Food doesn't affect drug absorption.	• Take with or without food.
zalcitabine (Hivid)	Any food reduces absorption.	• Take drug with or without food, although taking on an empty stomach may improve absorption.
zidovudine (Retrovir)	Food may have variable effects on drug absorption.	• Take with or without food.
Fusion inhibitor		
enfuvirtide (Fuzeon)	Administered parenterally.	• Take with or without food.
Non-nucleoside reverse transcriptase inhibitors		
delavirdine (Rescriptor)	Food doesn't affect drug absorption.	• Take with or without food. • Monitor for adverse effects or altered plasma drug concentrations if grapefruits or grapefruit juice are consumed. Avoid these foods if an interaction is suspected.
efavirenz (Sustiva)	High fat foods reduce drug absorption.	• Take with or without food, but avoid high fat foods. • Monitor for adverse effects or altered plasma drug concentrations if grapefruits or grapefruit juice are consumed. Avoid these foods if an interaction is suspected.

Combating food-drug interactions *(continued)*

Drug	Interaction	Patient education
Non-nucleoside reverse transcriptase inhibitors (continued)		
nevirapine (Viramune)	Food doesn't affect drug absorption.	• Take with or without food. • Monitor for adverse effects or altered plasma drug concentrations if grapefruit or grapefruit juice is consumed. Avoid these foods if an interaction is suspected.
Nucleotide analog reverse transcriptase inhibitor		
tenofovir (Viread)	Any food increases drug absorption.	• Take with food.

Total parenteral nutrition

Patients with severe diarrhea, bowel obstruction, or intractable vomiting and those at risk for aspiration sometimes require total parenteral nutrition (TPN). TPN allows the GI tract time to rest while providing the patient calories and other nutrients. However, TPN may not meet the nutritional needs of patients with over-whelming infection. These patients commonly experience HIV wasting despite TPN. TPN also places the patient at risk for infection.

I.V. lipid therapy should be used cautiously in patients with HIV disease because they typically have hyperlipidemia.

Food safety

Because patients with HIV disease have difficulty fighting infection, extra care must be taken in purchasing, storing, and preparing food. The patient should be encouraged to:
• select foods that pose the least risk of causing food poisoning
• use only pasteurized cheese and milk
• check the "sell by" or "use by" dates
• examine food packaging for defects
• use plastic cutting boards cleaned in the dishwasher or with sanitizing solution after use
• wash hands properly and frequently
• avoid raw foods, such as sushi, Caesar salad, and oysters on the half shell

- use a meat thermometer to ensure that adequate internal temperature is reached
- order foods well-done when eating in a restaurant
- avoid lightly steamed foods
- refrigerate foods immediately after purchase.

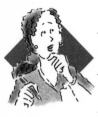

Quick quiz

1. Large doses of which two minerals should be avoided in patients with HIV disease?
     A.   Iron and chromium
     B.   Zinc and iron
     C.   Selenium and zinc
     D.   Iodine and iron

Answer: B. Large doses of zinc and iron can adversely affect immune function.

2. How much protein should a patient with HIV disease consume daily?
     A.   0.5 to 1 g/kg
     B.   1 to 2 g/kg
     C.   25 to 35 g/kg
     D.   35 to 45 g/kg

Answer: B. Patients with HIV disease should consume 1 to 2 g/kg of protein daily to replenish losses and help maintain lean body mass.

3. Safe food preparation by patients with HIV includes:
     A.   drinking unpasteurized milk.
     B.   eating lightly steamed foods.
     C.   refrigerating foods within 3 hours of purchase.
     D.   washing hands properly before preparing foods.

Answer: D. Proper hand washing before handling foods reduces the risk of infection in patients with HIV.

Scoring

✰✰✰   If you answered all three questions correctly, fantastic! You have no knowledge deficiency on this subject.

✰✰   If you answered two questions correctly, yippee! There's no need to stimulate your appetite for the facts.

✰   If you answered fewer than two questions correctly, relax, have a nutritious snack, and review the chapter.

Special conditions

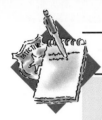

Just the facts

In addition to the health problems already presented in this book, various other conditions can also affect a patient's nutritional status. In this chapter, you'll learn:

♦ effects of severe stress on metabolism

♦ nutritional needs of patients with cancer, traumatic injuries, or burns

♦ indications for enteral or parenteral nutrition in cancer, trauma, and burn patients

♦ ways to maximize the nutritional status of cancer, trauma, and burn patients.

A look at special conditions

Patients with cancer, trauma, or severe burns experience changes in nutrient metabolism. Proper nutrition plays an indispensable role in helping these patients cope with changes and avoid or minimize complications.

The importance of being nutritious

In cancer, local disease effects may reduce the patient's oral intake, while systemic effects may increase energy expenditure and speed protein catabolism. Also, some cancerous tumors produce substances that alter nutrient absorption and metabolism.

Severe stress due to trauma and burns leads to hypermetabolism (increased energy expenditure) as well as protein catabolism. Starting nutritional support within the first 48 hours after injury can improve survival, decrease the risk of infection, and shorten the length of a hospital stay.

> Cancer takes a local and long distance toll on a patient's nutritional needs.

Stress response

In trauma and burns, hormonal and metabolic changes help the body adapt to stressors. This complex stress response has two major phases: ebb and flow. The ebb phase occurs soon after the stress occurs. As the patient's condition stabilizes, he enters the flow phase. (See *Exploring ebb and flow.*)

Adapting to the environment

After the initial stress response, protein catabolism peaks. During this adaptive phase, levels of stress hormones and blood glucose fall and metabolism returns to normal. Gradually, nitrogen balance is restored.

If adaptation succeeds, the patient recovers. If it fails, the body's inability to adapt to stress results in exhaustion and, possibly, death.

How stress affects nutritional status

Prolonged hypermetabolism and hypercatabolism accelerate the loss of energy and protein stores. As the body breaks down lean mass to meet increased protein demands, acute malnutrition may occur—even in a previously healthy patient.

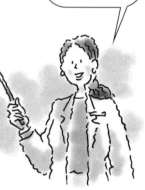

Stress response has its downs and ups — better known as *ebb* and *flow.*

Exploring ebb and flow

The body's response to stress can be broken down into two phases: ebb and flow.

Ebb

In the *ebb* phase—the first phase after exposure to severe stress when the patient is hemodynamically unstable—cardiac output, blood pressure, body temperature, and oxygen consumption all decrease. As the insulin level drops and catecholamine and glucagon levels rise, hyperglycemia occurs.

Flow

During the *flow* phase, as the patient's hemodynamic status stabilizes, the high metabolic demands of stress force the body to mobilize nutrients. As levels of glucocorticoids, catecholamines, and glucagon surge, the patient experiences:
• pronounced hypermetabolism
• accelerated protein catabolism
• persistent hyperglycemia
• increased urinary losses of potassium and nitrogen
• sodium and fluid retention
• slowed GI motility, possibly leading to abdominal distention, anorexia, nausea, vomiting, or constipation.

The body must break down its energy reserves to meet the high energy demands, and significant loss of protein and fat may occur.

Timing is everything

Once fluids and electrolytes are stabilized, early nutrition therapy, particularly enteral therapy, can reduce infectious complications. Other early goals of nutrition therapy include minimizing nutrient losses and preventing acute malnutrition. After the metabolic rate normalizes, nutrition therapy aims to promote a positive nitrogen balance and weight gain.

Nutrition administration methods

In patients with a functioning GI tract, oral or enteral nutrition is preferred because these methods help preserve GI functioning and stimulate GI associated lymphoid tissue.

Oral feedings are contraindicated if the patient isn't alert enough to eat, is receiving mechanical ventilation, or has a nasogastric tube. Enteral feedings aren't administered when conditions such as intestinal obstruction, ileus, or perforation are present. Parenteral nutrition may be indicated when enteral feedings aren't appropriate. Intestinal tube feedings typically can begin sooner than gastric feedings because the intestines regain motility much sooner than the stomach does.

Cancer

Although a cancer patient is more likely than other patients to become malnourished, appropriate nutrition therapy can maximize the effectiveness of cancer treatments, minimize adverse effects of the disease and treatments, and improve quality of life.

As a cancer patient undergoes treatment, he faces many nutritional challenges. He's also highly susceptible to claims made by proponents of unproven nutritional therapies.

Effects of cancer on nutritional status

Cancer patients typically have poor appetites, altered metabolism, and increased catabolism from direct and indirect tumor effects as well as from treatments and psychological factors (such as anxiety and depression).

Many cancer patients become full after just a few bites. This early satiety may result from:
• poorly understood mechanisms related to the cancer itself
• pressure from the tumor on the abdomen
• ascites (fluid accumulation in the abdomen).

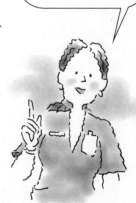

A cancer patient is more likely than any other patient to become malnourished.

Taste alterations also are common in cancer patients. Many report that food tastes bitter or metallic or that it isn't sweet or salty enough.

Wasting away

Commonly, the cancer patient consumes fewer—and expends more—calories. All too often, weight loss progresses to the point of *cachexia*, a wasting syndrome marked by a maladaptive metabolic rate, anorexia, muscle wasting, severe weight loss, and general debility.

Cachexia impairs wound healing and increases the risk of infections and other complications. It's associated with poor quality of life and shorter survival. In fact, cachexia causes more deaths than does cancer itself.

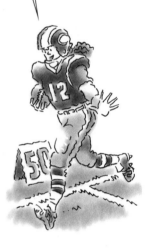

Here's the catch — cachexia causes more deaths than the cancer itself.

Local effects

The tumor itself may directly involve or interfere with GI tract function, causing dysphagia (difficulty swallowing), obstruction, nausea, vomiting, and malabsorption. Ovarian, hepatic, and genitourinary cancers may lead to ascites, which impairs oral intake by causing early satiety. Brain cancer, on the other hand, may alter the patient's mental status to the extent that oral intake decreases significantly.

Systemic effects

Various metabolic changes may impair the patient's nutritional status. These changes include:
• increased metabolic rate (particularly with lung and gastric cancer and sarcomas)
• increased protein catabolism
• peripheral insulin resistance, possibly caused by cytokines and tumor necrosis factor
• increased fat oxidation.

Effects of cancer treatments on nutritional status

Cancer treatments and their adverse effects commonly cause problems that jeopardize the patient's nutritional status.

Surgery

Effects of cancer surgery on nutrition vary with the surgical site:
• Head and neck surgery may alter chewing and swallowing ability.
• Surgery for esophageal cancer moves the stomach higher up in the chest. This limits the amount of food the patient can consume at one time and increases the risk of diarrhea and reflux.

• After gastrectomy, the patient must consume small, frequent meals and may develop severe diarrhea or dumping syndrome (nausea, weakness, sweating, palpitations, syncope) after eating.
• Pancreatic surgery may alter absorption, gastric emptying, and blood glucose levels.

Other potential adverse effects of surgery also can affect nutrition—for example, infection, fistulas, and short-gut syndrome (malabsorption after removal of part of the small intestine).

To help ensure adequate nutrition during the postoperative period, many patients have feeding tubes placed during surgery.

Radiation therapy

Like cancer itself, radiation may alter the patient's taste perception. Patients commonly complain that foods taste bitter and that they can't distinguish sweet from salty.

Simply radiating

Other adverse effects depend on the radiation dose and site. For instance, radiation to the abdominal area damages cells lining the GI tract, causing nausea, vomiting, and diarrhea. When such damage persists and intestinal inflammation becomes chronic, the condition is called *radiation enteritis*. The intestinal lining may remain inflamed for up to 10 years after radiation therapy. Besides vomiting and diarrhea, enteritis can cause intestinal narrowing, fistula development, poor absorption, and bowel obstruction.

Radiation to the head, neck, or esophagus may lead to sore throat, mucositis, and taste changes, resulting in anorexia and nausea. Radiation to the chest may cause esophagitis.

Chemotherapy

Chemotherapy drugs are highly toxic and damage not only cancer cells but also healthy cells. The rapidly growing cells of the GI tract, bone marrow, and hair are especially vulnerable.

On the side

Nausea and vomiting are among the most distressing adverse effects of chemotherapy. However, not all chemotherapeutic regimens cause these problems. Nausea and vomiting are more likely to occur with certain drugs and often can be prevented or minimized by administering antiemetics before the chemotherapy session.

Chemotherapy also may cause anorexia, diarrhea or constipation, malabsorption, mouth sores (stomatitis), mouth inflammation, taste changes, and infection. Signs or symptoms lasting more than 2 weeks are likely to significantly affect the patient's nutritional status.

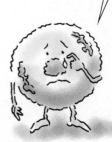

The healthy cells most likely to be damaged by chemotherapy are those of the GI tract, bone marrow, and hair.

Chemotherapy drugs that affect the bone marrow may lead to anemia and bleeding. Some also suppress the immune system, increasing the risk of serious infection.

Immunotherapy

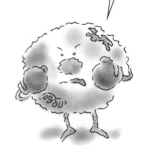

Immunotherapy uses the body's natural defenses to fight cancer.

Immunotherapy (also called *biologic response modifier therapy*) uses the body's natural defenses to fight cancer. Immunotherapies involving certain cytokines and antibodies have become part of standard cancer treatment. Other types of immunotherapy remain experimental. Interferon is the best known and most widely used biologic response modifier.

Depending on the specific agent used, immunotherapy may cause diarrhea, nausea, vomiting, appetite loss, abdominal pain, stomatitis, taste changes, and weight loss. It also may increase the patient's calorie and protein requirements.

Bone marrow transplantation

A patient with leukemia, lymphoma, or breast cancer may undergo bone marrow transplantation. Before transplantation, the patient receives high-dose chemotherapy and total body irradiation to suppress immune function and kill cancer cells. These treatments commonly cause nausea, vomiting, GI tract inflammation, taste changes, and anorexia. The transplantation itself may cause mucositis, stomatitis, esophagitis, and intestinal damage (leads to severe diarrhea).

Temporary TPN

Maximizing pain management and antiemetic therapy can improve the patient's ability to tolerate an oral diet. If severe GI dysfunction rules out oral or enteral intake, the patient may receive total parenteral nutrition (TPN).

Usually, GI dysfunction resolves about 30 days after transplantation and the patient can resume oral intake or tube feedings (if needed). To optimize nitrogen balance, the patient should receive 30 to 35 cal/kg/day and 1.5 to 2.5 g of protein per kg/day.

What to look for

Weigh the patient and ask if he has experienced recent unintentional weight loss. More than 10% weight loss within 6 months indicates severe malnutrition, a greater risk of complications, and a poorer prognosis. (At diagnosis, patients with stomach or pancreatic cancer typically show the greatest weight loss. Expect moderate weight loss in patients with lung, colon, esophageal, or prostate cancer.)

Also obtain other relevant history information. (See *Nutritional assessment in cancer patients*.)

Let's get physical

Then perform a physical examination, checking for classic signs of malnutrition, such as:

- edema
- subcutaneous fat loss
- muscle wasting
- dry, brittle hair
- pale skin
- skin rashes
- poor wound healing.

Also inspect the patient for ascites and for fluid buildup in other body cavities. Be sure to assess for complications of cancer treatments or surgery that may affect nutritional status.

Laboratory data

Serum protein levels may reflect skeletal muscle and visceral protein status. Expect the practitioner to order serum albumin, prealbumin, and transferrin tests. In malnutrition, serum albumin levels commonly measure less than 3.4 g/dl (SI, 34 g/L). Patients with marasmus (protein-energy malnutrition), however, have serum albumin levels within normal limits.

Levels of serum prealbumin, which serve as a marker for protein status, reflect the patient's response to stress or nutritional support earlier than do serum albumin levels. A level below 190 mg/dl indicates malnutrition.

Interfering with interpretation

When interpreting test results, keep in mind that they can be altered by various factors—the patient's hydration and iron status, infection, stress, other diseases, medications, and even bed rest. Ultimately, weight and diet history are the most important elements of nutritional assessment.

Nutritional requirements

Because of hypermetabolism and increased catabolism, the cancer patient has high protein and energy requirements. To spare protein for vital tissue building, he must receive adequate carbohydrates and fats.

Nutritional assessment in cancer patients

When assessing the nutritional status of a cancer patient, be sure to obtain:

- detailed weight history
- GI symptoms (such as nausea, vomiting, diarrhea, anorexia) lasting more than 2 weeks
- functional capacity (whether the patient can function normally, ambulates, or is bedridden)
- dietary history, including food preferences (if he's receiving oral intake)
- treatments received or scheduled (such as surgery, radiation, or chemotherapy)
- medication use
- type of cancer
- emotional status.

Calorie and protein needs vary with the cancer type and stage, presence of metastases, treatments administered, and the patient's nutritional status. When determining the patient's specific calorie and protein needs, consider such factors as:

- whether the patient needs to maintain, gain, or lose weight
- renal function
- presence of diabetes
- wound status
- patient's activity level.

Calories

A cancer patient who hasn't experienced significant weight loss needs 25 to 35 cal/kg/day to maintain weight. If he needs to gain weight, he requires higher calorie levels. A malnourished patient may need 35 to 40 cal/kg/day.

Be aware that breast cancer patients typically *don't* have a high calorie requirement. In fact, weight *gain* is relatively common among these patients.

Protein

To build tissue, the cancer patient needs nitrogen and essential amino acids, which promote healing and offset tissue breakdown. He should receive an optimal ratio of proteins to calories.

Specific protein needs hinge on nutritional status. A patient with a good nutritional status needs roughly 0.8 to 1.2 g/kg/day of high-quality protein to meet maintenance requirements. A malnourished patient needs 1.2 to 1.5 g/kg/day to combat deficits and regain a positive nitrogen balance.

Vitamins and minerals

Certain vitamins and minerals help regulate protein and energy metabolism. The cancer patient should receive optimal vitamin and mineral intake — at least the Recommended Dietary Allowance (RDA), but possibly higher.

Each patient's vitamin and mineral needs must be assessed individually. Factors that may influence requirements include the cancer type and stage, nutritional status, medications, and presence of such GI complications as malabsorption, diarrhea, and vomiting.

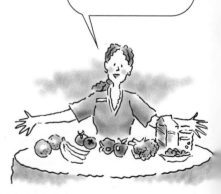

Cancer patients may need more than the Recommended Dietary Allowance of vitamins and minerals.

Fluids

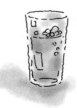

Adequate fluid intake is crucial—especially if the patient has been experiencing vomiting, diarrhea, fever, or infection. In addition to replenishing lost fluids, a high fluid intake of 2 qt/day (2 L/day) or more helps the kidneys eliminate metabolic breakdown products of toxic chemotherapy drugs and destroyed cancer cells.

Certain chemotherapy agents increase fluid needs even further. For instance, a patient who's receiving cyclophosphamide (Cytoxan) or ifosfamide (Ifex) may need up to 3 qt/day (3 L/day) of fluid to avoid hemorrhagic cystitis (bleeding from the bladder).

Nutrition therapy

Nutrition therapy is essential for combating cancer and boosting the immune system. Early nutritional intervention can improve the patient's tolerance for treatment, minimize adverse effects of treatment, and improve quality of life.

Goals of nutrition therapy are to prevent or reverse catabolism and help relieve side effects of the disease and treatments. In some patients, supplemental nutrition, which is rich in essential nutrients that aid in the metabolism and digestion of food, limits complications and allows completion of a course of chemotherapy or radiation therapy. (In terminally ill patients, however, it hasn't been shown to improve quality of life or outcome.)

Make a plan

For a patient who's receiving oral intake, develop a food plan in collaboration with the patient, family, and dietitian. The plan must account for the patient's food preferences and tolerances as well as any eating problems, such as anorexia, nausea or vomiting, or stomatitis. The food plan should emphasize high calorie levels and nutrient density in smaller volumes of food.

The backup plan

A patient who won't be able to receive adequate oral intake for a prolonged period needs nutritional support. If the GI tract is functioning, enteral nutrition is preferable to parenteral nutrition because it's safer, preserves GI function, and costs less.

If the GI tract isn't accessible or functional, parenteral nutrition may be given. Despite its risks, TPN can convert the patient's metabolic status from catabolism to anabolism and help prevent cancer cachexia.

> If the GI tract is functioning, enteral nutrition beats parenteral nutrition every time.

Improving intake

If your patient's oral intake is limited by anorexia, nausea and vomiting, stomatitis, or other problems, take steps to help him overcome these obstacles.

Food fight

Anorexia—the most common cause of malnutrition in cancer patients—may stem from:
• chemicals produced by the tumor
• pain
• early satiety
• depression
• mouth sores
• nausea and vomiting
• altered taste.
    You can help your patient fight anorexia by:
• providing small, frequent meals
• increasing the nutrient density of foods—for instance, adding instant milk powder to liquid milk
• encouraging family members to eat with the patient or bring his favorite foods from home
• asking the practitioner to prescribe an appetite stimulant, such as megestrol acetate (Megace), dronabinol (Marinol), or dexamethasone (Decadron)—if benefits don't appear after 2 to 6 weeks of drug therapy, the medication should be discontinued.
    To help promote adequate intake after discharge, review appropriate eating tips with the patient and family. (See *Overcoming anorexia.*)

Keep it down

Nausea and vomiting may result from the cancer itself, cancer treatments, pain, or certain pain medications. If your patient's undergoing chemotherapy, instruct him to take an antiemetic drug 6 hours before chemotherapy starts (if appropriate) and to continue taking it regularly as prescribed.
    Here are more suggestions for relieving nausea and vomiting:
• Serve small, frequent meals.
• Instruct the patient to eat slowly.
• Provide liquids for him to sip between meals, and advise him not to drink fluids with meals.
• Serve beverages cool or chilled.
• Instruct the patient to avoid foods that are fatty, greasy, fried, and spicy and foods with strong odors.
• Recommend low-fat foods, which are digested faster and leave less content in the stomach.

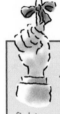

Memory jogger

To help your patient fight anorexia, remember Food Never Goes Away. Recommend:

Frequent, small meals

Nutrient-dense foods

Gathering family or friends for meals

Appetite stimulants.

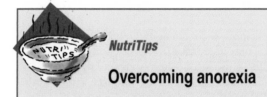

NutriTips

Overcoming anorexia

To help your anorexic patient maintain adequate oral intake after discharge, provide the following suggestions to the patient and family:
• Eat small, frequent meals or snacks (every 1 to 2 hours).
• Eat high-protein, high-calorie foods. Avoid low-calorie foods.
• Try to eat when you're feeling best. At other times, use nutritional supplements such as Ensure or Boost.
• Add extra calories and protein to food by preparing it with butter, margarine, honey, sugar, or dry milk powder.
• Make your eating environment as pleasant as possible.
• Experiment with different recipes, flavorings, spices, and food consistencies.
• To avoid strong food odors, which may cause nausea, have someone else prepare meals, cook outdoors on a grill, eat foods cold instead of hot, order take-out meals, and take tray covers off early.

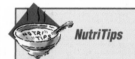

NutriTips

Resuming oral intake

If your patient has been vomiting, instruct him not to eat or drink. When the vomiting is under control, advise him to try eating small amounts of clear liquids, starting with 1 tsp every 10 minutes and increasing the amount gradually as tolerated.

Once the patient is able to tolerate clear liquids, instruct him to eat low-fat, nonspicy foods, such as hot cereal, crackers, pudding, and canned fruits. Suggest that he continue to take in small amounts as long as he can keep them down. Advise him to add new foods gradually.

• Encourage the patient to eat bland foods, such as toast, crackers, pretzels, rice cakes, hot cereal, sherbet, popsicles, and canned fruits.

For tips on eating after a bout of vomiting, see *Resuming oral intake.*

These are a few of my favorite foods

Some patients develop aversions to foods they ate just before a bout of nausea or vomiting. To prevent food aversions, instruct the patient to avoid favorite foods for 48 hours before and after chemotherapy or radiation therapy.

Fighting fatigue

Fatigue can result from the cancer itself or from radiation, chemotherapy, depression, poor nutrition, or dehydration. To counter fatigue, advise the patient to:
• choose healthy foods
• eat small, frequent meals
• use convenience foods and nutritional supplements to decrease energy demands
• drink plenty of fluids
• get adequate sleep and rest
• engage in light exercise, if possible.

A sore subject

Cancer treatment may cause stomatitis (sores in the mouth and throat), which certain foods may aggravate. To make eating less painful, instruct the patient to choose foods carefully and to practice good oral hygiene. To ease discomfort, advise him to use a topical anesthetic. (See *Coping with stomatitis.*)

A change in taste

Chemotherapy, radiation therapy, or cancer itself may alter taste perception. Some patients complain of a bitter, metallic taste when eating high-protein foods. Others become sensitive to sweets and prefer unsweetened foods and beverages. With radiation therapy, taste changes typically occur by the third week and resolve within 1 year after therapy ends.

To help your patient maintain adequate intake despite altered taste, advise him to:
• eat foods that look and smell good
• eat fish, chicken, turkey, eggs, dairy products, or tofu for protein if red meat tastes bad
• use small amounts of seasoning, such as basil, rosemary, or oregano
• consume tart foods and beverages, including oranges, lemonade, and lemon custard (unless he has stomatitis)

NutriTips

Coping with stomatitis

A patient with stomatitis may experience severe pain when he tries to eat. Provide the following tips to help him maintain adequate intake:

• Eat soft, mild foods and beverages, such as applesauce, bananas, canned fruits, cottage cheese, yogurt, milkshakes, nutritional supplements, milk, mashed potatoes, macaroni and cheese, custard, pudding, scrambled eggs, hot cereals, pureed or mashed vegetables, and pureed meats.

• Consume nutrient-dense foods and beverages, such as creamy soups and milk.

• Avoid foods that irritate the mouth, including citrus fruit and juices, spicy or salty foods, and rough, coarse, or dry foods.

• Mix food with butter, gravy, or sauce.

• Use a straw to drink beverages.

• Eat food cold or at room temperature. Cold foods have a numbing effect, whereas hot or warm foods can irritate mouth sores.

• Practice good oral hygiene to remove food and bacteria and promote healing. If necessary, use an anesthetic mouthwash.

- drink less-sweet liquid supplements, such as Isocal or Osmolite
- eat foods at room temperature
- drink liquids throughout the day to moisten the mouth and to flush metabolites from the body
- use plastic rather than metal utensils to counter a metallic taste
- rinse his mouth before eating.

Zinc deficiency also may lead to taste alterations. Supplemental zinc may help correct this problem.

Trauma

Like other severely stressed patients, trauma patients experience hypermetabolism and protein catabolism. These changes, combined with prolonged bed rest and inadequate nutrition, can lead to drastic loss of lean body mass. Adequate nutrition can minimize catabolic effects, help fight infection, and promote wound healing.

Nutritional requirements

Calorie needs vary among trauma patients, whereas protein needs are almost always high.

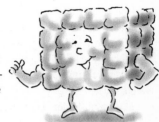

Nutritionally speaking, trauma patients need me, protein, the most.

Calories

The trauma patient should receive only enough calories to promote recovery. Giving excessive calories increases metabolism, oxygen consumption, and carbon dioxide production, placing a heavier burden on the heart and lungs.

Specific calorie requirements depend on the patient's condition. A sedated, paralyzed patient has very low resting energy expenditure. Other trauma patients, especially those with head injuries, may have high resting energy expenditures.

Ideally, indirect calorimetry should be used to measure the patient's actual energy expenditure. If this technology isn't available or practical, you can use one of several equations, such as the Harris-Benedict equation, to estimate energy expenditure. (See *Using the Harris-Benedict equation*, page 384.)

The Harris-Benedict equation can be time-consuming and inaccurate, though. It may overestimate calorie needs in some patients and underestimate them in others.

An easier way to estimate calorie needs is to multiply the patient's weight in kg by a specified calorie level—25 to 30 cal/kg/day for patients with mild to moderate stress and 30 to 35 cal/kg/day for those with moderate to severe stress. Generally, older patients should receive calories at the lower end of this

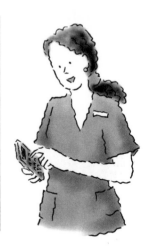

Using the Harris-Benedict equation

You can use the Harris-Benedict equation to estimate your patient's basal energy expenditure (BEE). This equation accounts for age, gender, height, and weight and makes adjustments based on the patient's stress and activity level.

For women: $BEE = 655 + (9.6 \times weight\ in\ kg) + (1.8 \times height\ in\ cm) - (4.7 \times age\ in\ years)$

For men: $BEE = 66 + (13.8 \times weight\ in\ kg) + (5 \times height\ in\ cm) - (6.8 \times age\ in\ years)$

Adjusting for stress

To find the patient's estimated calorie requirements, multiply BEE by the stress factor. The stress factor ranges from 0.7 in a patient suffering from starvation to 1.95 in a patient with burns affecting more than 40% of body surface area.

range because of their reduced metabolic rate. Patients who are obese or severely malnourished on admission should receive a lower level of calories.

Protein

Trauma patients have high protein requirements because of the presence of wounds, which need protein to heal, and the liver's preferential use of protein for energy during critical illness. Their protein requirements range from 1.5 to 2 g/kg/day — or up to 2.5 g/kg/day for patients with severe head injuries.

Vitamins and minerals

Experts aren't sure if trauma patients or other critically ill patients have special vitamin, mineral, or trace element requirements. Generally, however, they should receive adequate vitamins and minerals to meet established national standards. To maximize healing, patients with extensive wounds may receive extra zinc, vitamin C, and beta carotene.

Nutrition therapy

Nutrition therapy for trauma patients depends on such factors as injury type and severity, the patient's baseline nutritional status, and when the patient will be able to take adequate oral nutrition.

Usually, patients with minor injuries and those who can consume adequate oral intake (or are expected to within a few days) don't need enteral or parenteral nutrition. But they must receive an appropriate diet with adequate protein to promote healing. They may need liquid nutritional supplements, plus a multivitamin with minerals if oral intake is less than optimal.

Severe circumstances

For a trauma patient who's severely malnourished or isn't expected to take adequate oral nutrition for a prolonged period, enteral nutrition should begin as soon as the patient is hemodynamically stable. Starting tube feedings early is associated with fewer infectious complications and a shorter length of stay. (On the other hand, starting parenteral nutrition early probably isn't beneficial.)

> Check it out! Starting enteral nutrition early can help trauma patients be discharged sooner.

Burns

Severe burns cause a complex and extreme form of hypermetabolism. After a severe burn, energy expenditure increases and catabolism of lean body mass occurs. These changes result in muscle wasting, negative nitrogen balance, and depletion of protein and fat stores.

Many factors can influence the extent of these metabolic changes, including:
• burn depth and burn surface area
• evaporative losses from wounds
• fever
• sepsis
• serum catecholamine, glucagon, and cortisol levels
• surgery.

Nutritional requirements

Burn patients have extremely high fluid, protein, and calorie requirements. However, energy needs may vary from one patient to the next, and high amounts of calories may be inappropriate for some patients.

> Patients with burns over more than 15% of their bodies need I.V. fluid during the first 48 hours.

Fluids

Patients with burns affecting more than 15% of body surface area need I.V. fluid resuscitation during the first 48 hours to maintain adequate blood flow to vital organs. Immediate fluid administration helps offset fluid shifts and eliminate waste products produced by the burn injury. Fluids also help prevent gastric distention and paralytic ileus. The amount of fluid given depends on the burn extent, time elapsed since the injury, the patient's weight, and his response to fluid administration.

Here comes the flood

Once fluid resuscitation is completed, the patient should receive fluids in amounts that produce adequate urine output—30 to

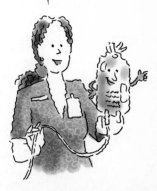

50 ml/hour in adults. Fluid requirements remain high for several weeks because water losses may be 10 times greater than normal during this period.

Calories

Hypermetabolism may double the patient's usual calorie needs. A high calorie intake spares the protein essential for tissue rebuilding and meets the dramatically increased metabolic demands. Also, burn patients are at high risk for sepsis — a condition that raises the metabolic rate even further. Most patients continue to have high calorie needs for several weeks or even longer after the burn injury.

Calorie requirements must be determined individually. Ideally, the patient's actual resting energy expenditure should be measured using indirect calorimetry. However, many practitioners use a formula, such as the Curreri formula, to estimate calorie requirements. (See *Estimating calorie needs in burn patients.*)

Protein

Burn patients need extremely large amounts of protein to promote wound healing and bolster the immune system. Requirements range from 2 to 3 g/kg of body weight/day, depending on burn extent and catabolic losses. Protein should account for 20% to 25% of total calories.

Much of the increased protein requirement comes from muscle breakdown for use in energy production. Although providing extra protein doesn't stop this breakdown, it provides the materials needed to synthesize lost tissue. Extreme hypercatabolism is compounded by protein losses from wound exudate. Nitrogen losses peak during the first 3 days after the injury, then taper off slowly until finally ending at about day 16. Even after that time, though, the patient must continue to receive large amounts of protein to promote wound healing.

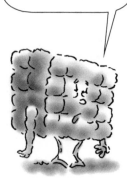

Being a protein is hard work! Burn patients need lots of protein to promote healing and boost immune function.

The nitrogen balancing act

Estimating the patient's nitrogen balance can help determine adequacy of protein intake. To estimate nitrogen balance, use this formula:

$$\text{Nitrogen balance} = \text{nitrogen intake} -$$
$$(\text{total urinary nitrogen} + \text{fecal nitrogen loss} +$$
$$\text{nitrogen loss from burn wounds})$$

Total urinary nitrogen, fecal nitrogen loss, and nitrogen loss from burn wounds are based on a 24-hour period. To achieve nitrogen balance, most adults need 2 to 3 g/kg. (See *Estimating nitrogen loss from wounds.*)

Estimating calorie needs in burn patients

The Curreri formula is the most commonly used formula for estimating calorie requirements in adult burn patients.

Here's the formula:

(25 cal × usual body weight in kg) + (40 × % total body surface area burned).

This formula yields the number of calories required daily.

Too generous?

Some experts think the Curreri formula overestimates calorie requirements. *Overfeeding* can lead to hyperglycemia and hyperosmolality which, in turn, result in osmotic diuresis, dehydration, and ketotic acidosis.

Children

In children with burn injuries, calorie requirements are based on weight or age, as shown here:

- Neonate to 6 months: 100 cal/kg
- 6 months to 2 years: 75 cal/kg (× 2 for burns of 15% or more)
- 2 years to 60 lb (27 kg): 50 cal/kg.

Estimating nitrogen loss from wounds

You can estimate nitrogen loss from your patient's wounds as described here:
- ≤ 10% open wound: 0.02 g of nitrogen/kg of body weight/day
- > 10% to < 30% open wound: 0.05 g of nitrogen/kg/day
- ≥ 30% open wound: 0.12 g of nitrogen/kg/day.

Estimate fecal nitrogen losses at about 2 g/day.

Total urinary nitrogen is determined by collecting a 24-hour urine specimen and determining the number of grams of urinary urea nitrogen present.

Carbohydrates and fats

The burn patient should get about 50% of daily calories from carbohydrates and roughly 25% to 30% from fat. Because excess fat intake may decrease immune function, fat intake must be monitored closely.

Vitamins and minerals

Many micronutrients are essential for optimal burn wound healing. Although specific requirements after severe burn injury haven't been determined, the patient should receive at least the RDA of each vitamin and mineral.

Thiamine, riboflavin, and niacin requirements may rise because of increased energy and protein metabolism. Some experts also recommend giving additional amounts of vitamins A and C and zinc to promote wound healing and limit oxidative damage.

Nutrition therapy

Without aggressive nutrition therapy, the burn patient is at high risk for malnutrition, weight loss and, possibly, death from tissue destruction and hypermetabolism. Early and aggressive nutrition therapy preserves lean body mass, promotes wound healing, and helps prevent infection. In many cases, it determines whether the patient will survive.

However, severe burns pose a serious challenge to nutrition therapy because the patient is likely to have fluid and electrolyte imbalances, pain, anorexia, gastric distention, paralytic ileus, infection, and emotional trauma. Also, he may need to undergo various medical procedures or surgery.

Nutrition administration routes

During the immediate postburn period, a patient with severe burns may be unable to receive oral intake because of paralytic ileus and other factors.

Experts disagree on the best time to begin feedings of any type. Some practitioners start tube feedings within 4 hours of the injury. Others start oral feedings (if tolerated) when normal bowel activity returns (usually 2 to 4 days after the injury).

Lip service

Whenever possible, oral intake is preferred. But even when oral feedings are possible, they usually must be augmented with concentrated liquids or oral supplements and, in some cases, periodic tube feedings.

Oral feedings begin with a clear or full liquid diet, with the diet progressing as tolerated. Typically, solid foods are added by the 2nd week. Provide small, frequent meals and assist in feeding as appropriate. Provide the patient's favorite foods, and encourage the family to bring food from home.

Try to schedule treatments and diagnostic procedures so they don't interfere with meals. (For tips on increasing protein and calorie intake, see *Boosting calorie and protein intake*.)

Enteral vs. parenteral nutrition

Enteral nutrition has become the preferred feeding method for all critically ill patients who can't tolerate oral intake. In the past, severe burn patients routinely received TPN. However, experts now believe TPN has no advantage over enteral nutrition. In fact, TPN is associated with an increased infection risk. Nonetheless, if GI function is absent, parenteral nutrition should be started within 3 to 4 days in severely burned patients.

Formula for success?

Because of the high risk of infection among burn patients, researchers are studying the use of immune-enhancing enteral nutrition formulas. These high-calorie, high-protein formulas contain extra glutamine, arginine, omega-3 fatty acids, ornithine, alpha-ketoglutarate, and other related compounds. At this time, though,

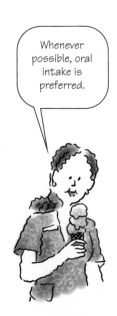

Whenever possible, oral intake is preferred.

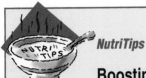

NutriTips

Boosting calorie and protein intake

Like other critically ill patients, burn patients have high protein and calorie requirements. To help these patients meet their increased needs, follow these guidelines:

- Add grated cheese to rice, pasta, casseroles, and soups.
- Spread raw fruit and vegetable slices with peanut butter.
- Add chopped hard-boiled eggs to soups, sauces, and casseroles.
- Use whole or evaporated milk in recipes instead of water.
- Serve egg- or milk-rich desserts, such as puddings, ice cream, and custard.
- Add butter to breads, pancakes, waffles, soups, vegetables, rice, and pasta.
- Top desserts and hot beverages with whipped cream.
- Provide high-calorie snacks, such as candy, nuts, dried fruit, cheese, and ice cream.

Memory jogger

Not sure when a burn patient may require enteral or parenteral nutrition? It's a SNAP. Just look for:

Significantly high calorie and protein needs

Neck or facial burns that make swallowing impossible

Anorexia

Paralytic ileus.

When the GI system is functioning, enteral nutrition should be used. When it isn't, choose parenteral nutrition.

researchers don't have strong evidence that the formulas improve outcome in burn patients.

Survey the situation

Nutrition therapy for a burn patient must be monitored and, as needed, adjusted continuously—increased if complications occur and decreased as wound healing progresses. Be sure to document daily calories consumed or administered by enteral or parenteral nutrition.

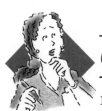

Quick quiz

1. For the trauma patient, which nutritional requirement is the highest?

    A   Protein
    B.   Fat
    C.   Carbohydrates
    D.   Vitamin E

Answer: A. Protein needs are the highest requirement for a trauma patient because of multiple physiologic compromises.

2.   Which metabolic changes occur in a cancer patient, impairing his nutritional status?
   A.   Decreased metabolic rate
   B.   Decreased protein catabolism
   C.   Decreased fat oxidation
   D.   Peripheral insulin resistance

Answer: D. Peripheral insulin resistance, possibly caused by cytokines and tumor necrosis factor, can adversely affect a cancer patient's nutritional status. Metabolic rate, protein catabolism, and fat oxidation all increase in cancer patients.

3.   To help make eating less painful for your patient with stomatitis, suggest that he eat:
   A.   hot foods.
   B.   soft, mild foods.
   C.   salty foods.
   D.   dry foods.

Answer: B. Eating soft, mild foods such as applesauce is less irritating to sore mouth tissue.

4.   How many grams of protein per kg of body weight does a burn patient require each day?
   A.   1 to 2 g
   B.   2 to 3 g
   C.   3 to 4 g
   D.   4 to 5 g

Answer: B. A burn patient requires 2 to 3 g/kg/day of protein to boost his immune system and promote healing.

5.   A malnourished cancer patient may require:
   A.   25 to 35 cal/kg/day.
   B.   20 to 30 cal/kg/day.
   C.   25 to 30 cal/kg/day.
   D.   35 to 40 cal/kg/day.

Answer: D. A malnourished patient may need 35 to 40 cal/kg/day to improve his nutritional status.

Scoring

☆☆☆   If you answered all five questions correctly, congratulations! One thing is for sure—you're certainly not nutrient dense.

☆☆   If you answered four questions correctly, good job! Your answers weighed in at the top of the class.

☆   If you answered fewer than four questions correctly, keep at it! With a second helping of studying, you'll see that nutrition can be as easy as pie.

Appendices and index

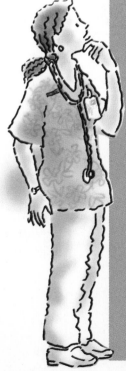

Fad diets

In an attempt to lose weight quickly, some patients try fad dieting. This chart provides information about many common fad diets, including their pros and cons.

Diet	Description	Pros	Cons
Atkins	• High-protein, low-carbohydrate diet to help body burn fat stores for energy • Initially limits carbohydrates to 20 to 40 g/day • Allows consumption of meat, eggs, cheese, butter, and cream	• Produces rapid weight loss (however, after 1 year, patients show no significant difference in weight loss compared to other popular diet plans) • Initially reduces cholesterol levels • Is easy to follow with no counting of calories or complicated meal plans to follow	• Has limited food choices, with carbohydrates being severely restricted • Is extremely high in saturated fat and protein • Limits fruit, vegetable, and fiber intake • Restricts foods that fight cancer • May damage the kidneys (due to long-term high-protein intake) • May be difficult to maintain long-term • Can cause ketosis, which may lead to nausea and fatigue
Cabbage soup	• Unlimited consumption of cabbage soup and water with limited amounts of other foods for 1 week	• Results in immediate weight loss • Is easy and affordable to follow	• Results in temporary weight loss • Offers little variety in diet • Results in very low intake of calories, protein, vitamins, and complex carbohydrates, which can adversely affect health • Can be used only short term
Eat more, weigh less	• High-carbohydrate, low-fat diet	• Emphasizes healthy eating, not amounts of foods • Promotes high fiber intake and limitation of processed foods • Promotes cholesterol and weight reduction • Promotes regular exercise	• Is time consuming to prepare • Limits foods, reducing long-term success • Restricts proteins from dairy and meats

Diet	Description	Pros	Cons
Eat right for your type	• Promotes eating foods that are compatible with blood type • Based on belief that each blood type reacts negatively to certain foods	• Doesn't require calorie counting • Promotes decreased calorie consumption, possibly resulting in weight loss • Provides lists of foods to avoid	• Restricts certain foods • Requires dieter to know blood type • Presents concerns for those eating high-protein, low-carbo-hydrate diets (recommended for type O blood) same as with oth-er similar diets
Glucose revolution	• Promotes foods with a low glycemic index	• Reduces consumption of refined carbohydrates • Provides lists of foods with high and low glycemic indexes	• Requires dieter to understand the concepts of "glycemic in-dex" and "glucose load" • Lacks unified glycemic lists for foods
Grapefruit	• Promotes consumption of grapefruit or grapefruit juice with meals in the belief that grapefruit contains fat-burning enzymes that promote weight loss	• Offers several diet plans • Is easy to follow	• Is based on special fat-burn-ing enzyme in grapefruit that has no scientific basis • May cause drug interactions (grapefruit juice interacts with many medications) • Offers limited choice of foods in small amounts • Results in very low intake of calories, proteins, fiber, and vit-amins and minerals, which can adversely affect health • Can only be used short term
Liquid protein	• Replaces breakfast, lunch, and snacks with shakes, bars, and other special foods	• Encourages portion control • Simplifies portion control by using special products • Provides structured diet plan	• Can be costly for special shakes • Offers limited food choices, making diet hard to maintain • Results in temporary weight loss • Shouldn't be followed long term

Diet	Description	Pros	Cons
Pritikin	• Low-fat, high-carbohydrate diet based on vegetables, grains, and fruits • Promotes belief that fat intake shouldn't exceed 10% of total daily calories	• Promotes foods with fewer calories per pound • Encourages exercise	• Requires dieter to calculate caloric density or refer to lists for food choices • Is difficult to maintain and promotes hunger (very-low-fat diet)
Scarsdale	• Rigid low-carbohydrate, low-fat, high-protein diet that's followed for 2 weeks, followed by a maintenance plan	• Requires no calorie counting	• Doesn't allow snacking, except for carrots, celery, and low-sodium broth • Encourages use of artificial sweeteners and herbal appetite suppressants to promote weight loss • Requires dieter to follow strict diet plan with very little substitutions and many rules
South Beach	• Initially carbohydrate restriction • After initial phase, refined carbohydrates restricted but whole grains, fruits, and vegetables allowed	• Promotes vegetable, fruit, and whole grain intake after initial ban of carbohydrates • Promotes intake of low saturated fat and high monounsaturated fats • Requires no calorie or carbohydrate counting • Encourages exercise	• Promotes very low carbohydrate intake during initial phase • Results in water loss during initial phase that may result in electrolyte imbalances • Requires dieter to understand glycemic index
Stop inflammation now	• Promotes a very-low-fat, low-protein diet	• Encourages intake of fruits, vegetables, whole grains, beans, and legumes • Connects inflammation with heart disease	• May result in insufficient calcium intake • Restricts protein from dairy and animal sources • Is very strict, making compliance difficult

Diet	Description	Pros	Cons
Sugar busters	• Promotes avoidance of simple sugars and refined grains • Promotes high-fiber carbohydrate, lean meat, and unsaturated fat intake • Based on belief that sugar is toxic to the body and leads to excess insulin levels and storage of excess sugar as fat	• Provides clear guidelines on foods to avoid • Uses the glycemic index to rank food	• Limits food portions • Requires dieter to understand glycemic index • Is difficult to follow
Volumetrics	• Promotes consumption of high-volume, low-calorie foods to produce feeling of fullness on fewer calories • Promotes portion control of high-density foods	• Allows all types of foods	• May result in slow weight loss • Involves much preparation time
Zone	• Divides meals into portions of 40% carbohydrates, 30% proteins, and 30% fats • Based on belief that "The Zone" is a state in which the body is at peak physical performance, mental focus, increased energy, and reduced illness and entering "the zone" is achieved by maintaining a specific insulin level, leading to a balance of eicosanoids	• Allows lean meats and fats • Emphasizes fruits and vegetables • Isn't as restrictive as other diets • Allows for a broad range of foods • Has a simple-to-follow eating plan • Promotes reduced caloric intake, which leads to weight loss	• Results in low fiber intake • Involves difficult "block" system

Commonly used herbs

If your patient is taking an herbal preparation, you'll need to know its intended use, adverse effects, and special considerations for use. Advise the patient to consult with his practitioner before taking any herbal preparation and to inform all practitioners and pharmacists about their use.

Herb	Use	Adverse reactions
Black cohosh	• Menopausal symptoms • Premenstrual syndrome • Dysmenorrhea	• Headache • GI complaints • Seizures • Weight gain
Chamomile	• Diarrhea • Anxiety • Restlessness • Stomatitis • Hemorrhagic cystitis • Flatulence • Motion sickness • Wound healing	• Conjunctivitis • Eyelid angioedema • Nausea • Vomiting • Contact dermatitis • Eczema • Anaphylaxis
Echinacea	• Stimulates the immune system • Acute and chronic upper respiratory infection • Urinary tract infection; wound healing • May prevent upper respiratory infection and the common cold	• GI complaints • Fever • Taste disturbance • Polyuria • Allergic reactions
Evening primrose oil	• Mastalgia, premenstrual syndrome • Cyclic mastitis • Neurodermatitis • Menopausal symptoms	• Headache • GI disturbances • Allergic reaction
Garlic	• Elevated cholesterol and triglyceride levels • Bacterial and fungal infections • Digestive problems • Hypertension	• Heartburn • Flatulence • Fatigue • Headache • Insomnia • Asthma • Shortness of breath • Contact dermatitis • Body odor • Facial flushing • Hypersensitivity reactions • Orthostatic hypotension

Practice pointers

• Avoid use in pregnant and breast-feeding women and those with breast cancer.
• Know that the drug may interact with antidepressants, antihypertensives, antiplatelets, anticoagulants, disulfiram, metronidazole, estrogen replacement therapy, iron preparations, sedatives, tamoxifen, and analgesics.
• Avoid confusion with blue or white cohosh.

• Know that the drug may interact with central nervous system (CNS) depressants, warfarin, alprazolam, atorvastatin, diazepam, ketoconazole, and verapamil.
• Know that the drug may cause anaphylaxis in patients who are sensitive to ragweed or feverfew and in those with a history of hayfever or asthma.
• Avoid use in pregnant or breast-feeding women and those with liver or kidney disorders.

• Avoid use in people with autoimmune diseases, human immunodeficiency virus, acquired immunodeficiency syndrome, tuberculosis, and pregnant and breast-feeding women.
• Limit use to no more than 8 weeks.
• Know that the drug may interact with protease inhibitors, disulfiram, metronidazole, immunosuppressants, and alcohol.

• Know that the drug may interact with phenothiazines and tricyclic antidepressants (TCAs).
• Know that the drug may be given with vitamin E to prevent toxic metabolites.
• Avoid use in pregnant and breast-feeding women and people with seizure disorder.

• Monitor for increased risk of bleeding.
• Know that the drug may interact with anti-inflammatory and nonsteroidal anti-inflammatory drugs.
• Avoid use in people following surgery or with diabetes, insomnia, pemphigus, organ transplants, or rheumatoid arthritis.

Herb	Use	Adverse reactions
Ginkgo biloba	• Enhances memory • Peripheral vascular disease	• Headache • Dizziness • GI disturbances • Palpitations • Allergic reaction • Bleeding
Ginseng	• Mental alertness • Energy enhancement • Atherosclerosis • Bleeding disorders • Colitis • Diabetes • Depression • Cancer	• Dizziness • Headache • Insomnia • Restlessness • Hypertension • Hypotension • Diarrhea • Vomiting • Estrogen-like effects, such as vaginal bleeding and mastalgia
Saw palmetto	• Benign prostatic hyperplasia • Congestion from colds, bronchitis, or asthma • Mild diuretic • Urinary antiseptic and astringent	• Dizziness • Headache • Hypertension • Urine retention • Abdominal pain • Diarrhea • Nausea
St. John's wort	• Depression • Anxiety • Seasonal affective disorder • Restlessness • Viral infections • Sleep problems	• Dry mouth • Dizziness • GI complaints • Fatigue • Headache • Pruritus • Neuropathies • Hypothyroidism • Delayed hypersensitivity • Photosensitivity

Practice pointers

• Know that the drug may interact with anticoagulants, aspirin, vitamin E, garlic supplements, trazodone, anticonvulsants, disulfiram, metronidazole, monoamine oxidase (MAO) inhibitors, TCAs, oral antidiabetic agents, and thiazide diuretics.
• Avoid use in people with diabetes and bleeding disorders.
• Explain that the components of ginkgo can vary significantly and should be obtained from a reliable source.

• Avoid use in people with untreated hypertension and women with history of breast cancer.
• Know that the drug may interact with MAO inhibitors, digoxin, insulin, CNS stimulants, estrogen, furosemide, ibuprofen, oral antidiabetic agents, warfarin, and ticlopidine.
• Monitor for ginseng abuse syndrome in those taking large amounts: increased motor and cognitive activity, diarrhea, nervousness, insomnia, hypertension, edema, and skin eruptions.

• Avoid use in people with bleeding disorders or scheduled for surgery and women who are pregnant, planning pregnancy, or breast-feeding.
• Know that the drug may interact with anticoagulants, adrenergics, aspirin, vitamin E, and gingko.
• Obtain baseline prostate-specific antigen level in men before starting this herb.

• Avoid use in people with photosensitivity, undergoing ultraviolet treatment, bipolar disorder, and women who are pregnant or want to become pregnant and their male partners.
• Stop herb several weeks before surgery.
• Know that the drug may interact with Ritalin, ephedrine, caffeine, protease inhibitors, digoxin, statins, warfarin, anesthetics, chemotherapy, hormonal contraceptives, TCAs, olanzapine, clozapine, theophylline, cyclosporine, and many over-the-counter drugs.

Toxic herbs

These herbs have been declared unsafe by the Food and Drug Administration because the plants contain poisonous components.

Common name	Botanical name
Arnica	*Arnica montana*
Belladonna	*Atropa belladonna*
Bittersweet	*Solanum dulcamara*
Bloodroot	*Sanguinaris canadensis*
Broom-tops	*Cytisus scoparius*
Buckeye	*Aesculus hippocastanum*
Heliotrope	*Heliotropium eropaeum*
Hemlock	*Conium maculatum*
Henbane	*Hyoscyamus niger*
Jimsonweed	*Datura stramonium*
Lily of the valley	*Convallaria majalis*
Lobelia	*Lobelia inflate*
Mandrake	*Mandragora officinarum*
Mayapple	*Podophyllum peltatum*
Mistletoe	*Phoradendron flavescens*
Periwinkle	*Vinca major, Vinca minor*
Snakeroot	*Eupatorium rugosum*
Tonka bean	*Dipteryx odorata, Coumarouna odorata*
Wahoo bark	*Euonymus atropurpureus*
Wormwood	*Artemisia absinthium*
Yohimbe	*Corynanthe yohimbe*

Selected references

Daniels, J. "Fad Diets: Slim or Good Nutrition?" *Nursing* 34(12):22-23, December 2004.

"Diagnosis and Classification of Diabetes Mellitus," *Diabetes Care* 28(Suppl 1):S37-S42, January 2005.

DiMaria-Ghalili, R.A., and Amella, E. "Nutrition in Older Adults," *AJN* 105(3):40-50, March 2005.

Dudek, S.G. *Nutrition Essentials for Nursing Practice*, 5th ed. Philadelphia: Lippincott Williams & Wilkins, 2006.

Elliot, K. "Nutritional Considerations after Bariatric Surgery," *Critical Care Nursing Quarterly* 26(2):133-38, April-June 2003.

Fischbach, F.T. *A Manual of Laboratory and Diagnostic Tests*, 7th ed. Philadelphia: Lippincott Williams & Wilkins, 2004.

Forbes, A. "Parenteral Nutrition: New Advances and Observations," *Current Opinions in Gastroenterology* 20(2):114-18, March 2004.

Giger, J.N., and Davidhizar, R.E. *Transcultural Nursing: Assessment & Intervention*, 4th ed. St. Louis: Mosby–Year Book, Inc., 2004.

Herbal Medicine Handbook, 3rd ed. Philadelphia: Lippincott Williams & Wilkins, 2006.

Johnson, C.A., et al. "Clinical Practice Guidelines for Chronic Kidney Disease in Adults: Part I. Definition, Disease Stages, Evaluation, Treatment, and Risk Factors," *American Family Physician* 70(5):869-76, September 2004.

Keithley, J.K., and Swanson, B. "Enteral Nutrition: An Update on Practice Recommendations," *MedSurg Nursing* 13(2):131-34, April 2004.

Legg, V. "Complications of Chronic Kidney Disease," *AJN* 105(6):40-49, June 2005.

Managing Chronic Disorders. Philadelphia: Lippincott Williams & Wilkins, 2006.

Miller, E.R., and Jehn, M. "New High Blood Pressure Guidelines Create New At-Risk Classification: Changes in Blood Pressure Classification by JNC 7," *Journal of Cardiovascular Nursing* 19(6):367-71, November-December 2004.

Nurse's Quick Check: Diseases. Philadelphia: Lippincott Williams & Wilkins, 2005.

Nursing2006 Drug Handbook, 26th ed. Philadelphia: Lippincott Williams & Wilkins, 2006.

Padula, C.A., et al. "Enteral Feedings: What the Evidence Says," *AJN* 104(7):62-69, July 2004.

Potyk, D. "Treatment of Alzheimer's Disease," *Southern Medical Journal* 98(6):628-35, June 2005.

Pull, C.B. "Binge Eating Disorder," *Current Opinions in Psychiatry* 17(1):4-48, 2004.

Reising, D.L. "Enteral Tube Flushing," *AJN* 105(3):58-63, March 2005.

Shils, M.E., et al. *Modern Nutrition in Health and Disease*, 10th ed. Philadelphia: Lippincott Williams & Wilkins, 2006.

"Standards of Medical Care in Diabetes," *Diabetes Care* 28(Suppl 1):S4-S36, January 2005.

Thibodeau, G.A., and Patton, K.T. *The Human Body in Health and Disease*, 4th ed. St. Louis: Mosby–Year Book Inc., 2005.

U.S. Department of Health and Human Services and U.S. United States Department of Agriculture. *Dietary Guidelines for Americans, 2005*. 6th ed, Washington, D.C: U.S. Government Printing Office, January 2005.

Index

i refers to an illustration; t refers to a table.

i refers to an illustration; t refers to a table.

i refers to an illustration; t refers to a table.